Self Assessment and Review of
OPHTHALMOLOGY

Self Assessment and Review of OPHTHALMOLOGY

Sixth Edition

Sudha Seetharam MBBS MS (Ophthal)
Consultant Ophthalmologist
Laxmi Eye Institute
Navi Mumbai, Maharashtra, India

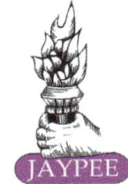

JAYPEE BROTHERS MEDICAL PUBLISHERS
The Health Sciences Publisher
New Delhi | London

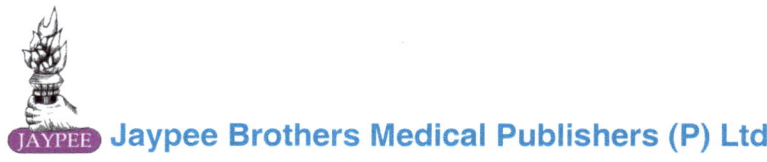

Headquarters
Jaypee Brothers Medical Publishers (P) Ltd
EMCA House, 23/23-B
Ansari Road, Daryaganj
New Delhi 110 002, India
Landline: +91-11-23272143, +91-11-23272703
+91-11-23282021, +91-11-23245672
Email: jaypee@jaypeebrothers.com

Corporate Office
Jaypee Brothers Medical Publishers (P)
Ltd 4838/24, Ansari Road, Daryaganj
New Delhi 110 002, India
Phone: +91-11-43574357
Fax: +91-11-43574314
Email: jaypee@jaypeebrothers.com

Overseas Office
J.P. Medical Ltd
83 Victoria Street, London
SW1H 0HW (UK)
Phone: +44 20 3170 8910
Fax: +44 (0)20 3008 6180
Email: info@jpmedpub.com

Website: www.jaypeebrothers.com
Website: www.jaypeedigital.com

© 2021, Jaypee Brothers Medical Publishers

The views and opinions expressed in this book are solely those of the original contributor(s)/author(s) and do not necessarily represent those of editor(s) of the book.

All rights reserved. No part of this publication may be reproduced, stored or transmitted in any form or by any means, electronic, mechanical, photocopying, recording or otherwise, without the prior permission in writing of the publishers.

All brand names and product names used in this book are trade names, service marks, trademarks or registered trademarks of their respective owners. The publisher is not associated with any product or vendor mentioned in this book.

Medical knowledge and practice change constantly. This book is designed to provide accurate, authoritative information about the subject matter in question. However, readers are advised to check the most current information available on procedures included and check information from the manufacturer of each product to be administered, to verify the recommended dose, formula, method and duration of administration, adverse effects and contraindications. It is the responsibility of the practitioner to take all appropriate safety precautions. Neither the publisher nor the author(s)/editor(s) assume any liability for any injury and/ or damage to persons or property arising from or related to use of material in this book.

This book is sold on the understanding that the publisher is not engaged in providing professional medical services. If such advice or services are required, the services of a competent medical professional should be sought.

Every effort has been made where necessary to contact holders of copyright to obtain permission to reproduce copyright material. If any have been inadvertently overlooked, the publisher will be pleased to make the necessary arrangements at the first opportunity. The **CD/DVD-ROM** (if any) provided in the sealed envelope with this book is complimentary and free of cost. **Not meant for sale.**

Inquiries for bulk sales may be solicited at: jaypee@jaypeebrothers.com

Self Assessment and Review of Ophthalmology

First Edition: 2016
Third Edition: 2018
Fifth Edition: 2020

Second Edition: 2017
Fourth Edition: 2019

Sixth Edition: 2021

ISBN: 978-93-5465-552-4

Dedicated to

My lucky charm;
Our son, Sreejit

PREFACE TO THE SIXTH EDITION

It gives me immense pleasure to introduce the sixth edition of my book *"Self-assessment and Review of Ophthalmology."* The questions from all the recently concluded examinations like NEET PG, INI-CET, FMGE have been included as a separate chapter in the beginning of the book for a quick revision just before the examination. Each chapter also includes clinical case scenario and image-based questions keeping in mind the recent trend. Constructive feedback from my students has helped to refine the content of the book and I would like to thank them for the same.

Sudha Seetharam

PREFACE TO THE FIRST EDITION

Dear Students,

Postgraduate medical entrance preparation is undoubtedly one of the most challenging phases in the life of a medico. There are over nineteen subjects to be covered, time is limited and the competition is tremendous. A PG seat in a subject and institution of choice is a dream for every MBBS graduate. But trust me; **this dream can become a reality for you.** What you need is organized preparation in the right direction; motivation to keep up the grueling task and most importantly, the belief that you will succeed.

Ophthalmology has always been a very scoring subject in entrance examinations. Over the past 4–5 years, the trend of questions in Ophthalmology has changed tremendously. The reason is that Ophthalmology is a rapidly evolving subject with new developments taking place at a very fast pace. Thus, diagnostic and treatment modalities keep changing too.

Keeping all this in mind, I have made an attempt to write this book. It is primarily intended for students preparing for PG medical entrance examinations. But it can be useful for MBBS students for a quick revision before their examination. It can also be used by Ophthalmology residents and practitioners as a ready reference.

In this book, I have attempted to include the theoretical discussions relevant for entrance examinations, with special emphasis on recent trends after referencing from standard textbooks like *Clinical Ophthalmology: Kanski, Ophthalmology: Yanoff and Duker* and *Comprehensive Ophthalmology: A K Khurana*. I have also provided MCQs from important examinations like AIIMS, PGI, COMEDK, State PG entrances, DNB. I have carefully chosen the representative questions from each topic so that after going through this book, the students should be able to answer not only the repeat questions but also any new questions that may be asked.

One common mistake that students make in this regard is trying to go through all questions of a particular subject that have been asked in the past 15–20 years. But many of these questions have actually no relevance today because that particular diagnostic or treatment modality may have changed. So those questions will never be asked again. Memorizing these only adds to the confusion and leads to waste of time. With this in mind, I have prepared a concise collection of representative questions mainly from recent examinations. I have also added a picture quiz as there is a rising trend of questions based on photographs. However, despite my best efforts there may be some inadvertent errors which I sincerely regret.

I sincerely hope that you will enjoy reading this book as much as I enjoyed writing it.

Best of luck for your exams and for life!

Sudha Seetharam

FROM THE AUTHOR'S DESK

Dear Students,

Postgraduate medical entrance preparation is undoubtedly one of the most challenging phases in the life of a medico. There are over nineteen subjects to be covered, time is limited and the competition is tremendous. A PG seat in a subject and the institution of choice is a dream for every MBBS graduate. But trust me; this dream can become a reality for you. What you need is organized preparation in the right direction; motivation to keep up the grueling task and most importantly, the belief that you will succeed.

Ophthalmology has always been a very scoring subject in entrance examinations. Over the past 4 to 5 years, the trend of questions in Ophthalmology has changed tremendously. The reason probably is that Ophthalmology is a rapidly evolving subject with new developments taking place at a very fast pace. Thus, diagnostic and treatment modalities keep changing too.

Keeping all this in mind, I have made an attempt to write this book. It is primarily intended for students preparing for PG medical entrance examinations. But it can be useful for MBBS students too for a quick revision before their examination. It can also be used by Ophthalmology residents and practitioners as a ready reference.

In this book, I have attempted to include the theoretical discussions relevant for entrance examinations, with special emphasis on recent trends after referencing from standard textbooks like Clinical Ophthalmology: Kanski, Ophthalmology: Yanoff and Duker and Peyman's Principles and Practices of Ophthalmology. I have also provided MCQs from important examinations like AIIMS, INI-CET, PGI, COMEDK, State PG entrances, DNB and NEET. I have carefully chosen the representative questions from each topic so that after going through this book, the student should be able to answer not only the repeat questions but also any new questions that may be asked. Special emphasis has been given to image-based questions as is the need of the hour.

I sincerely hope that you will enjoy reading this book as much as I enjoyed writing it.

Best of luck for your exams and for life!

Sudha Seetharam

ACKNOWLEDGMENTS

Writing this book was a big challenge, considering the amount of time, research and reading that it entailed. I was always skeptical as to whether I would be able to dedicate so much time for this endeavor within my busy schedule as a clinical practitioner. I would like to express my heartfelt gratitude to everyone who has helped me in my journey so far.

First and foremost, The Almighty God, whose blessings have always been with me in whatever I have done.

My parents: It is because of them that I am what I am today.

My husband: He has been a constant source of encouragement at every step in writing this book, never letting me give up. He has also helped me in typing out and arranging the text. Had it not been for him, I would not have seriously considered writing this book.

My parents-in-law: Their blessings and encouragement keep me going.

My brother: My childhood companion and perhaps, my greatest critic whose honest advice is priceless

My son: The greatest joy of my life whose smile is enough to make my day. I must acknowledge the many precious personal moments between us that were lost in this difficult task.

My grandparents and grandparents-in-law who, from somewhere in heaven, continue to shower their blessings on me even today.

My teachers at Guru Nanak Eye Centre, MAMC especially Dr Jawaharlal Goyal and Dr Ritu Arora, who have taught me almost all the ophthalmology that I know today. My teachers at Medical College, Kolkata and South Point School who have been instrumental in shaping me. My English teacher, Mrs Leena Guha Roy deserves special mention.

Dr Suhas Haldipurkar, Medical Director, Laxmi Eye Institute for initiating me into private practice and opening up a new arena of knowledge.

I sincerely thank Shri Jitendar P Vij and the team at Jaypee Brothers Medical Publishers (P) Ltd for their keen interest in publishing this book.

I sincerely thank Jaypee Brothers Medical Publishers (P) Ltd for allowing me to use few illustrations from its prestigious book 'Peyman's Principles and Practice of Ophthalmology' by Dr N Venkatesh Prajna.

And last but not least, my students who are the inspiration for this book.

HOW TO USE THIS BOOK

To make best use of this book, the student may follow these tips.
1. First read the text of each chapter with special emphasis on the points marked with superscript Q. This will cover all the theory that is relevant and important with respect to competitive examinations.
2. Next, try a self-assessment with the questions provided at the end of each chapter. The questions have also been divided into sections according to topics.
3. Read the explanation provided for each question. It will help you understand why a certain option has been chosen ahead of others. Then read through all the other allied information that has been discussed with the question.
4. Then try the image-based questions at the end of each chapter. When you look at each image, try to recall the theory you have read and apply it to identify the image.
5. When you read the explanation of the image-based questions, special emphasis is to be given to the salient identification points that have been given for the image.

UNIQUE FEATURES OF THIS EDITION

1. More than 150 high resolution ophthalmic images with image-based questions on clinical case scenarios
2. Explanation and tips for the identification of the images
3. Recent investigation modalities and their interpretation
4. Special emphasis on chapters like Retina and Neuro-ophthalmology which are important for MCQ and require in-depth understanding of concepts.
5. Full color edition

CONTENTS

	Recent Questions 2020-21	*xvii–xxviii*
1.	**Ocular Embryology** ★	1
2.	**Coats of the Eyeball** ★	3
3.	**Conjunctiva, Sclera and Cornea** ★★★	5
4.	**Lens** ★★★	36
5.	**Retina** ★★★	55
6.	**Uveal Tract** ★	93
7.	**Optics and Refraction** ★★	105
8.	**Strabismus** ★★	119
9.	**Glaucoma** ★★	132
10.	**Neuro-Ophthalmology** ★★★	154
11.	**Adnexae and Orbit** ★★	182
12.	**Assessment of Visual Function** ★	200
13.	**Ocular Manifestations of Systemic Diseases** ★	204
14.	**Miscellaneous** ★	205

★ Important
★★ Very important
★★★ Extremely important

RECENT QUESTIONS

This chapter contains questions from NEET 2021, INI-CET 2021, AIIMS 2020, PGI 2020, FMGE 2021 and FMGE 2020. These questions have been recalled from memory by students who have taken the examination, hence there may be some discrepancies in the questions and the options which cannot be avoided. But I believe that these questions will give the students an insight into the recent trend of questions so that they have a good understanding of what to expect in the upcoming examinations.

1. A 30-year-old female complains of diminution of vision on the right halves of both eyes. The visual field defect is given. What is the possible site of the lesion?   *(NEET 2021)*

   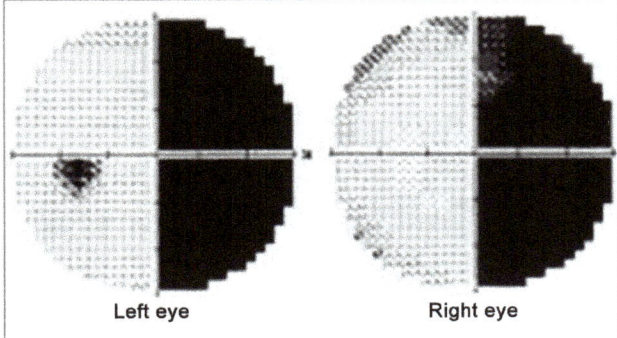

   a. Left optic tract
   b. Right occipital cortex
   c. Right optic nerve
   d. Optic chiasma

2. A patient presented with vision loss and on radiological examination, an aneurysm causing damage to the optic chiasma was noted. Which of the following may a possible cause?   *(NEET 2021)*
   a. Anterior communicating artery
   b. Middle cerebral artery
   c. Anterior choroidal artery
   d. Anterior cerebral artery

3. A child presenting with leucocoria underwent enucleation and histopathology shows Flexner-Wintersteiner rosette. What is the diagnosis?
   (NEET 2021)

   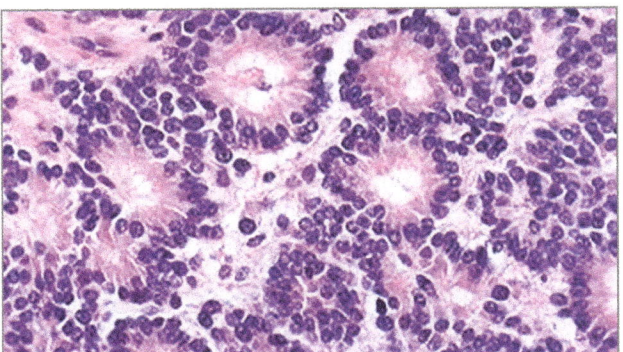

   a. Medulloblastoma
   b. Rhabdomyosarcoma
   c. Retinoblastoma
   d. Choroidal melanoma

4. A female with history of prolonged contact lens use presents with complains of foreign body sensation. The clinical picture is given. What is the possible diagnosis?   *(NEET 2021)*
   a. Spring catarrh
   b. Trachoma
   c. Acute follicular conjunctivitis
   d. Giant papillary conjunctivitis

   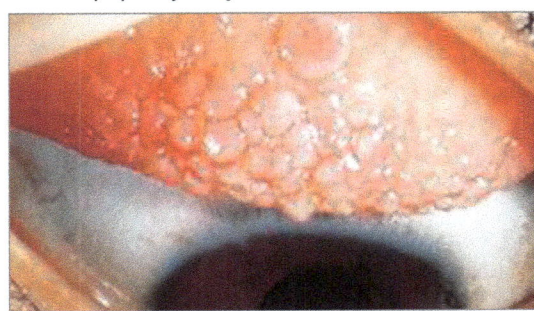

5. A patient of Primary Open Angle Glaucoma (POAG) has a known history of bronchial asthma. Which of the following should be prescribed as an anti-glaucoma drug in this patient?   *(NEET 2021)*
   a. Latanoprost
   b. Carboprost
   c. Gemeprost
   d. Alprostadil

6. An elderly female presents with gradually progressive decrease in vision. The clinical picture is given. What is the diagnosis?   *(NEET 2021)*

   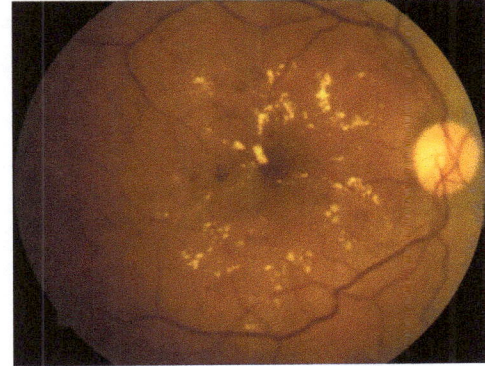

a. Hard exudates in diabetic retinopathy
b. Soft exudates in hypertension
c. Central retinal vein occlusion
d. Flame-shaped haemorrhages in hypertension.

7. A patient with history of ocular injury while working with chisel and hammer presents to the emergency. Which of the following investigations should not be performed for localisation of the intraocular foreign body (IOFB)? *(NEET 2021)*
   a. X-ray orbit
   b. CT scan orbit
   c. USG B-Scan
   d. MRI orbit

8. A patient presents with complaints of difficulty in vision in dim light with dryness of the ocular surface. Deficiency of which of the following may be associated with this condition? *(NEET 2021)*
   a. Protein
   b. Niacin
   c. Retinoic acid
   d. Iron

9. Acute red eye in a young male patient with history of back pain and morning stiffness. X-ray is likely to show which of the following? *(NEET 2021)*
   a. Rheumatoid arthritis
   b. Ankylosing spondylitis
   c. Psoriatic arthritis
   d. Osteoarthritis

10. A 15-year-old girl is not able to adjust or is not compliant to glasses for myopic astigmatism. What is the appropriate management for this patient? *(NEET 2021)*
    a. LASIK
    b. Femto LASIK
    c. ICL
    d. Spherical equivalent glasses

11. Corneal transparency is maintained by *(NEET 2021)*
    a. Keratan sulphate
    b. Chondroitin sulphate
    c. Heparan sulphate
    d. Hyaluronic acid

12. What is the most common complication associated with the condition in the clinical photograph? *(NEET 2021)*

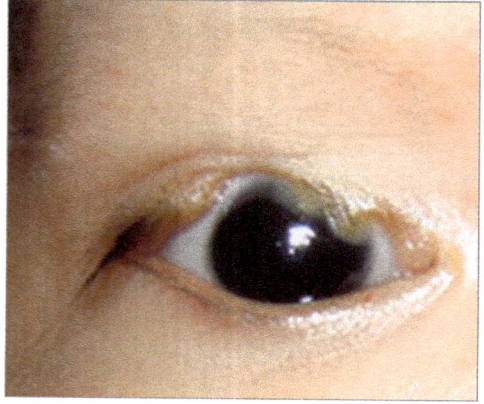

a. Cataract
b. Exposure keratopathy
c. Restriction of ocular movements
d. Amblyopia

13. A 2-month-old infant is brought with complaints of inability to open the eyes in bright light and excessive watering. The clinical picture is given. What is the possible diagnosis? *(NEET 2021)*

a. Ophthalmia neonatorum
b. Congenital glaucoma
c. Mucopolysaccharidosis
d. Cataract

14. The visual field defect of a patient is given. What is the site of the lesion? *(INI-CET July 2021)*

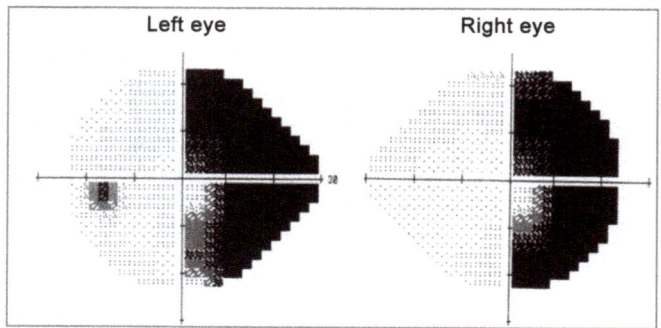

a. Right occipital lobe
b. Left occipital lobe
c. Right optic tract
d. Optic chiasma

15. What is the most common route of spread of retinoblastoma? *(INI-CET July 2021)*
    a. Direct spread
    b. Haematogenous spread
    c. Optic nerve invasion
    d. Lymphatic spread

16. Most common tumour of the lacrimal gland is: *(INI-CET July 2021)*
    a. Adenoid cystic carcinoma
    b. Pleomorphic adenoma
    c. Mucoepidermoid tumour
    d. Non-Hodgkin lymphoma

17. A patient presents with pain and redness in the right eye following trauma with vegetative matter. On examination, there is a corneal ulcer with hypopyon. The ulcer is dry looking with feathery margins. What is the diagnosis? *(INI-CET July 2021)*
    a. Bacterial corneal ulcer
    b. Fungal corneal ulcer
    c. Viral keratitis
    d. Acanthamoeba keratitis

Recent Questions

18. A patient presents with pain and redness in the right eye. On examination there are keratic precipitates with cells and flare in the anterior chamber. Her IOP is around 40 mm Hg. Which of the following anti-glaucoma drugs should not be used in this condition?
    (INI-CET July 2021)
    a. Mannitol
    b. β-Blockers
    c. Carbonic anhydrase inhibitors
    d. PG analogues

19. SAFE strategy for trachoma includes all *except*:
    (INI-CET July 2021)
    a. Surgery
    b. Antibiotics
    c. Facial cleanliness
    d. Evaluation of the control program

20. Diagnosis from the clinical photograph (INI-CET July 2021)

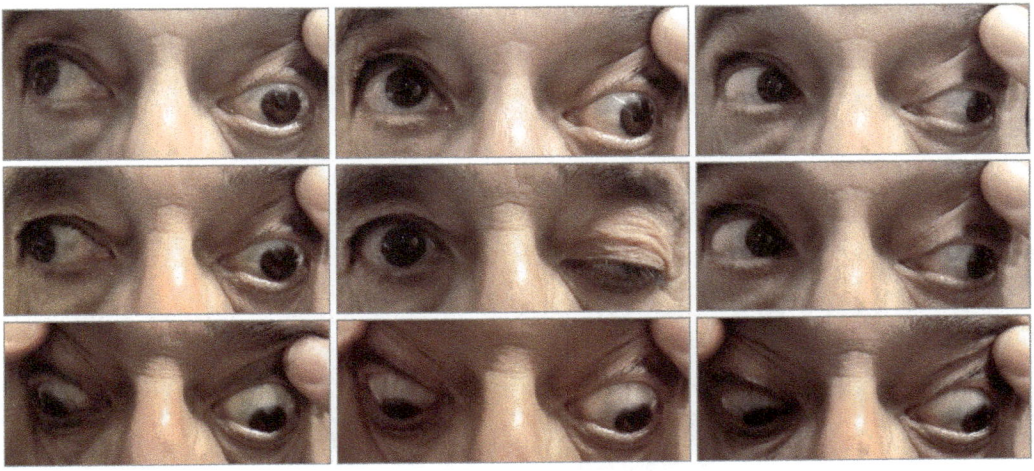

    a. Medial rectus palsy
    b. Trochlear nerve palsy
    c. Abducens nerve palsy
    d. Oculomotor nerve palsy

21. An 8-year-old child is diagnosed with amblyopia. What is the best treatment for the child?
    (FMGE June 2021)
    a. Occlusion
    b. Penalisation
    c. Observation
    d. None of the above

22. A 7-year-old boy presents with redness and itching in both eyes. The clinical photograph is given. What is the diagnosis? (FMGE June 2021)

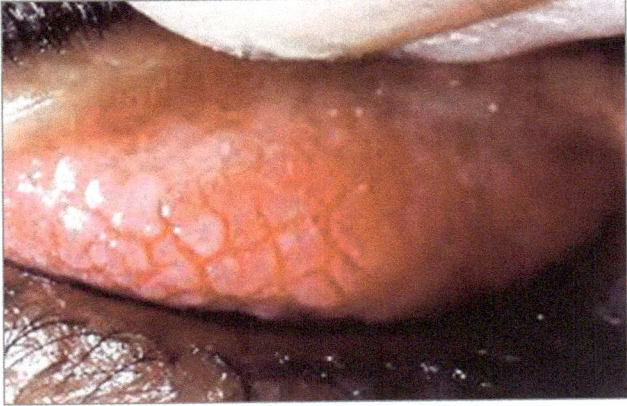

    a. Bacterial conjunctivitis
    b. Trachoma
    c. Vernal keratoconjunctivitis
    d. Angular conjunctivitis

23. A 3-month-old baby presents with mucoid fluid exuding from the eye on pressing over the lacrimal sac. What is the management? (June FMGE 2021)
    a. Syringing
    b. Sac massage
    c. Probing
    d. Dacryocystorhinostomy

24. All of the following are true about the following procedure *except*:
    (June FMGE 2021)

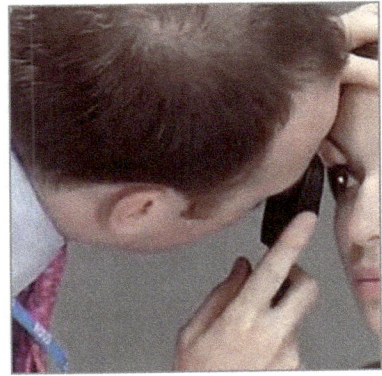

a. It can be done with patient in sitting position
b. There is no stereopsis
c. The retinal periphery cannot be examined.
d. Can be done in case of hazy ocular media

25. Treatment of recurrent pterygium: *(FMGE June 2021)*
    a. Observation
    b. Simple excision
    c. Excision with conjunctival autograft
    d. Excision with Mitomycin C

26. Which of the following is the gold standard for measuring IOP: *(FMGE June 2021)*
    a. Pulse-air tonometer
    b. Goldman applanation tonometer
    c. Tonopen
    d. Schiotz tonometer

27. A patient with jaundice and tremors presents with the given clinical photograph. What is the diagnosis? *(FMGE June 2021)*

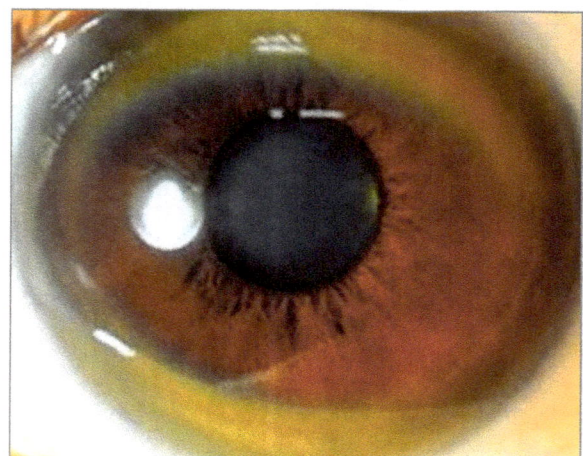

    a. Huntington's chorea
    b. Wilson's disease
    c. Heavy metal poisoning
    d. Sydenham's chorea

28. A tumour in the anterior pituitary causing compression of the optic chiasma will lead to *(FMGE December 2020)*
    a. Homonymous hemianopia
    b. Homonymous hemianopia with macular sparing
    c. Bitemporal hemianopia
    d. Monocular vision loss

29. The instrument in the picture is used for the surgery of: *(December FMGE 2020)*

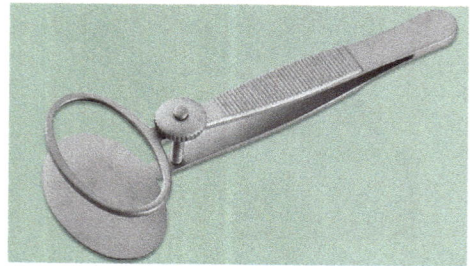

    a. Entropion
    b. Ectropion
    c. Chalazion
    d. Bitot's spot

30. β-Blockers should be avoided in all of the following conditions *except*: *(FMGE December 2020)*
    a. Glaucoma
    b. Chronic obstructive pulmonary disease
    c. Peripheral vascular disease
    d. Bradycardia

31. A patient with recurrent anterior uveitis presents to the OPD. Which of the following is likely to be associated with the patient? *(FMGE December 2020)*
    a. HLA B5
    b. HLA B27
    c. HLA DR4
    d. HLA B5

32. A patient presents with mild ptosis, miosis in the left eye and anhydrosis. Clinical image is given. What is the diagnosis? *(FMGE December 2020)*

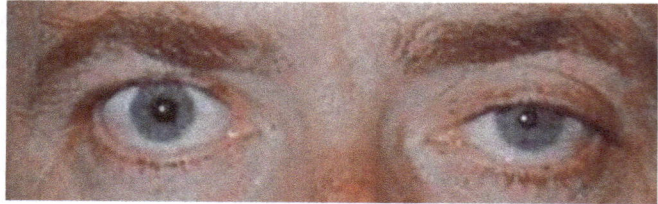

    a. Third cranial nerve palsy
    b. Horner syndrome
    c. Fourth cranial nerve palsy
    d. Sixth cranial nerve palsy

33. Which of the following is incorrect regarding the condition in the clinical photograph? *(FMGE December 2020)*

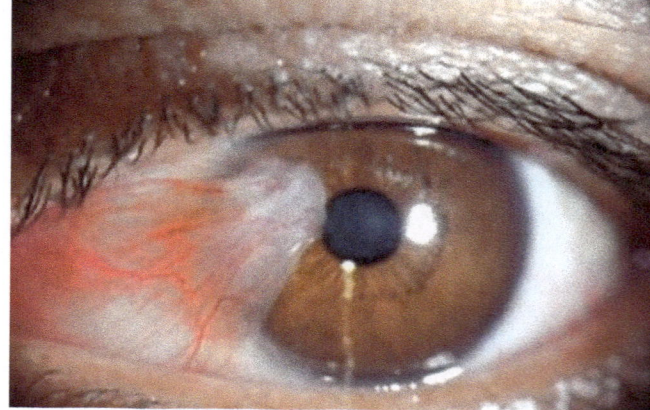

    a. More common in the nasal side
    b. Associated with sun exposure
    c. Iron deposition may be seen
    d. Causes myopia

34. From the clinical photograph, what is the possible diagnosis? *(FMGE December 2020)*

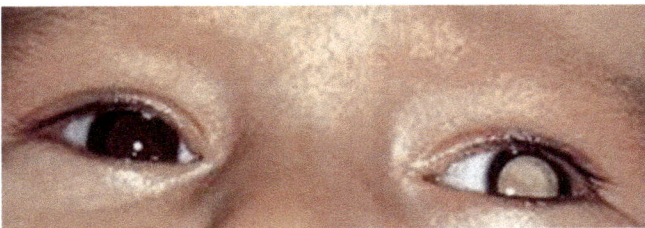

   a. Choroidal melanoma
   b. Retinoblastoma
   c. HSV keratitis
   d. Geographic ulcer

35. A 60-year-old woman presents with sudden onset pain and redness in the right eye associated with headache, nausea and vomiting. Examination reveals decreased visual acuity. The eye is congested with hazy cornea, shallow anterior chamber, dilated and fixed pupil. The eyeball is stony hard to touch. Clinical photograph is given. What is the diagnosis? *(FMGE August 2020)*

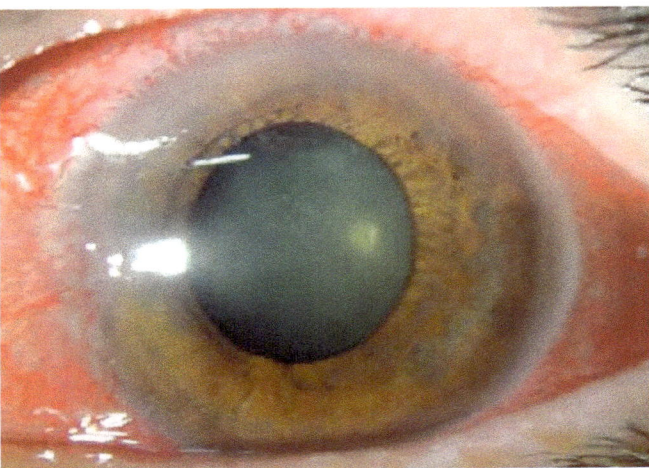

   a. Acute anterior uveitis
   b. Conjunctivitis
   c. Acute angle closure glaucoma
   d. Primary open angle glaucoma

36. A 2-year-old child presented with leucocoria in the right eye in the last 2 months. On examination total retinal detachment was present. Ultrasound B-Scan revealed a heterogonous sub-retinal mass with calcification. The most probable clinical diagnosis is: *(FMGE August 2020)*
   a. Coats' disease
   b. Retinoblastoma
   c. Toxocariasis
   d. Retinal tuberculoma

37. A patient was hit by a tennis ball and noted to have hyphaema. What is the source of bleeding? *(FMGE August 2020)*
   a. Anterior ciliary artery
   b. Posterior ciliary artery
   c. Major arterial circle of iris
   d. Minor arterial circle of iris

38. A 25-year-old man presented to the OPD for refraction. He is currently using glasses of -3DS in right eye and -2DS in the left eye. What is the expected movement of the retinoscopy reflex in the right eye? *(FMGE August 2020)*
   a. It moves in the same direction as the retinoscope
   b. It moves in the opposite direction as the retinoscope
   c. Moves in the opposite direction as the retinoscope only in the vertical axis
   d. There is no movement

39. All of the following are true about the cornea except: *(AIIMS June 2020)*
   a. Stratified squamous epithelium
   b. Bowman's membrane has regenerative potential
   c. Presence of microvilli
   d. Mitotic activity close to the limbus

40. A small pupil which does not increase in size in darkness. Possible diagnosis: *(AIIMS June 2020)*
   a. Argyll Robertson pupil   b. Adie's tonic pupil
   c. Blind eye   d. Horner syndrome

41. A nurse has to administer an eyedrop and eye ointment to the patient. What is the order in which this has to be administered? *(AIIMS June 2020)*
   a. Eye ointment followed by eye drop immediately
   b. Eye ointment followed by eye drop after 15 minutes
   c. Eye drop followed by eye ointment immediately.
   d. Eye drop followed by eye ointment after 15 minutes

42. Which of the following drugs causes visual field loss? *(AIIMS June 2020)*
   a. Phenobarbitone   b. Vigabatrin
   c. Ethosuximide   d. Levetiracetam

43. A 55-year-old patient who has a previous history of undergoing LASIK presents with cataract. Which is the best formula for IOL power calculation? *(AIIMS June 2020)*
   a. SRK II   b. Haigis L
   c. Hoffer Q   d. SRK- T

44. A patient presents with left head tilt. On examination, there is right hypotropia which worsens on dextroversion and right sided head tilt. What is the diagnosis? *(AIIMS June 2020)*
   a. Right Superior Oblique (SO) palsy
   b. Right Superior Rectus (SR) palsy
   c. Left Inferior Oblique (IO) palsy
   d. Left Superior Oblique (SO) palsy

45. Benign Intracranial Hypertension/Pseudotumour Cerebri is not caused by which of the following conditions? *(PGI June 2020)*
    a. Hypervitaminosis D
    b. Hypervitaminosis A
    c. Hypovitaminosis A
    d. Hypovitaminosis D
    e. Turner syndrome

46. Which of these tests are used for colour vision testing? *(PGI June 2020)*
    a. Pelli-Robson chart
    b. Ishihara chart
    c. Naegel's anomaloscope
    d. Lantern test
    e. Holmgren's wool test

47. Flow of aqueous humour takes place through which of the following structures? *(PGI June 2020)*
    a. Vitreous cavity
    b. Schlemm's canal
    c. Anterior chamber
    d. Posterior chamber
    e. Episcleral veins

ANSWERS AND EXPLANATIONS

1. **a. Left optic tract** *(Ref: Yanoff and Duker 4th edition, p 904-905)*
   The visual field defect is **Right Homonymous Hemianopia**. Hence the site of the lesion is left optic tract. (Please refer to the section "Visual Pathway" in the chapter "Neuro-ophthalmology" for further reading)

2. **a. Anterior communicating artery** *(Ref: Yanoff and Duker 4th edition, p 904-905)*
   Causes of optic chiasma involvement resulting in **bitemporal hemianopia** may be remembered as:
   - Pituitary adenoma
   - Craniopharyngioma
   - Anterior communicating artery aneurysm
   - Cavernous sinus thrombosis

3. **c. Retinoblastoma** *(Ref: Yanoff and Duker 4th edition, p 793-796)*
   The most common primary intraocular malignancy in children is Retinoblastoma.
   The most common presenting feature of retinoblastoma is leucocoria or white pupillary reflex. Flexner-Wintersteiner rosette in histopathology after enucleation is characteristic of retinoblastoma. (Please refer to the section "Retinoblastoma" in the chapter "Retina" for further reading.)

4. **d. Giant papillary conjunctivitis** *(Ref: Yanoff and Duker 4th edition, p 194)*
   Giant papillary conjunctivitis is a type of allergic conjunctivitis caused due to constant irritation of the conjunctiva by **contact lens, protruding sutures, ill-fitting prosthesis** etc.

5. **a. Latanoprost** *(Ref: Yanoff and Duker 4th edition, p 1117-1118)*
   Latanoprost is a **prostaglandin (PGF2α)** analogue used topically as an anti-glaucoma drug. It lowers IOP by increasing the aqueous humour outflow through the uveoscleral pathway.
   The other **PGF2α** analogues used as anti-glaucoma drugs are **Travoprost** and **Bimatoprost.**
   (Please refer to the section "Anti-Glaucoma Drugs" in the chapter "Glaucoma" for further reading)

6. **a. Hard exudates in diabetic retinopathy** *(Ref: Yanoff and Duker 4th edition, p 548)*
   The photograph shows **Clinically Significant Macular Oedema (CSME)** in Diabetic Retinopathy. One of the criteria for CSME is presence of hard exudates with 500 microns of the centre of the macula.
   (Please refer to the section on "Diabetic Retinopathy" in the chapter "Retina" for further reading)

7. **d. MRI orbit** *(Ref: Peyman's Principles and Practice of Ophthalmology, 2nd edition, p 1835-38)*
   Injury with chisel and hammer may result in metallic Intra-ocular Foreign Body (IOFB). MRI is contraindicated in metallic IOFB, hence the answer.
   The investigation of choice for a **metallic IOFB** is **CT Scan orbit** whereas for a **non-metallic IOFB** is **MRI Orbit.**

8. **c. Retinoic acid** *(Ref: National Program for Control of Blindness)*
   History of night-blindness and dryness or xerosis of the ocular surface suggests the diagnosis of **Xerophthalmia** caused by deficiency of **Vitamin A,** hence retinoic acid is chosen as the answer.
   (Please refer to the section "Xerophthalmia" in the chapter "Conjunctiva, Sclera, Cornea" for further reading.)

9. **b. Ankylosing spondylitis** *(Ref: Yanoff and Duker 4th edition, p 748)*
   Recurrent severe anterior uveitis in a young male patient should be investigated for **HLA B 27 associated Ankylosing Spondylitis**, hence the answer.

10. **d. Spherical equivalent glasses** *(Ref: Yanoff and Duker 4th edition, p 92-93)*
    According to the question it appears that the patient is unable to adjust to the glasses due to the astigmatism. Hence the alternative would be to provide spherical equivalent glasses.
    Example of spherical equivalent glasses:
    - Let us suppose there is a glass prescription with high astigmatism like -2DS/-6DS * 180. To get the spherical equivalent, half of the cylindrical power is algebraically added to the spherical power. So in this case half of -6DS that is -3DS is added to the spherical power -2DS. Thus the spherical equivalent becomes -5DS.

- The remaining options cannot be chosen because LASIK, Femto LASIK and ICL (Implantable Collamer Lens) are all different types of refractive surgery. The basic criteria for any refractive surgery are:
  - Age > 18 years
  - Stable refraction for at least 6 months

11. a. Keratan sulphate *(Ref: Yanoff and Duker, 4th edition, p 163-5)*

The **most common glycosaminoglycan (GAG)** present in the corneal stroma is the **keratan sulphate**, which is largely responsible for maintenance of its transparency.

12. b. Exposure keratopathy *(Ref: Skalicky SE et al. Microphthalmia, anophthalmia, and coloboma and associated ocular and systemic features: understanding the spectrum. JAMA Ophthalmol. 2013)*

The defect shown in the clinical photograph is a full- thickness defect of the upper eyelid or upper eyelid coloboma.
- Lid coloboma is a congenital full-thickness or partial thickness defect of the lid. It arises from defective eyelid development either during fusion of the lids in the third and fourth months of embryologic development, or during re-separation of the lids in the sixth or seventh month.
- **Upper lid colobomas** are usually present at the junction of the **medial one-third and lateral two-third** of the eyelid whereas **lower lid colobomas** are usually present at the junction of the **medial two-third and lateral one-third** of the eyelid.
- Lid coloboma may be associated with **Treacher Collins Syndrome, Goldenhar Syndrome** and **CHARGE syndrome**.
- Ocular anomalies associated with lid coloboma are **limbal dermoid,** symblepharon, corneal opacity, **iris coloboma, chorioretinal coloboma and optic nerve coloboma**.
- Coloboma causes incomplete closure of the lid resulting in corneal exposure and exposure keratopathy. Eyelid reconstruction is needed in large defects to prevent development of exposure keratopathy.

13. b. Congenital glaucoma *(Ref: Yanoff and Duker 4th edition, p 1102-03)*

The **triad of symptoms** in congenital glaucoma are:
- Lacrimation (excessive watering)
- Photophobia (intolerance to light)
- Blepharospasm.

The clinical photograph shows enlarged eyeball with hazy cornea or **Buphthalmos**, hence the answer.

Mucopolysaccharidosis may present with hazy cornea but the size of the eyeball is normal. Ophthalmia neonatorum presents with redness and discharge in the eyes.

(Please refer to the section "Congenital Glaucoma" in the chapter "Glaucoma" for further reading)

14. b. Left occipital lobe *(Ref: Yanoff and Duker 4th edition, p 904-905)*

The field defect given in the question is **Right Homonymous Hemianopia with Macular Sparing.** This is due to posterior cerebral artery (PCA) territory infarct with sparing of the middle cerebral artery (MCA) territory in the occipital lobe. Hence the site of the lesion is the left occipital lobe.

15. a. Direct spread *(Ref: Yanoff and Duker 4th edition, p 793-796)*

The most common route of spread of retinoblastoma is direct spread via the optic nerve or the sclera.

16. b. Pleomorphic adenoma

Important to remember
- Most common tumour or benign tumour of lacrimal gland: **Pleomorphic adenoma**
- Most common malignancy of the lacrimal gland: **Adenoid cystic carcinoma**

17. b. Fungal corneal ulcer *(Ref: Yanoff and Duker 4th edition, p 225-6)*

Corneal ulcer with **dry surface** and **feathery margins** following **trauma with vegetative matter** is typically suggestive of fungal ulcer.

(Please refer to section on "Corneal Ulcer" in the chapter "Conjunctiva, Sclera and Cornea for further reading)

18. d. PG analogues *(Ref: Yanoff and Duker 4th edition, p 1117-8)*

The clinical scenario is suggestive of **uveitic or inflammatory glaucoma**.

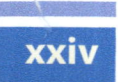

Answers and Explanations

Drugs contraindicated in uveitic glaucoma are:
- **PG analogues** (increase intraocular inflammation, may cause cystoid macular oedema)
- **Brimonidine** (increases intraocular inflammation, may cause cystoid macular oedema)
- **Pilocarpine** (causes miosis, increases ciliary spasm)

19. d. Evaluation of the control program *(Ref: National Program for Control of Blindness)*

SAFE Strategy in trachoma stands for
- Surgery
- Antibiotics
- Facial cleanliness
- **Environmental modification**

20. d. Oculomotor nerve palsy *(Ref: Yanoff and Duker 4th edition, p 929)*

The clinical photograph shows
- Left Eye: **Severe ptosis** with eyeball deviated **downwards and outwards in primary position.**
- All extraocular movements are limited in the left eye except abduction and depression.
- **Pupil is normal**

Therefore, the diagnosis is Left eye: **Pupil sparing third nerve palsy** suggestive of microvascular infarct.
(Please refer to the section "Cranial Nerve Palsies" in the chapter "Neuro-ophthalmology" for further reading)

21. a. Occlusion *(Ref: Yanoff and Duker 4th edition, p 1242)*

Occlusion of the good eye is the best management for amblyopia because it forces the child to use the amblyopic eye. Penalisation of the good eye with atropine may be considered as an alternative if the child is not co-operative for occlusion.

22. c. Vernal keratoconjunctivitis *(Ref: Yanoff and Duker 4th edition, p 192-3)*

The clinical photograph shows flat-topped elevations on the upper tarsal conjunctiva called as papillae. The appearance is called as **cobblestone appearance**. In a male child, history of bilateral redness and itching with cobblestone appearance is suggestive of Vernal Keratoconjunctivitis or Spring Catarrh.

23. b. Sac massage *(Ref: Yanoff and Duker 4th edition, p 1348)*
- The clinical scenario suggests the diagnosis of **Congenital Dacryocystitis.** The first line management of Congenital Dacryocystitis is **conservative** -Lacrimal sac massage or **Hydrostatic massage**.
- Syringing and probing may be done if the child is still symptomatic at around 1 year of age.
- Surgical management like Dacryocystorhinostomy may be considered in recurrent dacryocystitis or failure of probing. It is generally advised when the child is around 3 years of age.

24. d. Can be done in case of hazy ocular media *(Ref: Kanski 7th edition, p 692)*

The procedure shown in the photograph is **Direct Ophthalmoscopy**.
The main advantage of the Direct Ophthalmoscope is **high magnification**.
The drawbacks are:
- Field of view is limited to the central retina
- Non-stereoscopic view
- Not useful in hazy ocular media since the illumination is not as bright as the Indirect Ophthalmoscope.

25. c. Excision with conjunctival autograft *(Ref: Yanoff and Duker 4th edition, p 203-4)*

26. b. Goldman applanation tonometer *(Ref: Yanoff and Duker 4th edition, p 1020-21)*

27. b. Wilson's disease *(Ref: Yanoff and Duker 4th edition, p 415-16)*
- Wilson's disease is an inborn error of **copper metabolism** characterised by deficiency of **Ceruloplasmin**. Inheritance pattern is generally Autosomal Recessive.
- Deposition of copper in different tissues leads to **hepatic**, **neurological** and **ocular** manifestations.
- The important ocular features of Wilson's disease are **Kayser-Fleischer Ring (KF ring)** in cornea and **Sunflower Cataract.**
- The identification of KF ring is the most important clinical sign in the diagnosis of Wilson's disease. The ring is seen as a **greenish-yellow or golden-brown deposit** in the **Descemet's membrane** of the cornea due to Cu deposition.
- It starts in the **superior periphery**, then spreads **inferiorly** and finally becomes **circumferential**.

Self Assessment and Review of Ophthalmology

28. c. Bitemporal hemianopia *(Ref: Yanoff and Duker 4th edition, p 904-905)*

Compression of the centre of the optic chiasma leads to involvement of the nasal fibres of both eyes resulting in bitemporal hemianopia.

29. c. Chalazion *(Ref: Yanoff and Duker 4th edition, p 1304)*

The instrument in the picture is a **Chalazion Clamp** which is used in the **Incision and Curettage** of chalazion.
The other instrument used in the procedure is a **Chalazion Scoop**.

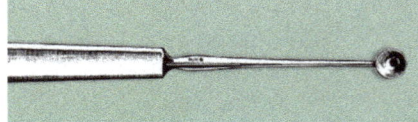

30. a. Glaucoma *(Ref: Yanoff and Duker 4th edition, p 1114-15)*

β-Blockers are used topically as **anti-glaucoma drug**. They **decrease aqueous humour** production by acting on the blood vessels of the ciliary body and the ciliary epithelium.

31. b. HLA B27 *(Ref: Yanoff and Duker 4th edition, p 748)*

HLA B27 associated uveitis presents with **recurrent/ chronic, severe, non-granulomatous anterior uveitis**. It is associated with diseases like:
- Ankylosing spondylitis
- Reiter's syndrome
- Psoriatic arthritis

32. b. Horner syndrome *(Ref: Kanski 6th edition, p 805)*

33. d. Causes myopia *(Ref: Yanoff and Duker 4th edition p 203-4)*
- The condition given in the clinical photograph is **Pterygium**. It is an elastotic degeneration of the conjunctiva.
- Pterygium generally causes **With the Rule Astigmatism** due to flattening of the horizontal axis of the cornea.
- Iron deposition close to the head of the Pterygium leads to the formation of **Stocker's Line**.

34. b. Retinoblastoma *(Ref: Yanoff and Duker 4th edition, p 796)*

The clinical photograph shows **leucocoria** or **white pupillary reflex** in the left eye of a child.
- Leucocoria is the **most common presenting feature** of Retinoblastoma
- Most common cause of leucocoria in a child is **congenital cataract**.

35. c. Acute angle closure glaucoma *(Yanoff and Duker 4th edition, p 1064)*

The important points in favour of the diagnosis are:
- Elderly female
- Sudden onset pain and redness in the eye
- Shallow anterior chamber
- Mid-dilated and fixed pupil
- Stony hard eyeball due to high IOP

(Please refer to the section "Primary Angle Closure Glaucoma" in the chapter "Glaucoma" for further reading)

36. b. Retinoblastoma *(Ref: Yanoff and Duker 4th edition, p 796-99)*

The important points in favour of the diagnosis:
- 2-year-old child
- White pupillary reflex or leucocoria
- **Intraocular mass with calcification on USG B-Scan**

37. c. Major arterial circle of iris

The major arterial circle of iris is formed by the anastomosis between the **long posterior ciliary arteries** and the **anterior ciliary arteries**. It is the most important source of blood supply in the anterior segment.

38. b. It moves in the opposite direction as the retinoscope *(Ref: Yanoff and Duker 4th edition, p 47-50)*

In the right eye, the refractive error is -3DS, meaning -3D in both principal meridians of the eye. As the **myopia is greater than -1D**, therefore **against movement** or movement of retinoscopy reflex opposite to the direction of retinoscope is observed.

(Please refer to the section "Retinoscopy" in the chapter "Optics and Refraction" for further reading.)

Answers and Explanations

39. b. Bowman's membrane has regenerative potential *(Ref: Yanoff and Duker 4th edition, p 163-5)*
Bowman's membrane has no regenerative potential.

40. d. Horner syndrome *(Ref: Kanski 6th edition, p 805)*
Adie's tonic pupil and Blind eye have dilated pupil, hence are automatically ruled out.
Argyll Robertson pupil has irregular small pupil but is an example of light-near dissociation.
Horner syndrome or **Oculo-sympathetic palsy** results in miosis due to loss of sympathetic nerve supply to the dilator pupillae muscle. Since dilatation of the pupil in darkness requires the stimulation of the dilator pupillae muscle, hence there is no increase in size of the pupil in darkness.

41. d. Eye drop followed by eye ointment after 15 minutes
Ointment has an oily base and may impair the absorption of the eye drop; hence the eye drop has to be administered first. After instilling the eye drop, one has to wait for about 10-15 minutes for it be absorbed before instilling the ointment. The basic rule is **two topical drugs should not be administered immediately** one after the other.

42. b. Vigabatrin

Side effects of some common medications			
Medication	**Used to treat**	**Side effects**	**Visual signs and symptoms**
Bisphosphonates	Osteoporosis, Paget's disease, metastatic bone disease, multiple myeloma	Scleritis, conjunctivitis, anterior uveitis	Blurred vision, ocular pain
Digoxin	Atrial fibrillation, congestive heart failure	Decreased visual acuity, central scotoma, color vision defects	Yellow vision, flashing lights, hazy vision, difficulty reading
Direct-acting oral anticoagulants	Venous thromboembolism, atrial fibrillation	Ocular toxicity	Blurred vision, keratoconjunctivitis, subconjunctival and retinal hemorrhage
Ethambutol	Tuberculosis	Optic neuropathy	Bilateral central vision loss, scotomas
Fingolimod	Multiple sclerosis	Possible cystoid macular edema	Blurry vision, central blind spot, sensitivity
Hydroxychloroquine	Rheumatoid arthritis, lupus erythematosus and Sjögren's syndrome	Retinal toxicity, bilateral bull's-eye maculopathy	Difficulty focusing, streaks or flashes, swelling, eye color changes
Isotretinoin	Acne and psoriasis	Meibomian gland dysfunction, intracranial hypertension	Blurred vision, headaches, tinnitus
Phosphodiesterase Inhibitors	Erectile dysfunction	Possible ischemic optic neuropathy (infrequent at low doses)	Bluish tinge to vision, light sensitivity
Tamoxifen	Metastatic breast cancer	Retinopathy, possibly cataract, intraretinal crystalline deposits	Corneal dryness, floaters, decreased visual acuity and color vision
Tamsulosin	Benign prostate hyperplasia	Floppy iris syndrome	Blurred vision
Topiramate	Migraines, seizures, bipolar disease, post-traumatic stress, obsessive-compulsive disorders	Ciliary body effusion and anterior rotation of the ciliary processes, angle-closure glaucoma, maculopathy	Blurred vision, diplopia, vision disturbances, myopic shift
Vigabatrin	Seizures not responding to other therapies	Progressive bilateral concentric visual-field constriction	Reduction of visual acuity

43. b. **Haigis L** *(Ref: Yanoff and Duker 4th edition, p 337-340)*

   (Please refer to the section "IOL power calculation formula" in the chapter "Lens" for further reading)

44. b. **Right Superior Rectus (SR) palsy** *(Ref: Yanoff and Duker 4th edition, p 929)*
   - Right eye hypotropia is equivalent to Left eye hypertropia
   - This may be due to paralysis of either the **elevators of the right eye (RSR/ RIO)** or the **depressors of the left eye (LIR/LSO).**
   - The question says that RE hypotropia/ LE hypertropia worsens in **right gaze.** This means that out of the four muscles (RSR/RIO/LIR/LSO), the muscles acting in right gaze should be faulty. Hence the defective muscle should be either **RSR or LSO.**
   - The question further says that it worsens on right head tilt. On right head tilt, the right eye extorts and the left eye intorts. So, to maintain the equilibrium, the intorters of the right eye and the extorters of the left eye must function.
   - Worsening on right head tilt indicates therefore that either the **intorter of the right eye or the extorter of the left eye** is defective. Out of these two muscles (RSR/ LSO), RSR is an intorter of the right eye. Hence it is the affected muscle.

45. a. **Hypervitaminosis D** *(Ref: Yanoff and Duker 4th edition, p8 75)*

46. b. **Ishihara chart, c. Naegel's anomaloscope, d. Lantern test, e. Holmgren's wool test**
   (Ref: Kanski 6th edition, p 20-21)

47. b. **Schlemm's canal, c. Anterior chamber, d. Posterior chamber, e. Episcleral veins**
   (Ref: Yanoff and Duker 4th edition, p 1012-1014)

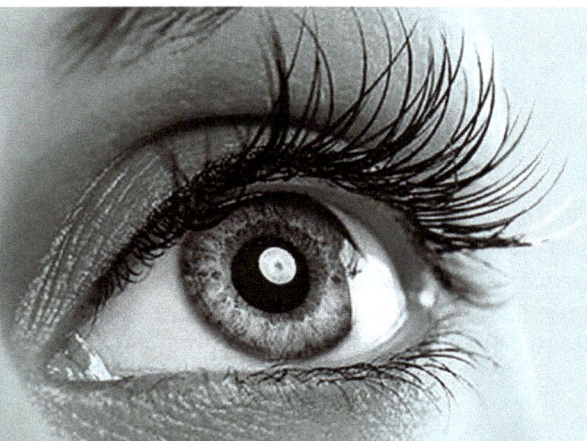

Ocular Embryology

The eye is formed from three different germ layers, namely neuroectoderm, surface ectoderm and mesoderm with contribution from the neural crest cells. The structures originating from the different layers are:

Neuroectoderm
• Optic nerve^Q
• Retina including the retinal pigment epithelium^Q
• Epithelium of ciliary body
• Epithelium of the iris
• Sphincter and dilator pupillae muscles^Q
• Ciliary zonules
• Secondary and tertiary vitreous
Surface ectoderm
• Epithelium of conjunctiva
• Epithelium of cornea

Contd...

Contd...

• Lens^Q
• Lacrimal glands
• Skin of eyelids
Mesoderm
• Sclera
• Walls of the orbit
• Extraocular muscles
• Connective tissue of the orbit
• Eyelids
Neural crest cells
• Stroma, Descemet's membrane and endothelium of the cornea
• Angle of anterior chamber^Q
• Stroma of the iris^Q
• Ciliary body and choroid
• Primary vitreous

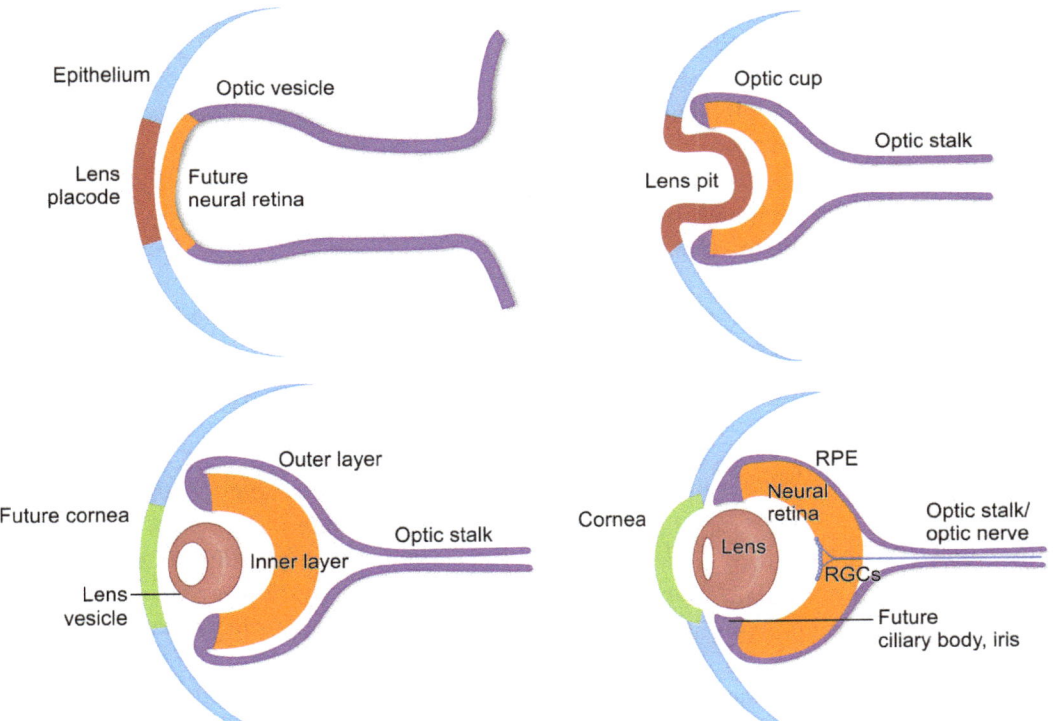

Fig. 1: Development of the eye
(RPE: Retinal pigment epithelium; RGCs: Retinal ganglion cells)

Self Assessment and Review of Ophthalmology

- The development of the eye starts at about **the third week of gestation.** The neural tube which forms the forebrain gives rise to one diverticulum on either side known as the **optic vesicle**[Q].
- The optic vesicle (neuroectoderm) meets the **surface ectoderm** which shows an area of thickening called the **lens placode**.
- The optic vesicle invaginates to form the two layered **optic cup**[Q]. Eventually, **the inner layer** of the cup forms the **neurosensory retina**[Q] whereas the **outer layer** forms the **retinal pigment epithelium**[Q]. It then continues backward as the **optic nerve** with its meninges to the brain. The anterior end of the cup later differentiates into the **ciliary epithelium, iris epithelium and muscles of the iris**[Q].
- The invagination of the optic cup however remains incomplete inferonasally in the form of a fissure known as the **embryonic fissure**[Q]. Through this fissure, the hyaloid artery passes to provide nutrition to the developing ocular structures. Eventually, the hyaloid artery disappears and the choroidal fissure closes. The space between the lens and optic cup becomes filled by a clear jelly called the vitreous which is mainly secreted by the neuroectoderm
- The lens placode invaginates into the optic cup and ultimately gets detached from the surface ectoderm to form **the lens vesicle**[Q]. This eventually forms **the crystalline lens**.
- After formation of the lens vesicle, there is migration of the waves of **neural crest cells**[Q]. These cells eventually differentiate into the **cornea, angle structures and stroma of the iris and ciliary body**[Q].
- While the ectodermal events are taking place, **the mesoderm** surrounding the optic cup differentiates to form the **sclera, extraocular muscles and orbital structures**[Q].

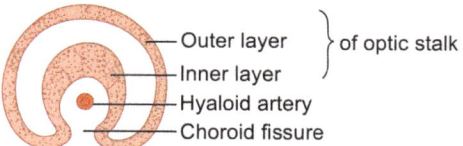

Fig. 2: Embryonic fissure

EMBRYONIC REMNANTS IN THE EYE

- *Mittendorf's dot*[Q]: It is the remnant of the anterior end of the hyaloid artery and remains attached to the posterior pole of the lens
- *Bergmeister papilla*[Q]: It is the remnant of the posterior end of the hyaloid artery. It remains attached to the optic disc associated with some glial tissue.
- *Persistent hyperplastic primary vitreous (PHPV):* Failure of the fetal vasculature to regress is called PHPV (explained in detail in the chapter on retina).
- *Coloboma:* Failure of the embryonic fissure to close gives rise to ocular coloboma

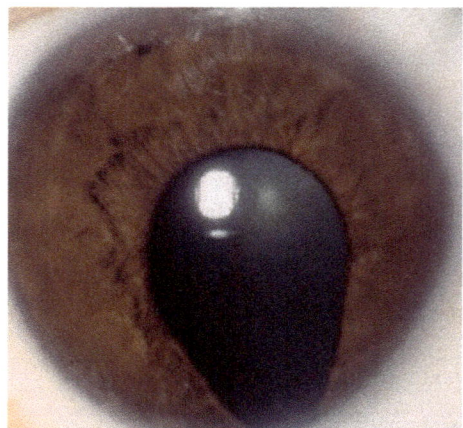

Fig. 3: Iris coloboma

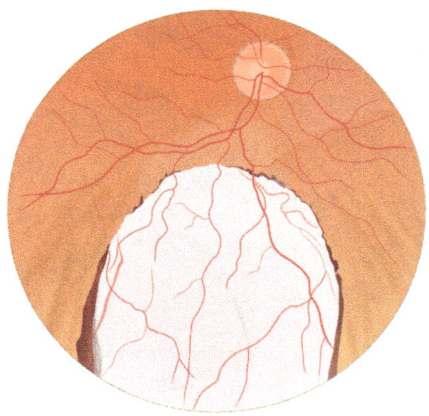

Fig. 4: Chorioretinal coloboma

> **Must Remember**
> - *Retinal Pigment Epithelium:* Derived from neuroectoderm
> - *Sphincter and dilator pupillae:* Derived from neuroectoderm
> - *Lens:* Derived from surface ectoderm
> - *Sclera:* Derived from mesoderm
> - *Angle of anterior chamber:* Derived from neural crest cells

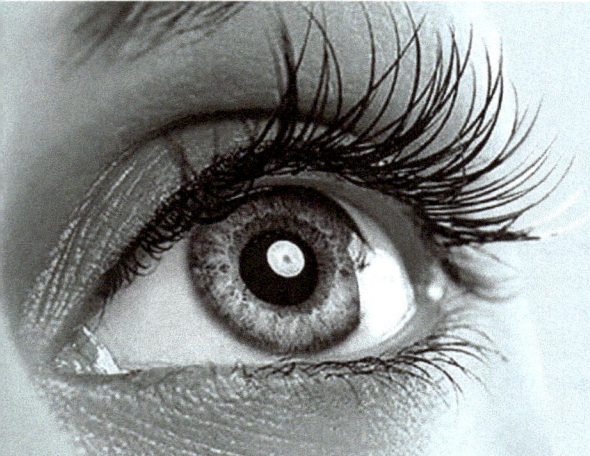

Coats of the Eyeball

The eyeball consists of three coats. From outside inwards, they are
- Outer fibrous coat
- Middle vascular coat
- Inner nervous coat.

OUTER FIBROUS COAT

It is the outermost coat of the eyeball which consists of:

Cornea
- It forms the **anterior one-sixth**[Q] of the fibrous coat
- It is transparent and **avascular**
- It functions as a **refractive medium**.

Sclera
- It forms the **posterior five-sixth**[Q] of the fibrous coat
- It is opaque
- It provides protection to the intraocular structures and provides insertion to the extraocular muscles
- The weakest point of the sclera is **just anterior to the insertion of the extraocular muscles**[Q]. This is the **commonest site of globe rupture in trauma**[Q].
- Posteriorly the sclera forms a circular mesh-like area called **lamina cribrosa** to transmit the nerve fibres which form the optic nerve
- The sclera is pierced by ciliary vessels and nerves and vortex veins

The junction of the cornea and sclera is called the **limbus** which contains the limbal **stem cells. The stem cells are responsible for migration and replacement of corneal epithelial cells in normal cell replacement and wound healing**[Q].

MIDDLE VASCULAR COAT

The middle coat, from anterior to posterior consists of:
- Iris
- Ciliary body
- Choroid

Iris
- It is a pigmented circular disc shaped structure with an aperture at the centre called the pupil.
- It is responsible for eye colour
- It **regulates the amount of light entering the eye** by constriction and dilatation of the pupil with the help of sphincter and dilator pupillae muscles.

Ciliary Body
- It is a wedge shaped structure which is divided into an anterior part called **pars plicata** and a posterior part called **pars plana.**

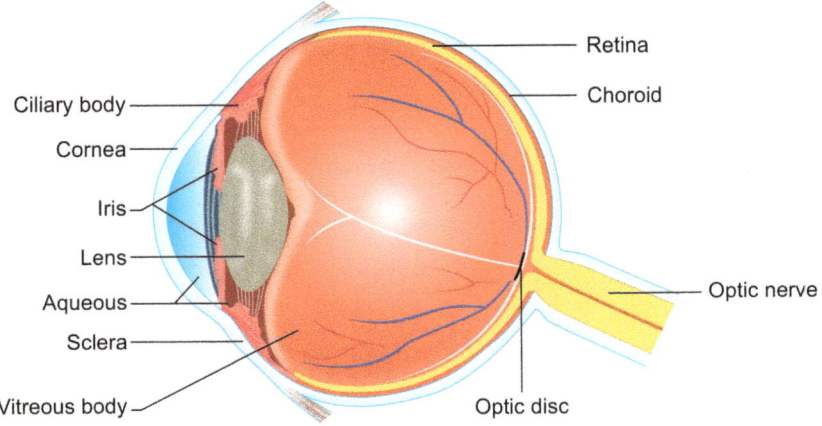

Fig. 1: Coats and contents of the eyeball

- The ciliary body contains ridge like projections called ciliary processes which are responsible for **production of aqueous humour**.
- It gives attachment to the **zonules** which help to keep the crystalline lens in normal position.
- The contraction of the ciliary muscles is responsible for **accommodation**.

Choroid

- It is a highly vascular structure lying in between the sclera and the retina
- Its main function is to provide nutrition and removal of excretory products.

INNER NERVOUS COAT

It consists of the **retina** which is responsible for neural perception. The ganglion cells of the retina continue posteriorly as the optic nerve which carries the visual impulse to the brain.

CONTENTS OF THE EYEBALL

Enclosed within the ocular coats are the contents of the eyeball. They are
- Crystalline lens
- Aqueous humour
- Vitreous humour

Crystalline Lens

- It is a **biconvex** structure suspended by the ciliary zonules
- It is located in a groove within the eyeball known as the **patellar fossa**[Q]
- It divides the eyeball into **anterior and posterior segment**. The anterior segment is further divided into anterior and posterior chamber by the iris.
- It is **transparent** and functions as **refractive medium**[Q]

Aqueous Humour

- It is the **transparent** watery fluid which fills the anterior segment of the eyeball
- It is produced by the ciliary body and drains out through the angle of anterior chamber.
- It acts as **refractive medium**
- It provides **nutrition** mainly to the **avascular cornea** and **crystalline lens**[Q]
- It is responsible for maintenance of **intraocular pressure**

Vitreous Humour

- It is the **transparent** gel that fills the posterior segment of the eyeball.
- It acts a **refractive medium**
- It maintains the shape and contour of the eyeball
- It also helps in the maintenance of intraocular pressure.

Refractive media of the eye

- Tear film
- Cornea
- Aqueous humour
- Lens
- Vitreous humour

Conjunctiva, Sclera and Cornea

CONJUNCTIVA

Conjunctiva is a translucent mucous membrane lining the posterior surface of the eyelids and anterior surface of the sclera. The parts of the conjunctiva are:

➤ *Palpebral*: It lines the posterior surface of the eyelid and is firmly attached to the tarsus
➤ *Forniceal*: It is the loose fold of conjunctiva at the fornix
➤ *Bulbar*: It covers the sclera

STRUCTURE OF CONJUNCTIVA

It has the following layers:
➤ *Epithelium*: It is **stratified squamous non keratinized epithelium**^{Q}
➤ *Adenoid layer*: It is also called the lymphoid layer and contains the lymphocytes.
➤ *Fibrous layer*: Consists of collagenous and elastic fibres, vessels and nerves

> **Glands of Conjunctiva**
> - *Mucin producing*: Goblet cells, Crypts of Henle and Glands of Manz
> - *Accessory lacrimal glands*: **Glands of Krause**^{Q} (in the fornices) and **Wolfring**^{Q} (along tarsal borders)

ALLERGIC CONJUNCTIVITIS

Vernal Keratoconjunctivitis

➤ It is an allergic keratoconjunctivitis seen in boys between 5 and 15 years of age
➤ It is a **Type I hypersensitivity**^{Q} reaction mediated by **IgE and mast cells**^{Q}
➤ It is also called as **spring catarrh**^{Q}
➤ *Symptoms*: **Itching**^{Q} associated with ropy discharge
➤ Signs
  ◆ Conjunctival features
    - Flat topped papillae are seen on the upper tarsal conjunctiva. The typical appearance is called **cobblestone appearance**^{Q}.
    - In the limbal variety, there is hypertrophy of the superior limbal conjunctiva. This gives rise to raised white nodules close to the upper limbus called **Horner-Tranta's spots**^{Q}
  ◆ Corneal features
    - Superficial punctate keratitis
    - **Shield ulcer**^{Q}
    - Curved white line close to the upper limbus called **pseudogerontoxon**^{Q}
    - **Keratoconus**^{Q} is an association
➤ Treatment
  ◆ *Acute episode*: The following drugs are given topically
    - Antihistaminics
    - Steroids
    - Cyclosporine
  ◆ *Prophylaxis*: The following drugs are given topically
    - **Sodium cromoglycate**^{Q}
    - Ketotifen
    - Olopatadine
    - Epinastine
    - Bepotastine

> **Phlyctenular Conjunctivitis**
> - It is a **Type IV hypersensitivity**^{Q} reaction, mainly to **tuberculous antigen**^{Q}. However in western countries, it is said to be mainly associated with **Staphylococcus**^{Q}.
> - It is seen in children (8–15 years)
> - It begins as a well-circumscribed nodule at the limbus but it may encroach upon the cornea. This is known as **fascicular ulcer**^{Q}
> - Treatment is topical steroids. Systemic evaluation and ATT is usually considered in our country

INFECTIVE CONJUNCTIVITIS

Acute Bacterial Conjunctivitis

This is a very common self-limiting condition seen mainly in children. The symptoms are redness, grittiness, discharge, sticking of lashes. On examination, there is conjunctival congestion, more in fornices, associated with purulent or mucopurulent discharge. **Follicles**^{Q} **may be seen (Follicles are collections of lymphocytes in the adenoid layer surrounded by blood vessels)**. The condition is usually self-limiting. Local antibiotics and lubricants may be prescribed. The different types of bacterial conjunctivitis are:

- *Membranous conjunctivitis*: This is caused by organisms of very high virulence like *Corynebacterium diphtheriae, Streptococcus haemolyticus*. A **thick yellowish-grey membrane** is formed in the palpebral conjunctiva which **bleeds on peeling**. The raw area left after sloughing of membrane may lead to complications like symblepharon and entropion due to cicatrisation. Systemic antibiotics and anti-diphtheric serum are also given in addition to local therapy
- *Pseudomembranous conjunctivitis*: This is the common variety where a pseudomembrane is seen on the palpebral conjunctiva due to organisation of the exudates. It is adhered loosely to the underlying conjunctiva and may bleed slightly on peeling but no raw area is seen beneath it. It is seen in conjunctivitis caused by *Staphylococcus aureus, Staphylococcus epidermidis, Streptococcus* of low virulence etc
- *Angular conjunctivitis*: This is a condition where the redness is limited to the inner and outer canthi and excoriation is seen at the lateral eye margins. It is caused by **Moraxella Axenfeld**^{Q}. It is treated with zinc and oxytetracycline topically.

Acute Viral Conjunctivitis

This is a common self-limiting condition seen in both children and adults. It presents with redness, watering and foreign body sensation. It is a **follicular conjunctivitis**^{Q} and may be associated with subconjunctival haemorrhage and pseudomembrane. **Pre-auricular lymphadenopathy is seen**^{Q}. It is self-limiting and lubricants are prescribed for relief. The different types are:

- *Haemorrhagic conjunctivitis*: It is associated with petechial haemorrhages in the conjunctiva. The causative organisms are **Adenovirus**^{Q}, **Enterovirus**^{Q}, **Echovirus**^{Q}, **Coxsackie**^{Q} **virus**
- *Keratoconjunctivitis*: This is commonly seen with **adenovirus** where nummular lesions are seen on the cornea associated with conjunctivitis. **It is associated with photophobia**^{Q} **and blurring of vision**. Nummular resolve spontaneously over a period of time but topical steroids are prescribed for quick resolution.

Adult Inclusion Conjunctivitis

- The causative organism is *Chlamydia trachomatis* **serotypes D-K**^{Q}.
- The primary source of infection is urethritis in males and cervicitis in females because these serotypes are sexually transmitted
- It may also be transferred through contaminated water of swimming pools. Hence it is also called **swimming pool conjunctivitis**^{Q}
- It is a type of **follicular conjunctivitis**^{Q} associated with preauricular lymphadenopathy

TRACHOMA

It is a specific type of keratoconjunctivitis which is characterized by formation of follicles and pannus followed by resolution by cicatrisation. The causative organism is **Chlamydia trachomatis serotypes A, B, Ba and C**^{Q}. It is seen in children < 5 years of age especially in areas of poverty, overcrowding and poor hygiene. Practices like applying surma, kohl and kajal increase transmission of disease among children.

Pathology

- Chlamydia is an epitheliotropic micro-organism which affects the conjunctival and corneal epithelium^Q.
- It can be seen in the epithelial cells as **HP inclusion bodies**^{Q}
- Trachoma is characterized by intense infiltration of lymphocytes in the adenoid layer of the conjunctiva. Aggregation of lymphocytes results in the formation of follicles. **Sago grain follicles are seen on the upper tarsal conjunctiva**^{Q}.
- Follicles seen close to the upper limbus are called as **Herbert's follicles**^{Q}
- On cicatrisation, a white line is seen on the upper tarsal conjunctiva known as **Arlt's line**^{Q}
- Herbert's follicles on scarring form **Herbert's pits**^{Q}

Prevalence

- *High endemic (50-70%)*: Punjab, Rajasthan, U.P.
- *Moderately endemic (20-50%)*: Gujarat, M.P. Bihar, Assam, Karnataka
- *Low endemic (<20%) J.K.A.P. Tamil Nadu Maharashtra*
- *Very low endemic (0-5%)*: West Bengal, Odisha

WHO Classification (1987)

F	(Follicles)	Presence of more than **5 follicles**^{Q}, larger than **0.5 mm diameter**^{Q} on the **upper tarsal conjunctiva**^{Q}
I	(Inflammation)	Intense inflammation with thickening of the conjunctiva obscuring more than 50% of the deep tarsal vessels
S	(Scarring)	Evidence of conjunctival cicatrisation with white lines, bands of fibrosis in the tarsal conjunctiva
T	(Trichiasis)	At least one trichiatic lash
O	(Opacity)	Corneal opacity obscuring the visual axis and causing a visual acuity <6/18.

Sequelae

- Trichiasis, entropion
- Ptosis, madarosis, tylosis
- Conjunctival and corneal xerosis
- Corneal ulcer and opacity
- Chronic dacryocystitis

Prevalence (in population 0–9 yrs)	Prophylaxis
>10%	Mass prophylaxis^Q
5–10%	Family prophylaxis
<5%	Only individual treatment

Safe Strategy^Q

- **S:** Surgery for trichiasis/entropion/corneal opacity
- **A:** Antibiotics for active infection **(Azithromycin 500 mg single dose)**^{Q}
- **F:** Facial cleanliness
- **E:** Environmental hygiene

Ophthalmia Neonatorum

- It is an acute inflammation of the conjunctiva seen in a new-born child within one month of birth. It is associated with catarrhal discharge (no tears are formed up to 4 weeks of life)
- The causes may be **chemical**, *Chlamydia*, **herpes simplex**, *Gonococcus*, other bacteria

CONJUNCTIVAL DEGENERATIONS

The different types of degenerations seen in conjunctiva are:
- **Pinguecula (most common)**^{Q}
- Pterygium
- Concretions
- Retention cyst

Pterygium

- It is an **elastotic degeneration**^{Q} of the conjunctiva
- A degenerated fold of conjunctiva grows on the surface of the cornea to **involve the superficial corneal layers up to the stroma**^{Q}
- It is associated with UV ray exposure
- More common on the **nasal side**^{Q}
- A pterygium has three parts: Head, neck and body. Close to the head of the pterygium is a pigmented line due to iron deposition called as **Stocker's line**^{Q}
- Pterygium may lead to
  - Visual disturbance when it encroaches the pupillary axis
  - *Astigmatism*: Usually, **with the rule**^{Q}
  - Diplopia due to restriction of ocular movements
  - Disturbance of tear film
  - Cosmetic blemish
- Treatment
  - **May be left alone if asymptomatic**^{Q}
  - Excision with bare sclera: Simple excision is associated with a high level of **recurrence**^{Q}
  - Excision with application of **Mitomycin C**^{Q} to the bed of pterygium
  - Excision with **conjunctival autograft**^{Q}
  - Excision with **amniotic membrane graft**^{Q}

SCLERA

EPISCLERITIS

- It is a common self-limiting disorder affecting young adults
- It is associated with mild redness and discomfort
- It may be nodular or diffuse
- It is treated with topical anti-inflammatory drugs

SCLERITIS

- It is a painful condition associated with severe redness and watering of the eye
- It is associated with connective tissue disorders like **Rheumatoid arthritis**^{Q}, Wegener granulomatosis, Polyarteritis nodosa and SLE.
- It may be associated with uveitis also
- Treatment is topical and systemic steroids. It may also need systemic immunosuppressants in severe cases

Classification

- Anterior
  - *Non-necrotizing*: It may be nodular or diffuse
  - *Necrotizing*: It may be with or without inflammation. **Scleromalacia perforans**^{Q} is a type of

necrotizing scleritis without inflammation, associated with long-standing **rheumatoid arthritis**[Q]
- Posterior
  - *Non-necrotizing*
  - *Necrotizing*: Surgically induced necrotizing scleritis (SINS)

Blue Sclera

- Osteogenesis imperfecta
- Paget's disease
- Ehler Danlos syndrome
- Marfan syndrome
- Staphyloma
- Healed scleritis

Staphyloma

It is an ectasia of the outer coats of the eyeball with incarceration of uveal tissue. It is of the following types
- **Anterior**: It is due to **perforated corneal ulcer**[Q]
- **Intercalary** (within 3 mm of the limbus): It is seen in **peripheral ulcerative keratitis**[Q]
- **Ciliary** (Posterior to 3 mm from the limbus) It is seen in **healed scleritis**[Q]
- **Equatorial**: It is seen in **high myopia, healed scleritis**[Q]
- **Posterior** (behind the equator): It is seen in **pathological myopia**[Q]

CORNEA

ANATOMY

The cornea is the transparent outermost coat which covers **the anterior one third of the eyeball**
- Refractive Index 1.376[Q]
- Refractive Power **43–44 Dioptres**[Q]
- *Thickness*:
  - Central 450–550 microns
  - Peripheral 700-900 microns
- Anterior surface of cornea is **elliptical**.
  - Vertical diameter 11.7 mm
  - Horizontal diameter 11 mm
- Posterior surface is circular. Diameter 11.7 mm
- *Microcornea*[Q]: Corneal diameter **<10 mm**
- *Megalocornea*[Q]: Corneal diameter **> or equal to 13 mm**
- *Radius of curvature*:
  - Anterior surface 7.84 mm[Q]
  - Posterior surface 6.4 mm[Q]

It is composed of five layers. From outside inwards, they are
- *Epithelium*: Stratified squamous non-keratinized epithelium
- Bowman's layer
- *Stroma*: **Thickest layer**[Q]
- *Descemet's membrane*: **Toughest layer**[Q]
- *Endothelium*: **Most metabolically active layer**[Q]. It is composed of a single layer of hexagonal cells.
- A sixth layer called **Dua's layer** has been recently identified. It lies between stroma and Descemet's membrane

Maintenance of Corneal Transparency

The factors responsible for the maintenance of corneal transparency are
- The smooth texture of the epithelium and the tear film
- **Arrangement of stromal lamellae**[Q]: The regular arrangement of the stromal lamellae ensure that all the scattered light is lost by mutual interference
- **Avascularity**[Q]
- Unmyelinated nerve fibres
- **Endothelial pump mechanism**: The endothelial pump (Na+/K+ ATPase) ensures an optimum level of corneal hydration by pumping out excess water from the cornea. **This relative dehydration of the cornea is responsible for its transparency**[Q]. Optimum hydration of cornea is 80%
- Intraocular pressure: Increase in intraocular pressure affects the endothelial pump activity leading to increased hydration of cornea

Important Investigations Related to Cornea

- *Pachymetry*: **To measure corneal thickness**[Q]
- *Keratometry*: To measure the corneal curvature[Q]
- *Corneal topography*: **Measures corneal curvature, shape and thickness**
- *Specular microscopy*: **To assess the corneal endothelium**[Q]
- Anterior segment ocular coherence tomography (AS-OCT): To assess different corneal layers
- Vital stains:
  - **Fluorescein stain**[Q]: To identify epithelial defect
  - Rose Bengal stain: It stains the degenerated epithelial cells. It causes severe stinging, hence rarely used

Conjunctiva, Sclera and Cornea

INFECTIVE KERATITIS

The different types of infectious keratitis are bacterial, fungal, *Acanthamoeba* and viral.

Bacterial and Fungal Keratitis

The corneal epithelium is usually resistant to infection but if the integrity of the epithelium is disturbed, keratitis may result.

> **Factors Predisposing for Development of Ulcer**
> - Corneal abrasion
> - Trauma and foreign body
> - Dry eyes
> - Contact lens misuse
> - Misuse of anaesthetic drops
> - Prolonged steroid use
> - Neurotrophic/Exposure keratopathy
> - Bullous keratopathy
> - Chronic blepharitis or dacryocystitis
> - Immunosupression due to any cause

But there are certain bacteria capable of invading an intact epithelium. These are
- *N. gonorrhoea, N. meningitis*^{Q}
- *Corynebacterium diphtheriae*^{Q}
- *Listeria*^{Q}

Clinical Features of Corneal Ulcer

	Bacterial ulcer	Fungal ulcer
History	Presence of predisposing factors	Predisposing factors especially **trauma with vegetable matter**^{Q}
Symptoms	Pain, redness, photophobia and lacrimation	Same symptoms but **less pronounced**^{Q}
Ulcer margins	Well-defined	**Indistinct and feathery**^{Q}
Base of the ulcer	Clean	**Necrotic**
Number of ulcers	Usually single	Multiple small ulcers surround the main ulcer. Known as **satellite ulcers**^{Q}
Associated features	None	Surrounded by a ring called **immune ring**
Hypopyon	**Sterile** and **mobile**^{Q}	**Non-sterile**^{Q}, contains fungal hyphae **Fixed**^{Q}

Contd...

Investigation	Corneal scraping and staining with **Gram stain.** Inoculation in **blood agar**	Corneal scraping and **KOH mount.** Inoculation in **Sabouraud's dextrose agar**
Treatment (Medical)	Fortified antibiotics Cefazoline (50 mg/ml) Tobramycin (14 mg/ml Atropine^Q	Anti-fungal drops **Natamycin (50 mg/ml)**^{Q} Amphotericin B (1.5 mg/ml) Voriconazole (10 mg/ml) Oral Ketoconazole Atropine^Q
Treatment (Surgical)	Debridement Therapeutic keratoplasty	Debridement Therapeutic keratoplasty

> **Things to Remember**
> - Hypopyon corneal ulcer with rapid progression and perforation: *Pseudomonas*^{Q}
> - **Ulcer serpens:** *Pneumococcus*^{Q}
> - Most common causative organism causing fungal ulcer in India: Aspergillus
> - **Drug of choice for fungal corneal ulcer (filamentous): Natamycin**^{Q}
> - Drug of choice for fungal corneal ulcer (non-filamentous): Amphotericin B
> - **Steroids are absolutely contraindicated in both bacterial and fungal ulcers**
> - Atropine must be given in all cases to relieve ciliary spasm^Q
> - Ulcer resembling fungal ulcer is caused by **Nocardia asteroides**^{Q}, a filament acid-fast bacterium. The ulcer has feathery margins with satellite lesions. The typical appearance is called **cracked windshield appearance**^{Q}. It usually follows trauma associated with contamination with soil. Other organisms causing similar ulcer are *Mycobacteria,* and *Actinomyces*

Complications of Corneal Ulcer
- *Thinning and bulging of cornea*
- *Bulging of Descemet's membrane called **Descemetocele**^{Q} due to thinning or necrosis of the overlying layers. Desmetocoele is treated with tissue adhesive like **Cyanoacrylate glue** and **bandage contact lens**^{Q}*
- Corneal opacity due to healing of the ulcer
  - *Nebular opacity*: This is due to involvement of the superficial stroma (<1/3). It is the **most visually disturbing**^{Q} type of corneal opacity because it causes scattering of light

- *Macular opacity*: This is seen when up to 1/2 of the thickness of the corneal stroma is involved.
- *Leucomatous opacity*: This is see due to involvement of ½ to full thickness of the corneal stroma
- Perforation of cornea may lead to
  - Small perforation is usually plugged by iris resulting in adherent leucoma
  - Large perforation leads to iris prolapse. Exudation forms a pseudocornea over it
  - Anterior staphyloma: Protrusion of the cornea with incarcerated iris tissue

Acanthamoeba Keratitis

- *Acanthamoeba* is a **fresh water protozoan**^{Q} which capable of causing corneal infection. It is **seen in contact lens users**^{Q} who use outdated solutions, tap water to clean their lenses
- However the **most common infectious keratitis in contact lens user is caused by *Pseudomonas*** ^{Q}

Clinical Features

- Severe pain, out of proportion to the degree of inflammation is the distinctive feature. **Most painful type of keratitis**^{Q}
- Redness, photophobia and lacrimation
- Starts as a **dendritic ulcer**^{Q} but soon becomes **a ring ulcer**^{Q}
- Involves the adjoining limbus causing **limbitis**
- Inflammation of the corneal nerves called **radial keratoneuritis**^{Q}

Investigation

- *Acanthamoeba* is basically a diagnosis of exclusion
- Corneal scraping and staining with **Calcoflour white stain**^{Q}
- Inoculation of scraped material in **Non-nutrient agar enriched with *E. coli***^{Q}

> **Drugs used in the Treatment of Acanthamoeba Keratitis**
> - **Polyhexamethylene Biguanide (0.02%)**^{Q}
> - Chlorhexidine (0.02%)
> - **Propamidine**^{Q}
> - Neomycin

Viral Keratitis

Viral keratitis may be by either **Herpes simplex keratitis (HSV)** or **Herpes zoster ophthalmicus (HZO)**

Herpes Simplex Keratitis

It may be either primary or secondary

- *Primary infection*: This is the first infection by the virus seen in children less than 5 years of age. The features are
  - Vesicles are seen on the lids and periorbital area which heal without scarring
  - Acute follicular conjunctivitis
  - Mild superficial punctuate keratitis: (SPK)
  - It is treated with **Acyclovir ointment (3%)**^{Q} 5 times/day for 2 weeks
- *Secondary infection/Reactivation stage*: This may have varied presentation
  - Epithelial keratitis
    - This is due to the **direct invasion of the epithelium by the virus**^{Q}.
    - It starts as a **dendritic ulcer with marked decrease in corneal sensitivity**^{Q}. Later, the multiple dendrites may join together to form a **geographical ulcer.**
    - Due to decrease in corneal sensitivity, the ulcer is relatively **painless**^{Q}.
    - Treatment is **Acyclovir (3%) ointment**^{Q} for 7–10 days.
    - **Steroids are absolutely contraindicated**^{Q}.
  - *Stromal keratitis*: This is an **immune response to the viral antigen**^{Q}. Characterized by stromal oedema which may progress to necrosis of the underlying bed. **Treatment is topical steroids**^{Q}. Oral acyclovir may be prescribed depending on the severity of the disease and in recurrent cases
  - *Disciform keratitis*: This is an **immune response to the viral antigen**^{Q}. It presents with localized stromal oedema, Descemet's folds and keratic precipitates. **Treatment it is topical steroids**^{Q}. Oral acyclovir may be prescribed in recurrent cases.
  - *Endothelitis*: This is also an **immune response to the viral antigen**^{Q}. It presents with stromal oedema, Descemet's folds and endothelial exudates. Keratic precipitates with anterior uveitis may be present. **Treatment of it is topical steroids**^{Q} Oral acyclovir may be prescribed in severe and recurrent cases.
  - *Metaherpetic keratitis*: This is a type of epithelial ulceration where there is **no active virus**. It results from inability of the epithelium to heal even after the virus has been eliminated. It may be due to loss of underlying innervation (neurotrophic), toxicity due to multiple medications or underlying low-grade inflammation.

Herpes Zoster Ophthalmicus

- This is a reactivation of the chickenpox or **Varicella zoster virus** in conditions where the immune system is suppressed like in elderly, chemotherapy, corticosteroid or immunosuppressive therapy.

Conjunctiva, Sclera and Cornea

- After the initial exposure, the virus remains latent in the sensory ganglion. When reactivated, it migrates down the sensory nerve and causes skin vesicles in that particular dermatome.
- **HZO with ocular involvement** is seen when the virus involves the **nasociliary division**^{Q} of the **ophthalmic branch**^{Q} of the **Trigeminal nerve**^{Q}. (However, **the most commonly** involved division of ophthalmic nerve is **frontal nerve**^{Q} but it does not lead to ocular manifestations.)
- The distribution of the skin lesions helps to fairly predict the occurrence of ocular features in HZO. This is known as **Hutchison's sign**^{Q} which states that if the lesions involve the tip and sides of the nose, the chance of ophthalmic involvement is high.

Clinical Features of HZO

- Vesicles on the lids
- Blepharitis
- Acute follicular conjunctivitis
- Episcleritis and Scleritis
- Keratitis: This may be of different types
  - Punctate epithelial keratitis
  - **Pseudodendritic keratitis**^{Q}: These are different from the true dendrites seen in Herpes simplex because they are **devoid of terminal bulbs**^{Q} and are more peripheral in location
  - Stromal keratitis
  - Disciform keratitis
  - Endothelitis
- Iridocyclitis, choroiditis
- Acute retinal necrosis
- Neuroretinitis
- In the chronic cases, due to decrease in corneal sensation, the patient may develop **neurotrophic keratitis**^{Q}

Treatment

- Oral Acyclovir 800 mg 5 times daily for 14 days
- Topical steroids with cycloplegics

Interstitial Keratitis

- This is a very distinctive entity characterized by stromal keratitis with no involvement of epithelium or endothelium
- It is associated with **tuberculosis**^{Q}, **leprosy**^{Q} and **syphilis**^{Q}
- The basis of the disease is essentially an immune reaction to the foreign antigen

Contd...

Interstitial Keratitis

- It is a dense keratitis associated with deep corneal vascularisation
- The pinkish discolouration of the cornea associated with the condition is called **Salmon patch of Hutchinson**^{Q}
- Treatment is topical steroids. Therapy for the associated systemic disease has to be initiated

NON-INFECTIOUS KERATOPATHIES

Peripheral Ulcerative Keratitis (PUK)

- This is an immunological ulcer associated with disorders like **rheumatoid arthritis, SLE, PAN, Wegener's granulomatosis, etc**^{Q}
- Ulcer involves the periphery of the cornea, extending up to the limbus. It may lead to thinning and perforation. Healed ulcer gives rise to irregular astigmatism^Q
- Treatment is **topical steroids**. **Corneal patch grafting** may be done in cases of severe thinning

Mooren's Ulcer

- Mooren's ulcer is, by definition, an idiopathic PUK where no systemic association can be identified^Q.
- May be unilateral or bilateral and is **severely painful**
- Response to topical steroids is not very good
- Treatment
  - Systemic steroids and immunosuppressants
  - **Conjunctival resection and cautery**^{Q}: It is assumed that the antibodies responsible for corneal destruction and ulceration are brought by the conjunctival vessels. Hence conjunctival resection is done
  - Corneal patch graft

Neurotrophic Keratopathy

- This type of keratopathy is seen in patients with **decreased corneal sensation**
- **Causes may be Herpes, Diabetes, Leprosy, Trigeminal nerve palsy**^{Q}, brain tumours, cerebrovascular accidents, etc
- Decreased sensation leads to decrease in reflex tearing. This leads to epithelial breakdown and poor healing
- It is an indolent, **painless ulcer** which does not respond to conventional management
- Treatment is **artificial tears and tarsorrhaphy**

Exposure Keratopathy

- This type of keratopathy is seen in patients of **lagophthalmos^Q or proptosis**
- Evaporation of tears is increased, leading to excessive drying of the cornea. This leads to epithelial breakdown and poor healing.
- Treatment is **artificial tears and tarsorrhaphy**

Drug-induced Keratopathy

- This is also called **Vortex Keratopathy^Q or Cornea Verticillata^Q**
- It consists of whorl shaped deposits in the cornea
- The important drugs causing this type of keratopathy are
    - **Chloroquine^Q**
    - Chlorpromazine
    - **Amiodarone^Q**
    - Indomethacin
    - Tamoxifen

CORNEAL ECTASIA

Corneal ectasia refers to a group of disorders where protrusion of the cornea is associated with thinning. The different disorders are
- Keratoconus
- Keratoglobus
- Pellucid marginal degeneration
- Inflammatory ectasias due to trauma, corneal ulcer, etc

Keratoconus

- It is a non-inflammatory corneal ectasia where **conical protrusion of a part of the cornea is seen, associated with thinning.** It is bilateral but asymmetrical where one eye is more affected than the other
- It presents in the adolescent age group. The common complaint is frequent change of refraction and lack of clarity with the prescribed glasses
- **Irregular myopic astigmatism is seen^Q**
- **Scissoring Reflex^Q** is seen on retinoscopy
- Slit lamp examination shows a conical protrusion of the cornea. **Fine vertical folds (Vogt's striae)^Q are seen in the deep stroma or Descemet's membrane.** Prominent corneal nerves are seen due to associated thinning of the cornea. At the base of the cone, a pigmented line (**Fleischer's ring^Q**) is seen due to iron deposition
- *Munson's sign^Q*: In advanced cone, the protruded cornea indents the lower lid when the patient is asked to look down
- **Corneal Topography** is used for confirmation of the diagnosis
- *Complication*: Tear in the Descemet's membrane may occur due to excessive stretching. This leads to inflow of aqueous into the cornea. Over hydration leads to corneal oedema and loss of transparency. This is called **acute hydrops^Q**
- Treatment:
    - Spectacles followed by **rigid gas permeable contact lenses^Q**
    - **Collagen cross linking (C3R)^Q**— Application of **riboflavin followed by U-V ray** exposure causes cross-linkage of the corneal collagen which leads to flattening of the cornea
    - **Keratoplasty** is done in advanced cases

Associations of Keratoconus
- Down's Syndrome
- Vernal Catarrh
- Turner's Syndrome
- Blue Sclera
- Marfan's Syndrome
- Aniridia
- Ehler Danlos Syndrome
- Retinitis Pigmentosa
- Leber's Congenital Amaurosis
- Osteogenesis Imperfecta

Keratoglobus

- It is a rare condition where the entire cornea is abnormally protruded and thin
- High Myopia is seen
- May be associated with **Leber's congenital amaurosis^Q**
- **Scleral contact lenses^Q** and Keratoplasty are treatment options

Pellucid Marginal Degeneration

- It is a bilateral progressive thinning disorder **involving the inferior peripheral cornea^Q**
- A crescent shaped band of corneal thinning is present from 4 o'clock to 8 o'clock position. It is separated from the limbus by a zone of normal cornea
- **Irregular myopic astigmatism** is seen
- **Rigid gas permeable contact lenses** are Keratoplasty are the treatment options

CORNEAL DYSTROPHIES

This is a group of disorders where some layer of the cornea is affected from birth. The presentation of the disease

Conjunctiva, Sclera and Cornea

however may be later in life. Depending upon the layer of the cornea which is affected corneal dystrophies are classified as follows

Anterior Dystrophies

➢ Anterior dystrophies do not have much effect on vision. In these conditions, the adhesion of the epithelium to the underlying basement membrane is weak. Hence the epithelium gets eroded from time to time. These are subdivided into:

Epithelial dystrophies	Bowman's membrane dystrophies
Cogan microcystic dystrophy/ Map-dot-fingerprint dystrophy Messman and Stocker dystrophy	Reis-Bucklers dystrophy Thiel-Behnke dystrophy

➢ The presentation of anterior dystrophies is **recurrent corneal erosions**[Q].
➢ Treatment is **Phototherapeutic Keratectomy (PTK)**[Q] or superficial keratectomy

Stromal Dystrophies

➢ In these dystrophies there is deposition of a foreign substance within the corneal stroma.
➢ Stromal dystrophies usually present with **diminution of vision.**
➢ Treatment is **keratoplasty**

Name of dystrophy	Substance deposited	Test
Lattice dystrophy	Amyloid[Q]	Congo-red[Q]
Granular dystrophy	Hyaline[Q]	Masson's trichrome[Q]
Avellino (Combination of Lattice and Granular dystrophy)	Amyloid and Hyaline	Congo-red and Masson's trichrome
Macular dystrophy	Mucopoly-saccharide[Q]	Alcian blue[Q]
Schnyder's Crystalline dystrophy	Phospholipids[Q]	Oil-red O
Gelatinous drop like dystrophy	Amyloid	Congo-red

Posterior Dystrophies

They are the endothelial dystrophies namely
➢ Congenital hereditary endothelial dystrophy
➢ Fuchs' endothelial dystrophy
➢ Posterior polymorphous dystrophy

These conditions present with diminution of vision and bullous keratopathy due to corneal oedema.
Treatment is Keratoplasty

CORNEAL DEGENERATIONS

This is a group of disorders where degenerative changes take place in a corneal tissue that was normal at the time of birth. The important degenerations are:

Arcus Senilis

➢ It is the **most common corneal degeneration**[Q]. It is present in about 50% individuals above 60 years of age
➢ If present in children or young adults, it is called **arcus juvenilis** and it may be a feature of **systemic hyperlipidemias**[Q]
➢ Arcus is a bilateral lipid deposition which starts in the superior and inferior perilimbal cornea. It progresses circumferentially to form a band which is about 1 mm wide
➢ The peripheral border is separated from limbus by a clear zone of cornea.
➢ Lipid is first deposited in anterior part of the Descemet's membrane and the stroma

Climatic Droplet Keratopathy

➢ It is also known as **spheroidal degeneration**[Q] or **Labrador keratopathy**[Q]
➢ Prolonged exposure to UV rays is the cause
➢ Golden yellow spherules are seen in the interpalpebral area. It may cause visual impairment in advanced cases
➢ Treatment is phototherapeutic keratectomy (PTK)[Q] or superficial keratectomy

> **Band-shaped Keratopathy**[Q]
>
> - This type of degeneration is due to deposition of **Ca^{++} salts**[Q] in the **Bowman's layer** [Q] of the cornea
> - It is seen as a white band in the interpalpebral area with clear space separating it from the limbus
> - Causes
>   - Local: Chronic uveitis, silicon oil in the anterior chamber
>   - Systemic causes: Hyperparathyroidism, Hypervitaminosis D, Multiple Myeloma
>   - Treatment is **chelation with of calcium with EDTA after scraping the epithelium**[Q]. Phototherapeutic Keratectomy (PTK) and superficial keratectomy are further options

KERATOPLASTY

Keratoplasty is a procedure where a part or entire diseased cornea is replaced by cadaveric donor cornea.

Corneal Preservation and Eye Banking

Corneal donor tissue collection and preservation technique is of prime importance in order to maintain endothelial viability.

Ideal death enucleation time is **6 hours**^Q

There are different types of storage media

- *Refrigerated Moist chamber*: Eyes are stored in a special bottle with sterile solution placed at the bottom of a jar to produce a moist chamber. The eye is supported by a metal holder with the cornea facing up. The jar is kept in a refrigerator at 4°C. The tissue can be stored for 24–48 hours. This is **short-term preservation**.
- **Modified M.K. Medium**^Q (McCarey Kaufman Medium)— (i) 5% Dextran 40 (ii) HEPES buffer, (iii) Phenol Red as pH indicator (iv) Gentamycin (v) Sodium bicarbonate. Most surgeons prefer using the stored tissue within 3-4 days. This is **intermediate preservation**
- *Long-term preservation*: Cryopreservation or tissue culture

Contraindications for use of Donor Tissue^Q

- Infections like HIV, Hepatitis B, Hepatitis C
- Intraocular malignancies like retinoblastoma, choroidal melanoma
- Head and neck malignancies
- Rabies^Q
- Septicemia^Q
- Prion diseases
- Death from unexplained cause^Q

Types of Keratoplasty

Keratoplasty may be either full thickness or partial thickness. The different types are

- *Penetrating keratoplasty*^Q *(Full-thickness keratoplasty)*: The entire tissue from epithelium to endothelium is transplanted. Indications are
  - Tectonic graft is done to restore globe integrity in perforated corneal ulcer
  - Optical graft is done to improve vision in full-thickness cornel opacities, adherent leucoma etc
- *Deep anterior lamellar keratoplasty (DALK)*: In this procedure, transplantation of epithelium and stroma is done over the host endothelium and Descemet's membrane. Possible indications are keratoconus, stromal dystrophies, corneal opacities^Q etc
- *Descemet stripping automated endothelial keratoplasty (DSAEK)*: In this procedure, only the Descemet's membrane and endothelium is transplanted.

Indications are endothelial dystrophies and bullous keratopathy^Q

Complications of Keratoplasty

- *Graft refection*: The donor tissue suffers immunological rejection from the host. Rejection may be epithelial, stromal or endothelial. **Krachmer's spots**^Q are seen in epithelial rejection. Endothelial rejection presents with a typical rejection line called **Khodadoust line**^Q.
- Graft infection
- Secondary glaucoma
- *Graft failure*: Primary failure is due to poor viability of the host tissue. Secondary failure may be due to infection, rejection, etc

Crystalline Keratopathy

This is a typical entity where refractile crystals are seen in the epithelium and **anterior stroma**^Q of the cornea. It may be infectious or non-infectious

Infectious crystalline keratopathy (ICK) is usually seen after corneal graft and refractive surgeries. The most common causative organism is ***Streptococcus viridians***. Other organisms may be *Staphylococcus epidermidis*, *Pneumococcus*, *Haemophilus* and *Candida*.

Non-infectious causes

- **Schnyder's crystalline dystrophy**^Q
- **Cystinosis**^Q
- Lymphoproliferative disorders
- Topical fluoroquinolones

XEROPHTHALMIA

It is the term used to cover all the ocular manifestations of vitamin A deficiency. Nightblindness occurs because of disturbance in the visual cycle involving rhodopsin. **The ocular surface features are due to metaplasia of the non-keratinized epithelium to keratinized epithelium**^Q

WHO Classification (1982)

- XN: Night blindness
- XIA: Conjunctival xerosis
- XIB: **Bitot's spots**^Q— triangular, foamy, grey, sharply demarcated patch
- X2: Corneal xerosis
- X3A: Corneal ulceration/keratomalacia < 1/3 corneal surface
- X3B: Corneal ulceration/keratomalacia > 1/3 corneal surface
- XS: Corneal scar or opacity
- XF: Xerophthalmia fundus

Conjunctiva, Sclera and Cornea

Treatment

- Children < 1 year of age or weighing < 8 kg: 1 lakh IU orally on days 0, 1 and 14^Q
- Children equal to or > 1 year of age or weighing > 8 kg: 2 lakh IU orally on days 0, 1 and 14^Q
- IM dose is half of the oral dose

Corneal Tattooing is a procedure used to provide cosmesis in case of corneal opacities when there is practically no useful vision. The materials used in tattooing are **gold** chloride, **platinum** chloride or **silver** nitrate reduced by **hydrazine hydrate**. These chemicals are applied directly to the corneal stroma after peeling off the epithelium. Direct injection of coloured pigments into the stroma by multiple punctures can also be done. The materials used are Indian ink, Chinese ink and organic colours

Must Remember

- *Stocker's sign:* Pterygium
- *Cobblestone appearance of conjunctiva:* Vernal Keratoconjunctivitis (VKC)
- *Horner Tranta's spots:* Vernal Keratoconjunctivitis (VKC)
- *Herbert's pits:* Trachoma
- *Munson's sign:* Keratoconus

QUESTIONS

Infective/Allergic Conjunctivitis

1. Which of the following is not true of acute viral conjunctivitis? *(AIIMS 2013)*
   a. Vision is not affected
   b. Corneal infiltration is seen
   c. Antibiotics are the mainstay of treatment
   d. Pupil remains unaffected

2. Which of the following causes acute haemorrhagic conjunctivitis? *(DPG 2010)*
   a. Adenovirus   b. *Staphylococcus*
   c. Herpes simplex   d. *Haemophilus*

3. Which of the following does not cause haemorrhagic conjunctivitis? *(AIPG)*
   a. Adenovirus   b. Coxsackie virus
   c. Enterovirus   d. Papilloma virus

4. Angular conjunctivitis is caused by: *(DNB 2013)*
   a. *Haemophilus*   b. Adenovirus
   c. *Moraxella*   d. *Bacteroides*

5. Angular conjunctivitis is caused by *Moraxella* which is typically: *(APPG 2013)*
   a. Gram-positive diplococcus
   b. Gram-negative diplococcus
   c. Gram-positive diplobacillus
   d. Gram-negative diplobacillus

6. Inclusion conjunctivitis is caused by: *(AIPG 2000/ PGI 2008)*
   a. *Chlamydia trachomatis*
   b. *Chlamydia psittaci*
   c. Herpes simplex
   d. *Gonococcus*

7. In the grading of trachoma, follicular stage is defined as the presence of : *(AIIMS)*
   a. Five or more follicles in the lower tarsal conjunctiva
   b. Three or more follicles in the lower tarsal conjunctiva
   c. Five or more follicles in the upper tarsal conjunctiva
   d. Three or more follicles in the upper tarsal conjunctiva

8. Herbert's pits are seen in: *(Maharashtra PG 2010)*
   a. Spring catarrh   b. Trachoma
   c. Phlyctenular conjunctivitis d. Sarcoidosis

9. Arlt's line is seen in: *(AIPG/DNB 2013)*
   a. Vernal keratoconjunctivitis b. Pterygium
   c. Trachoma   d. Ocular pemphigoid

10. SAFE strategy is used for: *(AIIMS)*
    a. Trachoma   b. Diabetic retinopathy
    c. Onchocerciasis   d. Glaucoma

11. Which of the drugs is not effective against trachoma? *(APPG 2013)*
    a. Azithromycin   b. Erythromycin
    c. Ivermectin   d. Rifampicin

12. A recurrent bilateral conjunctivitis occurring with the onset of hot weather in young boys with symptoms of burning, itching and lacrimation with polygonal raised areas on the palpebral conjunctiva is: *(AIPG 2004)*
    a. Trachoma
    b. Phlyctenular conjunctivitis
    c. Mucopurulent conjunctivitis
    d. Vernal keratoconjunctivitis

13. Features of Vernal keratoconjunctivitis is/are: *(PGI)*
    a. Papillary hypertrophy   b. Follicular hypertrophy
    c. Herbert's pits   d. Trantas' spots
    e. Ciliary congestion

14. Cobblestone appearance of the conjunctiva is seen in: *(APPG 2013)*
    a. Trachoma   b. Spring catarrh
    c. Ophthalmia nodosum
    d. Long-term use of miotics

15. Pseudogerontoxon is seen in: *(NEET 2016)*
    a. Vernal Keratoconjunctivitis b. Trachoma
    c. Retinoblastoma   d. Choroidal melanoma

16. Shield ulcer is seen in: *(DNB 2015)*
    a. Phlyctenular conjunctivitis b. Spring catarrh
    c. Herpetic keratitis   d. Fungal keratitis

17. Topical sodium chromoglycate is used in the treatment of : *(COMEDK)*
    a. Phlyctenular conjunctivitis
    b. Vernal keratoconjunctivitis
    c. Trachoma
    d. Subconjunctival haemorrhage

18. Phlyctenular conjunctivitis, false is: *(Manipal 2009)*
    a. It is most commonly associated with tuberculosis
    b. The lesions are typically found near the limbus
    c. It predominantly affects children
    d. It is a type IV hypersensitivity reaction

19. Giant papillary conjunctivitis is caused by: *(COMEDK 2008/ APPG 2006)*
    a. Contact lens
    b. Ocular prosthesis
    c. Protruding corneal sutures
    d. All of the above

Xerophthalmia

20. Changes seen in the conjunctiva in vitamin A deficiency: *(AIIMS 2013)*
    a. Actinic degeneration
    b. Hyperplasia of goblet cells
    c. Hyperkeratosis of the squamous epithelium
    d. Stromal infiltration

Conjunctiva, Sclera and Cornea

21. A child of weight 8 kg has Bitot's spots in both eyes. Which is the most appropriate schedule of vitamin A for the child? *(AIPG)*
    a. 2 lakh units IM on days 0,14
    b. 1 lakh units IM on days 0, 14
    c. 2 lakh units IM on days 0,1,14
    d. 1 lakh units IM on days 0,1,14

22. Bitot's spots are seen in: *(Bihar PG 2014)*
    a. Conjunctiva   b. Cornea
    c. Retina   d. Vitreous

23. Which of the following is true about pterygium? *(AIIMS 2013)*
    a. Probe can be passed underneath the pterygium at the limbus
    b. Associated with exposure to infrared radiation
    c. Bare sclera technique has 30–80% recurrence
    d. Elastotic degeneration with distortion of the Descemet's membrane is seen

Pterygium

24. The histology of pterygium is: *(Manipal 2009)*
    a. Elastotic degeneration
    b. Epithelial inclusion bodies
    c. Precancerous changes
    d. Squamous metaplasia of the epithelium

25. Most common cause of visual disturbance in pterygium is: *(DNB 2013)*
    a. Retinal detachment b. Corneal perforation
    c. Astigmatism   d. Myopia

26. True about pterygium is: *(DNB 2014)*
    a. More common on the temporal side
    b. Associated with exposure to UV rays
    c. It is a neoplastic condition
    d. All pterygia need to be operated

27. Stocker's line is seen in: *(AIIMS 2010)*
    a. Pinguecula   b. Pterygium
    c. Conjunctival melanosis d. Conjunctival naevus

28. Iron deposition close to the head of the pterygium is known as: *(NEET 2016)*
    a. Stocker's line   b. KF ring
    c. Fleischer's ring d. Ferry's line

29. Which of the following may be used to prevent recurrence after pterygium excision? *(APPG)*
    a. Natamycin   b. Mitomycin C
    c. Amphotericin   d. Chloromycetin

30. Subconjunctival haemorrhage is seen in all except: *(JIPMER)*
    a. Passive venous congestion
    b. Pertussis
    c. Trauma
    d. High intraocular pressure

31. Goblet cells are seen in: *(DNB 2016)*
    a. Cornea   b. Conjunctiva
    c. Retina   d. Vitreous

Sclera

32. Most common cause of scleritis is: *(DNB 2015)*
    a. Rheumatoid arthritis b. SLE
    c. Sjögren's syndrome   d. Behçet's disease

33. Most common cause of anterior staphyloma is: *(DNB 2013)*
    a. Corneal ulcer   b. Myopia
    c. Hypermetropia   d. Herpetic Keratitis

34. Most common cause of posterior staphyloma is: *(DNB 2012)*
    a. Corneal ulcer   b. Degenerative myopia
    c. Uncontrolled glaucoma d. Scleritis

35. The sclera is the thinnest at: *(DNB 2016)*
    a. Limbus
    b. Insertion of extraocular muscles
    c. At the optic nerve
    d. On the nasal side

36. Sclera is thinnest at: *(AIIMS)*
    a. Limbus
    b. Equator
    c. Anterior to the attachment of superior rectus
    d. Posterior to the attachment of superior rectus

37. The most common systemic association of scleritis is *(AIIMS 2005)*
    a. Ehler-Danlos   b. Systemic sclerosis
    c. Rheumatoid arthritis d. Giant cell arteritis

38. In scleritis, all are true except: *(Manipal 2009)*
    a. Scleromalacia perforans is commonly associated with systemic disease
    b. Pain is not a prominent feature
    c. Retinal detachment is a known complication
    d. Glaucoma may occur

39. Most common cause of anterior staphyloma is: *(APPG 2013)*
    a. Perforated corneal ulcer b. Scleritis
    c. Myopia   d. Glaucoma

40. Ciliary staphyloma is due to: *(APPG)*
    a. Scleritis   b. Myopia
    c. Iridocyclitis   d. Choroiditis

41. Blue sclera is seen in : *(COMEDK/ PGI 2014)*
    a. Alkaptonuria
    b. Osteogenesis imperfecta
    c. Ehler-Danlos
    d. Kawasaki disease

42. Which of the following may present as a bluish red nodule resembling conjunctival haemorrhage? *(APPG 2013)*
    a. Kaposi sarcoma   b. Ciliary staphyloma
    c. Lymphoma   d. Limbal dermoid

43. Parenchymatous xerosis of the conjunctiva is seen in: *(PGI)*
    a. Trachoma   b. Vitamin A deficiency
    c. Vernal conjunctivitis
    d. Phlyctenular conjunctivitis
    e. Alkali burns

17

Self Assessment and Review of Ophthalmology

Anatomy and Physiology of Cornea

44. **True about cornea is/are:** *(PGI 2010)*
    a. Power is 43D
    b. Majority of the refraction occurs at the air-cornea interface
    c. With the rule astigmatism is seen because the vertical meridian is steeper than the horizontal
    d. Spherical in shape
    e. Refractive index is 1.334

45. **In which of the following tissues is long spaced collagen seen?** *(AIIMS 2013)*
    a. Diaphragm
    b. Cornea
    c. Basement membrane
    d. Tympanic membrane

46. **Where are stem cells present in the corneöa?** *(DNB 2016)*
    a. Limbus
    b. Epithelium
    c. Stroma
    d. Descemet's membrane

47. **Avascular structure of the eye is:** *(DNB 2014)*
    a. Conjunctiva
    b. Cornea
    c. Retina
    d. Ciliary body

48. **In hypoxic injury, the cornea becomes edematous due to the accumulation of** *(AIIMS 2014)*
    a. Carbon dioxide
    b. Lactate
    c. Pyruvate
    d. Glycogen

49. **Which of the following is not true regarding the cornea?** *(PGI 2015)*
    a. Endothelium helps to maintain the cornea in a dehydrated state
    b. Oxygen is derived by the corneal epithelium from the air through the tear film
    c. Glucose supply for the cornea is derived from the aqueous
    d. Thickness of the cornea is more at the centre than the periphery
    e. Richly vascular

50. **The nerve supply to the cornea is:** *(DNB 2015)*
    a. Maxillary branch of trigeminal nerve
    b. Facial nerve
    c. Auriculotemporal nerve
    d. Ophthalmic branch of trigeminal nerve

51. **Contact lens wear has been shown to have deleterious effects on the corneal physiology. Which of the following statements is incorrect?** *(AIPG)*
    a. The level of glucose availability in the corneal epithelium is reduced
    b. There is reduction in the density of hemidesmosomes
    c. There is increased production of CO_2 in the epithelium
    d. There is reduction in the glucose utilization by the corneal epithelium

52. **Corneal transparency is maintained by all except:** *(AIIMS 2005)*
    a. Relative hydration of the cornea
    b. Arrangement of collagen fibres
    c. Unmyelinated nerve fibres
    d. Mitotic figures at the centre of cornea

53. **Corneal transparency is maintained by** *(AIIMS 2007)*
    a. Keratocytes
    b. Bowman's membrane
    c. Descemet's membrane
    d. Endothelium

54. **Corneal thickness is best measured by:** *(APPG 2013)*
    a. Ophthalmometer
    b. Lensometer
    c. Pachymeter
    d. Focimeter

Infective Keratitis

55. **A patient with conjunctival infection led to corneal perforation. Swabs showed gram-negative cocci which had translucent colonies and were oxidase positive. What would be the most probable causative organism?** *(AIIMS 2013)*
    a. *Moraxella catarrhalis*
    b. *Neisseria gonorrhoeae*
    c. *Pseudomonas aeruginosa*
    d. *Acietobacter actinatus*

56. **Which of the following can penetrate the intact cornea** *(PGI)*
    a. Gonococcus
    b. *Pseudomonas*
    c. *C. diphtheriae*
    d. *Streptococcus*
    e. *Staphylococcus epidermidis*

57. **Ulcer serpens is caused by:** *(DPG 2009)*
    a. *Pseudomonas*
    b. *Pneumococcus*
    c. Gonococcus
    d. *C. diphtheriae*

58. **Which of the following can cause corneal perforation in just 48 hours?** *(AIIMS)*
    a. *Staphylococcus*
    b. *Pseudomonas*
    c. *C. diphtheriae*
    d. *Aspergillus*

59. **Which of the following is not a feature of fungal corneal ulcer?** *(AIIMS 2014)*
    a. Fixed hypopyon
    b. Ulcer with sloughing margins
    c. Symptoms are more pronounced than signs
    d. Fungal hyphae are seen on KOH mount

60. **Satellite nodule with corneal ulcer is seen in:** *(AIPG/ UPPG 2008)*
    a. Fungal ulcer
    b. Viral keratitis
    c. Bacterial ulcer
    d. Acanthamoeba keratitis

61. **A young man aged 30 years presents with difficulty in vision in the left eye for the past 10–15 days. He gives history of trauma to the eye with vegetative matter 15 days back. On examination there is an ulcerative lesion in the cornea whose base has a soft creamy infiltrate. The margins are feathery with a few satellite lesions. Which is the most probable etiological agent?** *(AIIMS 2002)*
    a. Acanthamoeba
    b. *Corynebacterium diphtheriae*
    c. *Fusarium*
    d. *Streptococcus pneumoniae*

62. A 33-year-old male came with pain and watering in the right eye for 36 hours. On examination, a 3 × 2 mm corneal ulcer is seen with elevated margins, feathery

finger-like projections and minimal hypopyon. What is the likely causative organism? *(May AIIMS 2016)*
a. HSV
b. Aspergillus
c. Pseudomonas
d. Acanthamoeba

63. Microscopy of a corneal ulcer showed branched septate hyphae. The probable diagnosis is *(AIIMS)*
a. Candida
b. Aspergillus
c. Mucormycosis
d. Histoplasma

64. Which of the following is the drug of choice for fungal corneal ulcers caused by filamentous fungi? *(AIPG 2005)*
a. Itraconazole
b. Natamycin
c. Nystatin
d. Fluconazole

65. Which of the following is used in the treatment of fungal keratomycosis? *(AIIMS 2014)*
a. Silver sulfadiazine
b. Linezolid
c. Vancomycin
d. Doxycycline

66. Which of the following is the most important adjuvant therapy for fungal corneal ulcer? *(AIPG 2004)*
a. Atropine sulphate
b. Dexamethasone
c. Pilocarpine
d. Lignocaine

67. Steroids are contraindicated in: *(AIPG)*
a. Phlyctenular conjunctivitis
b. Mooren's ulcer
c. Vernal keratoconjunctivitis
d. Dendritic ulcer

68. Corneal ulcer resembling fungal ulcer is seen due to infection with: *(May AIIMS 2016)*
a. Nocardia asteroides
b. Mycobacterium
c. Chlamydia trachomatis
d. Klebsiella pneumoniae

69. Corneal sensation are decreased in: *(DNB 2014)*
a. Herpes simplex
b. Fungal infection
c. Trachoma
d. Mooren's ulcer

70. Which of the following is an important feature of herpes simplex keratitis? *(COMEDK 2013)*
a. Circumciliary congestion
b. Corneal infiltrate
c. Pannus
d. Decrease in corneal sensation

71. All of the following are true about herpetic keratitis except: *(DNB 2016)*
a. Topical steroids are given in dendritic keratitis
b. Topical steroids are given in disciform keratitis
c. Geographic ulcer is a type of epithelial keratitis
d. Metaherpetic ulcer is not active disease

72. A 56-year-old man has painful rashes over the forehead and upper eyelid along with punctate keratopathy for the past two days. About a year ago, he underwent chemotherapy for Non-Hodgkin's lymphoma. What is the most probable diagnosis? *(AIIMS)*
a. Impetigo
b. SLE
c. Herpes zoster
d. Pyoderma gangrenosum

73. In a patient presenting with herpes zoster ophthalmicus, all of the following are true except: *(WBPG 2010)*
a. It is caused by varicella zoster
b. The virus is lodged in the Gasserian ganglion and travels down the trigeminal nerve
c. Corneal involvement is seen when the tip and sides of the nose are involved
d. Punctate keratitis may coalesce to form dendritic ulcers like herpes simplex

74. A 17-year-old girl with severe painful keratitis came to the hospital and *Acanthamoeba* keratitis was suspected. Which of the following is not a risk factor for the same? *(AIIMS)*
a. Extended wear contact lens
b. Exposure to dirty water
c. Corneal trauma
d. Squamous blepharitis

75. Which of the following statements regarding *Acanthamoeba* keratitis is true? *(AIPG 2008)*
a. For isolation of the causative agent, the corneal scrapings should be cultured on a nutrient agar plate
b. The causative agent *Acanthamoeba* is a helminth whose normal habitat is the soil
c. Keratitis due to *Acanthamoeba* is not seen in immunocompromised host
d. *Acanthamoeba* does not depend upon human host for the completion of its life cycle

76. A patient using contact lens develops corneal infection. Laboratory diagnosis of *Acanthamoeba* keratitis is made. The following is the best drug for treatment: *(AIPG 2003)*
a. Propamidine
b. Neosporine
c. Ketoconazole
d. Polyhexamethylene biguanide

77. Kallu, a 25-year-old male patient presented with red eye and complains of pain, photophobia, watering and blurred vision. He gives history of trauma with vegetable matter. Corneal examination shows a dendritic ulcer. Microscopy shows macrophage like cells. On culture in Non-nutrient agar enriched with *E. coli*, there are plaque formations. Which is the most likely organism? *(AIIMS)*
a. Herpes simplex
b. Acanthamoeba
c. Candida
d. Adenovirus

78. A person with prolonged usage of contact lens presented with irritation of the left eye. After examination a diagnosis of keratitis was made and corneal scrapings revealed the growth of *Pseudomonas aeruginosa*. The organisms were found to be multidrug resistant. Which of the following best explains the mechanism of antibiotic resistance in these organisms? *(AIPG)*
a. Ability to transfer resistance genes from adjacent flora
b. Improper contact lens hygiene
c. Frequent and injudicious use of antibiotics
d. Ability of *Pseudomonas* to produce biofilm

79. Pain which is out of proprtion to signs is seen in which type of corneal ulcer? *(NEET 2016)*
    a. Herpetic keratitis
    b. Fungal ulcer
    c. *Acanthamoeba* keratitis
    d. Bacterial ulcer

80. Salmon patch appearance is seen in *(CET JUNE 2017)*
    a. Subconjunctval hemorrhage
    b. Interstitial keratitis
    c. Retinitis Pigmentosa
    d. Buphthalmos

81. Which of the following is/are caused by bacterial infection? *(PGI 2013)*
    a. Phlyctenular conjunctivitis
    b. Marginal keratitis
    c. Mooren's ulcer
    d. Vogt-Koyanagi Harada's disease
    e. Hypopyon corneal ulcer

Non-infectious Keratitis

82. Treatment of Mooren's ulcer is: *(NEET 2016)*
    a. Antibiotics
    b. Immunosuppressive agents
    c. Debridement
    d. Antifungals

Keratoconus

83. Recurrent corneal erosions are seen in: *(PGI 2007)*
    a. Keratoglobus
    b. Keratoconus
    c. Glaucoma
    d. Corneal dystrophy

84. In Keratoconus, all are seen except: *(PGI 2000)*
    a. Munson's sign
    b. Thinning of cornea at the centre
    c. Distortion of the corneal reflex
    d. Hypermetropic refractive error

85. Keratoconus is associated with all except: *(Manipal 2009)*
    a. Down's syndrome
    b. Marfan's syndrome
    c. Ehler-Danlos syndrome
    d. Usher syndrome

86. True about Keratoconus is/are: *(PGI 2014)*
    a. Increased curvature of the cornea
    b. Astigmatism is seen
    c. Kayser-Fleischer ring is seen
    d. Cornea is thick
    e. Soft contact lenses are used

87. Acute hydrops is seen in: *(APPG 2013)*
    a. Keratoglobus
    b. Bullous keratopathy
    c. Keratoconus
    d. Buphthalmos

88. Fleischer's ring is seen in: *(WBPG /Punjab 2011)*
    a. Pterygium
    b. Chalcosis
    c. Keratoconus
    d. Trauma

89. Early Keratoconus may be diagnosed by: *(APPG 2014)*
    a. Corneal topography
    b. Keratometry
    c. Pachymetry
    d. Ophthalmoscopy

90. KISA index is used in the diagnosis of: *(CET JUNE 2017)*
    a. Keratoconus
    b. Keratoglobus
    c. Terrien marginal degeneration
    d. Pellucid marginal degeneration

91. Enlarged corneal nerves may be seen in all of the following except: *(AIPG)*
    a. Keratoconus
    b. Herpes simplex keratitis
    c. Leprosy
    d. Neurofibromatosis

Corneal Dystrophy and Degeneration

92. Band-shaped keratopathy is due to the deposition of: *(AIIMS 2013)*
    a. Calcium
    b. Amyloid
    c. Iron
    d. Melanin

93. Band-shaped keratopathy is treated by: *(APPG 2008)*
    a. Propamidine isethionate
    b. EDTA
    c. Polyhexamethylene biguanide
    d. Chlorhexidine

94. Corneal dystrophies are: *(AIIMS 2012)*
    a. Primarily unilateral
    b. Primarily bilateral
    c. Primarily unilateral with systemic disease
    d. Primarily bilateral with systemic disease

95. Which of the following dystrophies is an autosomal recessive condition? *(AIPG 2006)*
    a. Lattice dystrophy
    b. Granular dystrophy
    c. Macular dystrophy
    d. Fleck dystrophy

96. Which of the following is the least common corneal dystrophy? *(AIPG 2010)*
    a. Macular dystrophy
    b. Lattice type I dystrophy
    c. Lattice type II dystrophy
    d. Granular dystrophy

97. Which of the following stains is used in granular dystrophy of cornea? *(AIIMS 2015)*
    a. Masson's trichrome
    b. Congo-red
    c. Colloidal iron
    d. PAS

Miscellaneous

98. A 12-year-old girl with tremors has golden brown discolouration of the Descemet's membrane. The most likely diagnosis is: *(WBPG 2006)*
    a. Fabry's disease
    b. Wilson's disease
    c. Glycogen storage disease
    d. Acute rheumatic fever

99. KF ring is seen in: *(NEET 2016)*
    a. Chalcosis
    b. Siderosis
    c. Tuberous sclerosis
    d. VKH syndrome

Conjunctiva, Sclera and Cornea

100. A 28-year-old male complains of glare in both eyes. The cornea shows whorl like opacities in the epithelium. He gives history of long-term treatment with Amiodarone. The most likely diagnosis is *(COMEDK 2008)*
    a. Terrian's marginal degeneration
    b. Cornea verticillata
    c. Band-shaped keratopathy
    d. Arcus juvenilis

101. Pigment deposition on cornea is seen in toxicity of: *(PGI)*
    a. Chloroquine   b. Digoxin
    c. Amiodarone   d. Ranitidine
    e. Diclofenac

102. Which of the following does not result in amorphous whorl like deposits in the cornea? *(AIIMS 2015)*
    a. Chloroquine   b. Amiodarone
    c. Indomethacin   d. Chlorpromazine

103. Dellen is: *(Manipal 2006)*
    a. Localized thinning of peripheral cornea
    b. Raised lesion at the limbus
    c. Marginal keratitis
    d. Age-related corneal degeneration

104. Neurotrophic keratopathy is caused by: *(AIPG)*
    a. Bell's palsy   b. Facial nerve palsy
    c. Trigeminal nerve palsy d. None of the above

105. Exposure keratopathy is due to paralysis of: *(APPG 2010)*
    a. Trigeminal nerve   b. Facial nerve
    c. Abducens nerve   d. Occulomotor nerve

106. Photophthalmia or Snow blindness is caused by: *(AIPG 2000)*
    a. Ultraviolet rays   b. Infrared rays
    c. Gamma rays   d. X-rays

107. Welder's flash is due to: *(DNB 2016)*
    a. Infra-red rays
    b. Ultra-violet rays
    c. Light in the visible spectrum
    d. None of the above

108. Treatment of photophthalmia includes: *(PGI)*
    a. Irrigation with saline
    b. Cold compress
    c. Pad and bandage
    d. Analgesics
    e. Lubricant eye drops

109. Universal marker for limbal stem cells is: *(AIIMS 2015)*
    a. Elastin   b. Keratin
    c. Collagen   d. ABCG2

Keratoplasty

110. In human corneal transplantation, the donor tissue is: *(AIIMS 2005)*
    a. Synthetic polymer
    b. Donor tissue from cadaveric human eyes
    c. Donor tissue from live human eyes
    d. Monkey eyes

111. Donor cornea is harvested from cadaveric donors with what time interval of death? *(Kerala PG 2015)*
    a. 3 hours   b. 6 hours
    c. 2 days   d. 16 hours

112. Which of the following is not an absolute contraindication for corneal transplantation? *(AIIMS 2014)*
    a. TB Meningitis
    b. Rabies
    c. Death due to unknown cause
    d. SSPE

113. Which of the following statement regarding corneal transplantation is true: *(AIPG)*
    a. Whole eye is preserved in tissue culture
    b. Donor is not accepted if age is more than 60 years
    c. Specular microscopy is used to assess endothelial cell count
    d. HLA matching is mandatory

114. Signs of graft rejection are all except: *(PGI)*
    a. Krachmer's spots   b. Khodadoust line
    c. Graft oedema   d. Epithelial rejection line
    e. Foster's spots

115. Khodadoust line indicates: *(DNB 2016)*
    a. Sympathetic ophthalmia
    b. Rejection in corneal graft
    c. Acute congestive glaucoma
    d. Lesion in optic chiasma

116. Percentage of endothelial cell loss after Descemet's Stripping Automated Endothelial Keratoplasty (DSAEK) is: *(AIIMS)*
    a. 5%   b. 10-20%
    c. 30-40%   d. 50-60%

Chemical Injury

117. A patient presents with history of 'chuna' particles falling in the eye. Which of the following should not be done? *(AIIMS 2014)*
    a. Repeated irrigation of the conjunctival sac with normal saline
    b. Frequent instillation of Na- citrate drops
    c. Thorough slit lamp examination
    d. Double eversion of the lids to remove the chuna particles

21

Self Assessment and Review of Ophthalmology

ANSWERS AND EXPLANATIONS

1. c. **Antibiotics are the mainstay of treatment** *(Ref: Yanoff & Duker 4th edition p184-5)*
   The mainstay of treatment in viral conjunctivitis is only lubricants
2. a. **Adenovirus** *(Ref: Yanoff & Duker 4th edition p 184-5)*
   Acute haemorrhagic conjunctivitis is caused by Adenovirus, Echovirus, Enterovirus and Coxsakie virus
3. d. **Papilloma virus** *(Ref: Yanoff & Duker 4th edition p 184-5)*
4. c. *Moraxella* *(Ref: Yanoff & Duker 4th edition p 184)*
5. d. **Gram-negative diplobacillus** *(Ref: Yanoff & Duker 4th edition p 184)*
6. a. *Chlamydia trachomatis* *(Ref: Yanoff & Duker 4th edition p 186)*
7. c. **Five or more follicles in the upper tarsal conjunctiva**
   (Ref: Solomon A et al. Diagnosis and Assessment of Trachoma: Clin Microbiol Rev. Oct 2004; 17(4): 982-1011)
8. b. **Trachoma** *(Ref: Yanoff & Duker 4th edition p 186)*
9. c. **Trachoma** *(Ref: Yanoff & Duker 4th edition p 186)*
10. a. **Trachoma** *(Ref: Solomon A et al. Diagnosis and Assessment of Trachoma: Clin Microbiol Rev. Oct 2004; 17(4): 982-1011)*
11. c. **Ivermectin** *(Ref: Solomon A et al. Diagnosis and Assessment of Trachoma: Clin Microbiol Rev. Oct 2004; 17(4): 982-1011)*
    The main drug for trachoma is Azithromycin (500 mg single dose). Other drugs which have been found to be useful are Tetracyclines, Erythromycin and Rifampicin
12. d. **Vernal keratoconjunctivitis** *(Ref: Yanoff & Duker 4th edition p 192-3)*
13. a. **Papillary hypertrophy d. Tranta's spots** *(Ref: Yanoff & Duker 4th edition p 192-3)*
14. b. **Spring catarrh** *(Ref: Yanoff & Duker 4th edition p 192-3)*
15. a. **Vernal Keratoconjunctivitis** *(Ref: Yanoff & Duker 4th edition p 192-3)*
    It is a whitish area close to the superior limbus also called as Cupid's bow outline.
16. b. **Spring catarrh** *(Ref: Yanoff & Duker 4th edition p 192-3)*
17. b. **Vernal keratoconjunctivitis** *(Ref: Yanoff & Duker 4th edition p 192-3)*
18. a. **It is most commonly associated with tuberculosis.** *(Ref: Yanoff & Duker 4th edition p 194)*
    In our country, Phlyctenular conjunctivitis is most commonly associated with tuberculosis. But in western countries, it is associated with staphylococcus
19. d. **All of the above** *(Ref: Yanoff & Duker 4th edition p 194)*
    Giant papillary conjunctivitis is a type of allergic conjunctivitis caused due to constant irritation of the conjunctiva by contact lens, protruding sutures, ill-fitting prosthesis etc
20. c. **Hyperkeratosis of the squamous epithelium** *(Ref: National Program for Control of Blindness)*
    The ocular surface changes associated with Xerophthalmia are due to metaplasia of the non-keratinized epithelium into keratinized epithelium
21. c. **2 lakh units IM on days 0,1,14** *(Ref: National Program for Control of Blindness)*
22. a. **Conjunctiva** *(Ref: National Program for Control of Blindness)*
23. c. **Bare sclera technique has 30-80% recurrence** *(Ref: Yanoff & Duker 4th edition p 203-4)*
    Probe can be passed beneath a pseudopterygium but not a true pterygium.
    It is associated with exposure to UV rays
    Pterygium is an elastotic degeneration but it does not reach up to the Descemet's membrane. It encroaches only up to the stroma of the cornea
24. a. **Elastotic degeneration** *(Ref: Yanoff & Duker 4th edition p 203-4)*
25. c. **Astigmatism** *(Ref: Yanoff & Duker 4th edition p 203-4)*
26. b. **Associated with exposure to UV rays** *(Ref: Yanoff & Duker 4th edition p 203-4)*
27. b. **Pterygium** *(Ref: Yanoff & Duker 4th edition p 203-4)*
28. a. **Stocker's line** *(Ref: Yanoff & Duker 4th edition p 203-4)*

Conjunctiva, Sclera and Cornea

29. b. Mitomycin C (Ref: Yanoff & Duker 4th edition p 203-4)

   Since bare sclera technique of pterygium has high recurrence, the methods used are Pterygium excision with Mitomycin C, amniotic membrane graft or conjunctival autograft

30. d. High intraocular pressure

   Causes of subconjunctival haemorrhage:
   - **Trauma**^Q
   - Foreign body
   - **Hypertension**^Q
   - Pertussis
   - Bleeding disorders
   - Pneumococcus
   - **Haemorrhagic viral conjunctivitis**^Q

31. b. Conjunctiva (Ref: Yanoff & Duker 4th edition p 203-4)
32. a. Rheumatoid arthritis (Ref: Yanoff & Duker 4th edition p 209-2011)
33. a. Corneal ulcer
34. b. Degenerative myopia
35. b. Insertion of extraocular muscles

   The sclera is actually weakest or thinnest just posterior to the insertion of the extraocular muscles

36. d. Posterior to the attachment of superior rectus
37. c. Rheumatoid arthritis (Ref: Yanoff & Duker 4th edition p 212)
38. b. Pain is not a prominent feature. (Ref: Yanoff & Duker 4th edition p 210)

   Scleritis is associated with moderate to severe pain

39. a. Perforated corneal ulcer
40. a. Scleritis
41. b. Osteogenesis imperfecta, c. Ehler-Danlos
42. a. Kaposi sarcoma
43. a. Trachoma, b. Vitamin A deficiency, e. Alkali burns (Ref: Yanoff & Duker 4th edition p 275)
44. a. Power is 43D, b. Majority of the refraction occurs at the air-cornea interface, c. With the rule astigmatism is seen because the vertical meridian is steeper than the horizontal (Ref: Yanoff & Duker 4th edition p 163-4)
45. b. Cornea (Ref: Yanoff & Duker 4th edition p 163-4)
46. a. Limbus (Ref: Yanoff & Duker 4th edition p 163-4)
47. b. Cornea (Ref: Yanoff & Duker 4th edition p 163-5)
48. b. Lactate (Ref: Yanoff & Duker 4th edition p 280)

   The cornea derives its nutrition from the aqueous humour and the limbal blood vessels. Oxygen supply to the cornea comes mainly from the air. Contact lenses may decrease the oxygen supply to the cornea. As a result, there is increase in anaerobic glycolysis leading to accumulation of lactic acid

49. d. Thickness of the cornea is more at the centre than the periphery, e. Richly vascular (Ref: Yanoff & Duker 4th edition p 163-5)
50. d. Ophthalmic branch of Trigeminal nerve (Ref: Yanoff & Duker 4th edition p 163-5)
51. d. There is reduction in the glucose utilization by the corneal epithelium (Ref: Yanoff & Duker 4th edition p 280-6)
52. a. Relative hydration of the cornea (Ref: Yanoff & Duker 4th edition p 163-5)

   It is the relative dehydration of the cornea that is responsible for transparency, not the hydration

53. d. Endothelium (Ref: Yanoff & Duker 4th edition p 163-5)
54. c. Pachymeter (Ref: Yanoff & Duker 4th edition p 61)
55. b. *Neisseria gonorrhoeae* (Ref: Yanoff & Duker 4th edition p 217)

   The question hints at an organism which causes conjunctivitis and penetrates through an intact cornea. Hence the answer is *Neisseria*

56. a. *Gonococcus*, c. *C. diphtheriae* (Ref: Yanoff & Duker 4th edition p 217)
57. b. *Pneumococcus* (Ref: Yanoff & Duker 4th edition p 218)
58. b. *Pseudomonas* (Ref: Yanoff & Duker 4th edition p 220)
59. c. Symptoms are more pronounced than signs (Ref: Yanoff & Duker 4th edition p 225-6)
60. a. Fungal ulcer (Ref: Yanoff & Duker 4th edition p 225-6)
61. c. *Fusarium* (Ref: Yanoff & Duker 4th edition p 225-6)
62. b. *Aspergillus* (Ref: Yanoff & Duker 4th edition p 225-6)
63. b. *Aspergillus* (Ref: Yanoff & Duker 4th edition p 225-6)
64. b. Natamycin (Ref: Yanoff & Duker 4th edition p 226-7)

Self Assessment and Review of Ophthalmology

65. a. **Silver sulfadiazine**
    Though not commonly used, silver sulfadiazine and iodine also have been shown to be effective in fungal infections in cornea
66. a. **Atropine sulphate**
67. d. **Dendritic ulcer** *(Ref: Yanoff & Duker 4th edition p 234-6)*
68. a. *Nocardia asteroides* *(Ref: Yanoff & Duker 4th edition p 219, 221)*
    Actually both *Nocardia* and *Mycobacteria* are correct but *Nocardia* is the better option
69. a. **Herpes simplex** *(Ref: Yanoff & Duker 4th edition p 247)*
70. d. **Decrease in corneal sensation** *(Ref: Yanoff & Duker 4th edition p 247)*
71. a. **Topical steroids are given in dendritic keratitis** *(Ref: Yanoff & Duker 4th edition p 235-6)*
    Topical steroids are absolutely contraindicated in dendritic and geographic ulcers, both of which are forms of active epithelial keratitis. Steroids are indicated in stromal, disciform and endothelial keratitis.
72. c. **Herpes zoster** *(Ref: Yanoff & Duker 4th edition p 180)*
73. d. **Punctate keratitis may coalesce to form dendritic ulcers like herpes simplex**
    Ref: Yanoff & Duker 4th edition p 180
    Herpes Zoster forms Pseudodendrites which look similar to the dendritic ulcers of Herpes simplex. But dendrites have a small terminal bulb at the end of the shaft of the ulcer whereas pseudodendrites are devoid of this terminal bulb
74. d. **Squamous blepharitis** *(Ref: Yanoff & Duker 4th edition p 228)*
75. d. ***Acanthamoeba* does not depend upon human host for the completion of its life cycle**
    (Ref: Yanoff & Duker 4th edition p 228-9)
    Acanthamoeba are free-living protozoa, not helminth living in water and soil.
    They do not require any host for completion of their life cycle but may cause infection in humans and animals.
    They cause infection in both immunocompetent and immunocompromised hosts.
    Culture should be done in non-nutrient agar enriched with *E. coli*
76. d. **Polyhexamethylene biguanide** *(Ref: Yanoff & Duker 4th edition p 229)*
77. b. *Acanthamoeba* *(Ref: Yanoff & Duker 4th edition p 229)*
78. d. **Ability of *Pseudomonas* to produce biofilm** *(Ref: Yanoff & Duker 4th edition p 220)*
79. c. *Acanthamoeba* **keratitis** *(Ref: Yanoff & Duker 4th edition p 228-9)*
    Acanthamoeba causes inflammation of corneal nerves or keratoneuritis which is the cause of severe pain in this type of keratitis
80. b. **Interstitial keratitis**
81. e. **Hypopyon corneal ulcer** *(Ref: Yanoff & Duker 4th edition p 218)*
    Phlyctenular conjunctivitis is an allergic keratoconjunctivitis. Marginal keratitis and Mooren's ulcer are immunological in etiology. VKH disease is a panuveitis, also immunological in etiology
82. b. **Immunosuppressive agents**
    Mooren's ulcer is a PUK which is immunological in etiology, hence the answer
83. d. **Corneal dystrophy** *(Ref: Yanoff & Duker 4th edition p 256-7)*
    Recurrent corneal erosions are seen in anterior corneal dystrophies, fingernail trauma etc
84. d. **Hypermetropic refractive error** *(Ref: Yanoff & Duker 4th edition p 252-3)*
85. d. **Usher syndrome** *(Ref: Yanoff & Duker 4th edition p 253)*
86. a. **Increased curvature of cornea, b. Astigmatism is seen** *(Ref: Yanoff & Duker 4th edition p 252-3)*
87. c. **Keratoconus** *(Ref: Yanoff & Duker 4th edition p 252-3)*
88. c. **Keratoconus** *(Ref: Yanoff & Duker 4th edition p 252-3)*
89. a. **Corneal topography** *(Ref: Yanoff & Duker 4th edition p 252-3)*
    Keratometry, Pachymetry, Topography and Retinoscopy are all used in the diagnosis of Keratoconus. But early diagnosis is done by Corneal Topography.
90. a. **Keratoconus**
    KISA index is a complex value calculated from multiple parameters on videokeratography to make a diagnosis of keratoconus

Conjunctiva, Sclera and Cornea

91. a. **Keratoconus** *(Ref: Kim et al: Causes of enlarged corneal nerves: Int Ophthalmol Clin. 2001; 41(1):13-23)*

Causes of enlarged corneal nerves
• **Neurofibromatosis**^{Q}
• **MEN 2B**^{Q}
• Refsum's disease
• Amyloidosis
• Ichthyosis
• **Leprosy**^{Q}
• HSV keratitis
• ***Acanthamoeba* keratitis**^{Q}

Causes of prominent corneal nerves
- Keratoconus
- Buphthalmos
- Reis-Buckler dystrophy

92. a. **Calcium** *(Ref: Yanoff & Duker 4th edition p 270)*
93. b. **EDTA** *(Ref: Yanoff & Duker 4th edition p 270)*
94. b. **Primarily bilateral** *(Ref: Yanoff & Duker 4th edition p 259)*
95. c. **Macular dystrophy** *(Ref: Yanoff & Duker 4th edition p 261)*
96. a. **Macular dystrophy** *(Ref: Yanoff & Duker 4th edition p 259-261)*

Most common stromal dystrophy is **Lattice dystrophy**

97. a. **Masson's trichrome** *(Ref: Yanoff & Duker 4th edition p 261)*
98. b. **Wilson's disease** *(Ref: Yanoff & Duker 4th edition p 294)*

Deposition of Cu in the **Descemet's membrane of the cornea**^{Q} in Wilson's disease gives rise to Kayser-Fleischer (KF) ring. **It first appears close to the superior limbus**^{Q}

99. a. **Chalcosis** *(Ref: Yanoff & Duker 4th edition p 294)*

KF ring is classically described in Wilson's disease where there is increase in copper levels (Chalcosis)

100. b. **Cornea verticillata** *(Ref: Parson 21st edition p 214)*
101. a. **Chloroquine, c. Amiodarone** *(Ref: Parson 21st edition p 214)*
102. **None** *(Ref: Parson 21st edition p 214)*

All the mentioned drugs may cause whorl like deposits on the cornea or vortex keratopathy

103. a. **Localized thinning of cornea at the limbus**
104. c. **Trigeminal nerve palsy** *(Ref: Yanoff & Duker 4th edition p 247)*
105. b. **Facial nerve** *(Ref: Kanski 6th edition p 281)*
106. a. **Ultraviolet rays** *(Ref: Khurana 4th edition p 111)*

Photophthalmia or snow blindness refers to corneal epithelial erosions due to exposure to intense UV rays. It was seen due to reflection of UV rays from snow in extremely cold areas and hence the name.

Treatment is reassurance, tranquilizers and analgesics. Locally, cold compress, pad and bandage, lubricants and cycloplegics are given

107. b. **Ultraviolet rays** *(Ref: Khurana 4th edition p 111)*
108. b. **Cold compress, c. Pad and bandage, d. Analgesic, e. Lubricant eye drops** *(Ref: Khurana 4th edition p 111)*
109. d. **ABCG2**
110. b. **Donor tissue from cadaveric human eyes** *(Ref: Yanoff & Duker 4th edition p 299)*
111. b. **6 hours** *(Ref: Yanoff & Duker 4th edition p 299)*
112. a. **TB meningitis** *(Ref: Yanoff & Duker 4th edition p 299)*
113. c. **Specular microscopy is used to assess endothelial cell count** *(Ref: Yanoff & Duker 4th edition p 299)*

Specular microscopy is used to assess the endothelium of the donor tissue prior to transplantation. HLA matching is not mandatory for cornea transplant. Usually only donor cornea is preserved in preservation media. Age is not a criterion for discarding donor tissue

114. e. **Foster's spots** *(Ref: Yanoff & Duker 4th edition p 301-2)*

Graft rejection is an immunological response of the host to the donor tissue. It may lead to graft failure if not properly treated. The clinical features of rejection in a graft are

Self Assessment and Review of Ophthalmology

- Decrease in vision
- Graft oedema
- **Krachmer's spots**[Q] in the epithelium and anterior stroma suggestive of epithelial/ stromal rejection
- **Khodadoust line**[Q] in the endothelium suggestive of endothelial rejection
- Foster Fuch's spots are seen in the retina in myopia

115. b. Rejection in corneal graft *(Ref: Yanoff & Duker 4th edition p 301-2)*

116. c. 30–40% *(Ref: Yanoff & Duker 4th edition p 318-9)*

117. c. Thorough slit lamp examination *(Ref: Yanoff & Duker 4th edition p 296-8)*

Chemical injury to the eye is an ophthalmic emergency. **Alkali injury due to lime or chuna** is very common in children especially in the rural areas. If not treated properly it may have serious consequences. The features of alkali injury are

- Necrosis of the conjunctival and corneal epithelium.
- **Loss of limbal stem cells leads to conjunctivalisation and vascularisation of the cornea with loss of corneal transparency**[Q]
- Deep stromal necrosis may lead to perforation of the cornea
- Intraocular inflammation may also be seen

Treatment includes

- **Thorough irrigation with normal saline for 15–30 minutes till the pH becomes normal**[Q]
- **Double eversion of the lids**[Q] to remove all the lime particles
- Debridement of the necrotic epithelium to allow proper epithelialisation
- Antibiotics
- **Topical steroids are given for 7–10 days**[Q] to decrease inflammation and encourage epithelialisation. They should be stopped after 10 days because they impair the healing process.
- **Ascorbic acid**[Q] to promote healing
- **Tetracyclines**[Q] may be given because they have anti-collagenase activity
- Citrates are given as they have anti-neutrophilic activity and decrease inflammation

Thorough slit lamp examination may not be possible in acute stage due to severe pain and hence the answer

Rehabilitation of these patients may involve surface reconstruction procedures like **amniotic membrane grafting followed by keratoplasty**[Q].

Keratoprosthesis[Q] is the final option when keratoplasty is not possible due to severely damaged ocular surface.

IMAGE BASED QUESTIONS

1. The clinical photograph of a patient is given in the question. What is the refractive error expected in the patient?

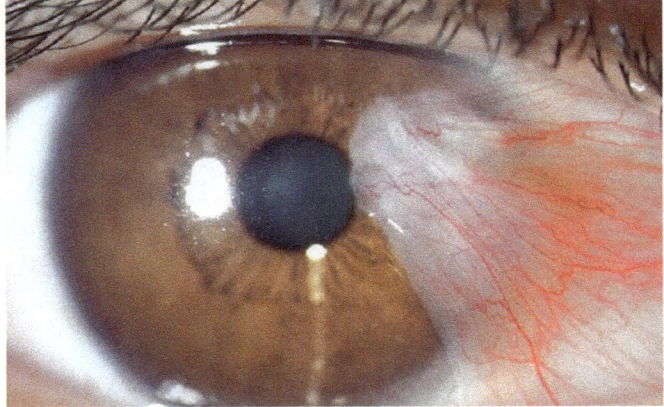

   a. Myopia
   b. Hypermetropia
   c. With the rule astigmatism
   d. Against the rule astigmatism

2. A child with history of lime injury few years back presents to the OPD. The clinical photograph is given below. What is the diagnosis? *(NEET Pattern)*

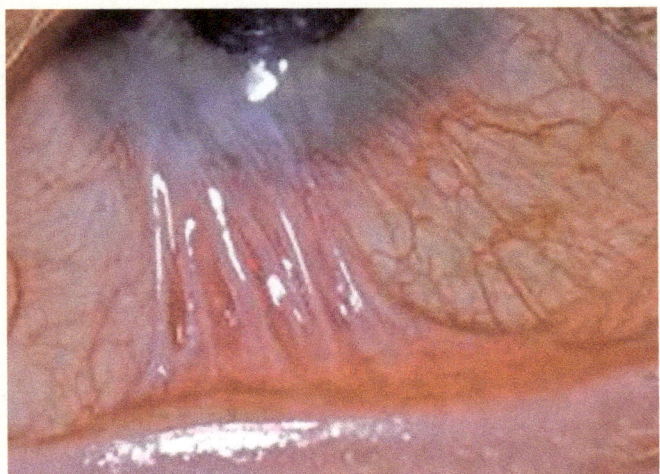

   a. Entropion
   b. Ectropion
   c. Symblepharon
   d. Blepharophimosis

3. A 10-year-old boy presented with complaints of recurrent episodes of itching and redness in both eyes. The symptoms are worse in summer. The photograph shows the appearance of the upper tarsal conjunctiva. What is the diagnosis?

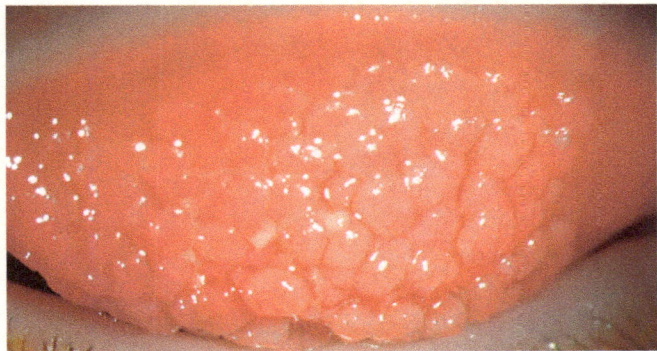

   a. Trachoma
   b. Vernal keratoconjunctivitis
   c. Phlyctenular conjunctivitis
   d. Viral conjunctivitis

4. A 10-year-old girl presents with redness in right eye. On examination, a nodular lesion close to the limbus is seen as shown in the photograph. Lymph nodes are palpable in the neck. What is the possible diagnosis?

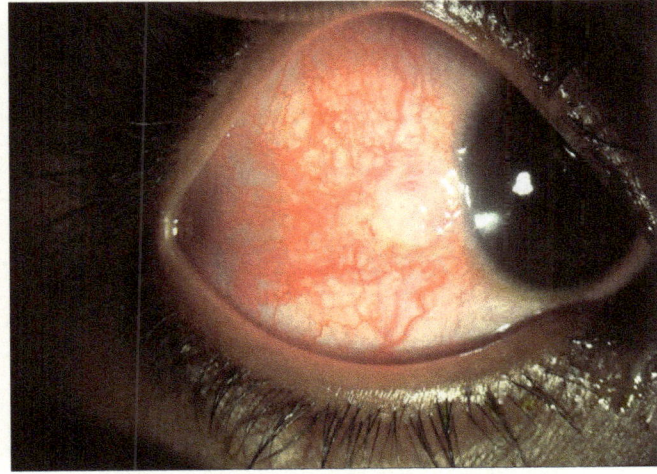

   a. Vernal keratoconjunctivitis
   b. Adenoviral conjunctivitis
   c. Trachoma
   d. Phlyctenular conjunctivitis

Answer Key: 1. c 2. c 3. b 4. d

5. From the picture identify the diagnosis:
   (Nov AIIMS 2017)

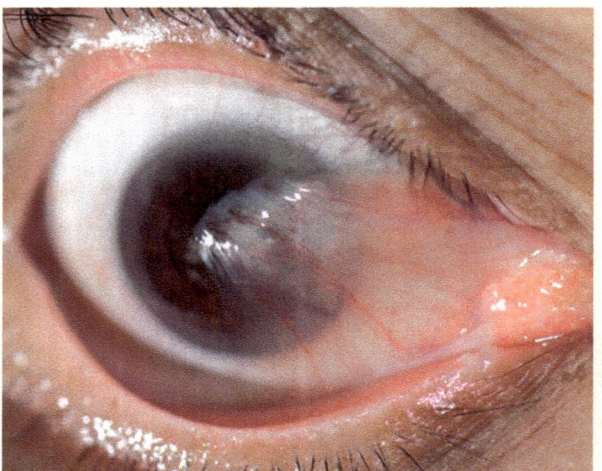

   a. Pterygium
   b. Limbal dermoid
   c. Ocular surface squamous neoplasia (OSSN)
   d. Pinguecula

6. A farmer presented to the ophthalmology emergency with blurred vision, redness, tearing, photophobia, pain and foreign body sensation following injury to the eye. Examination reveals a corneal ulcer with fuzzy margins and redness. A picture of the eye is shown. How will you manage the patient?
   (Nov AIIMS 2016)

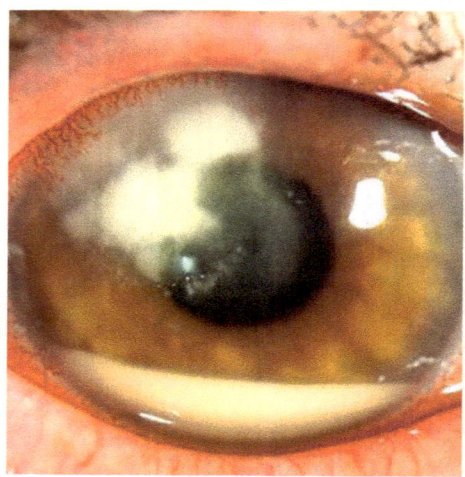

   a. Topical antibiotics and drainage of hypopyon
   b. Topical Natamycin and drainage of hypopyon
   c. Topical natamycin only, no need to drain the hypopyon
   d. Topical Steroids

7. A patient presents with complain of pain, redness, photophobia and decrease in vision. From the clinical photograph, what is the provisional diagnosis?

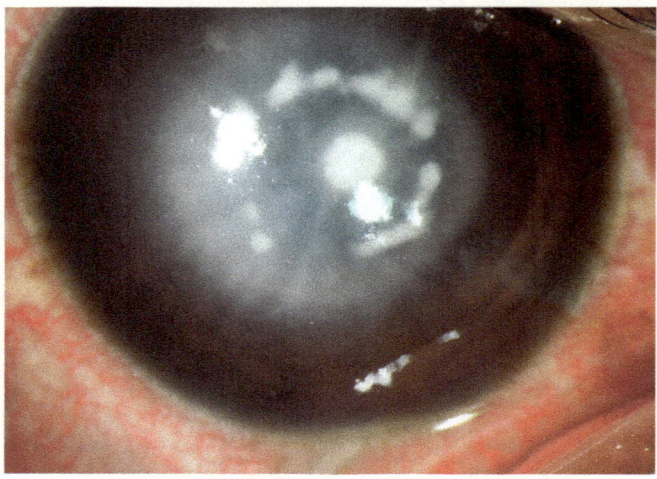

   a. Bacterial keratitis
   b. Fungal keratitis
   c. Viral keratitis
   d. Mooren's ulcer

8. A patient, with history of prolonged contact lens use, presents with an indolent ulcer not responding to conventional medication. From the clinical photograph, what may be the provisional diagnosis?

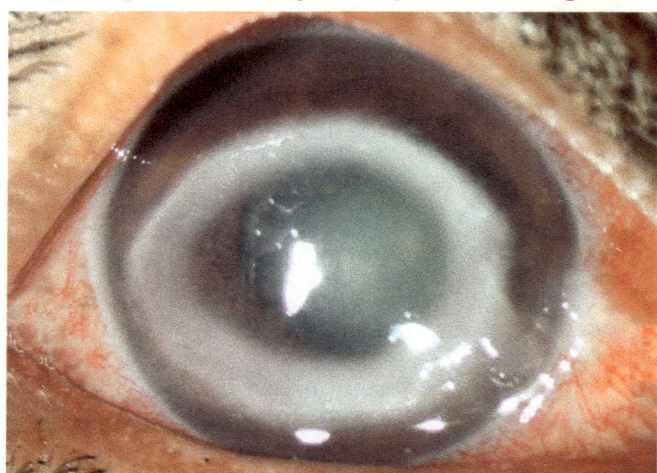

   a. Fungal keratitis
   b. *Acanthamoeba* keratitis
   c. Viral keratitis
   d. Vernal keratoconjunctivitis

Answer Key: 5. a   6. c   7. b   8. b

Conjunctiva, Sclera and Cornea

9. A patient presents with complain of photophobia and irritation in the right eye. From the clinical photograph, what is the diagnosis?

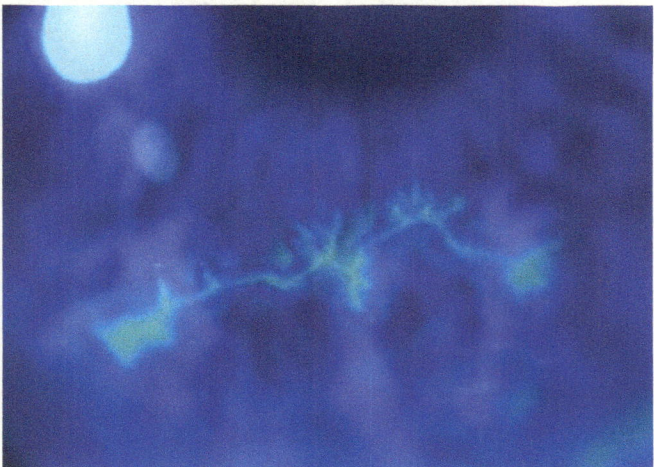

   a. Bacterial keratitis
   b. Viral keratitis
   c. Fungal keratitis
   d. *Acanthamoeba* keratitis

10. The clinical photograph of a patient with corneal ulcer is given. What is the line of management of the patient?

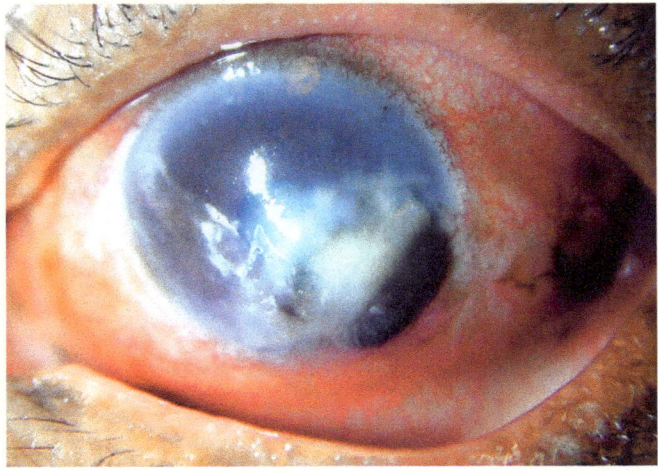

   a. Symptomatic treatment
   b. Antibiotics
   c. Therapeutic penetrating keratoplasty
   d. Debridement of the ulcer

11. A 50-year-old male patient presented with severe pain and redness in the right eye for the past two weeks. On examination, an ulcer as shown in the photograph above was seen. Scraping and culture from the ulcer bed showed no organism. Systemic work up was also normal. What may be the likely diagnosis?

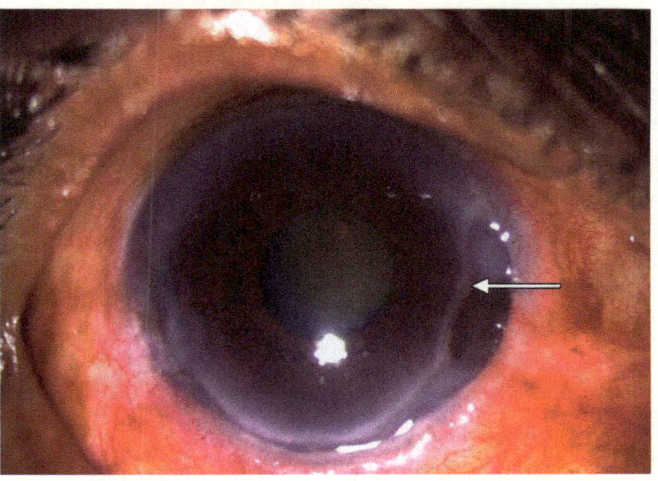

   a. Marginal keratitis
   b. Terrien's marginal degeneration
   c. Mooren's ulcer
   d. Fungal corneal ulcer

12. A 50-year-old patient presents with gradually progressive decrease in vision in both eyes associated with glare. The clinical photograph is given. What is the diagnosis?

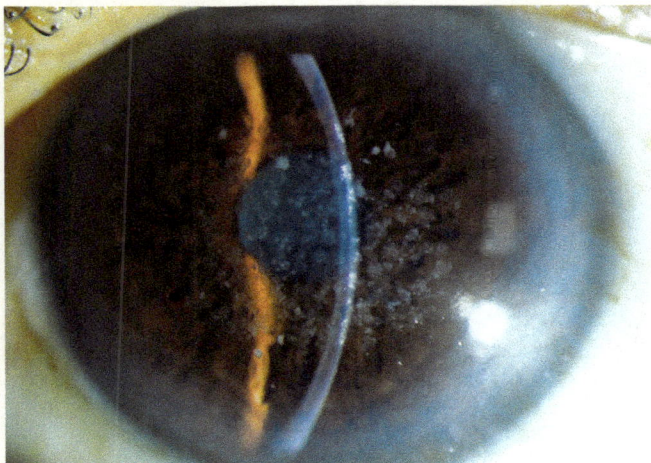

   a. Lattice dystrophy
   b. Granular dystrophy
   c. Fuchs' dystrophy
   d. Posterior polymorphous dystrophy

Answer Key: 9. b   10. c   11. c   12. b

13. A 30-year-old patient presents with progressive loss of vision in both eyes. From the photograph, what is the diagnosis?

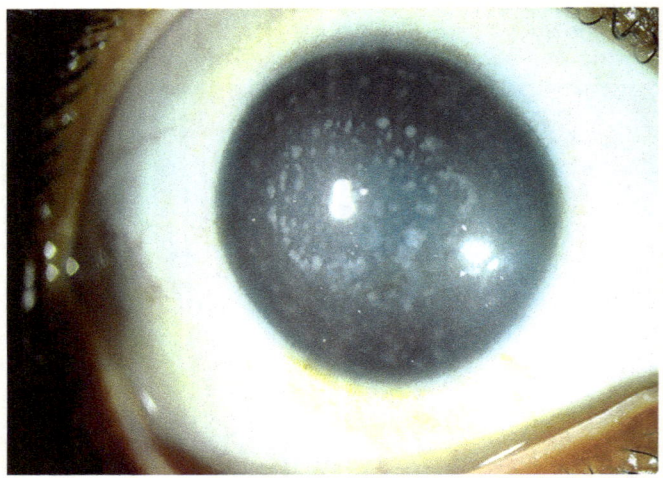

a. Lattice dystrophy
b. Granular dystrophy
c. Macular dystrophy
d. Fuchs' dystrophy

14. From the clinical photograph, what is the diagnosis?

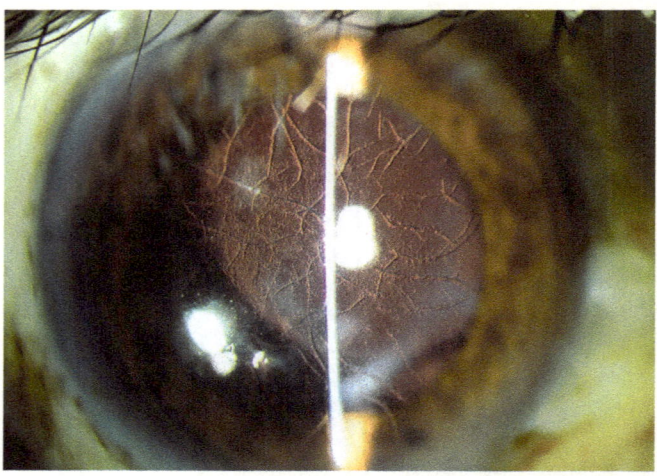

a. Lattice dystrophy
b. Granular dystrophy
c. Macular dystrophy
d. Fuchs' dystrophy

15. Identify the type of corneal opacity

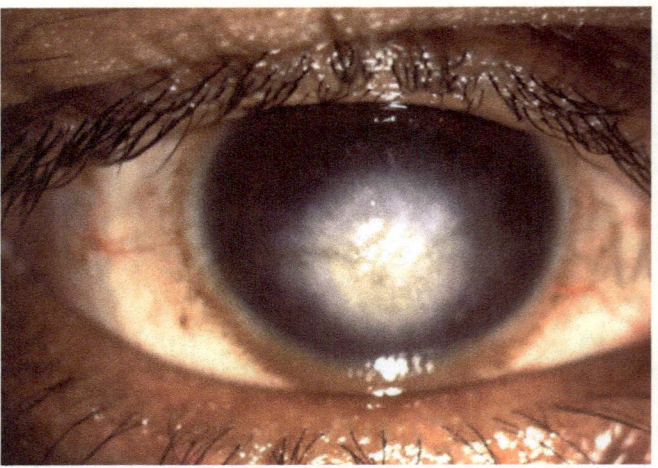

a. Nebular
b. Macular
c. Leucomatous
d. None of the above

16. This is the photograph of a patient who has undergone a certain corneal surgery. What is the name of the surgery?

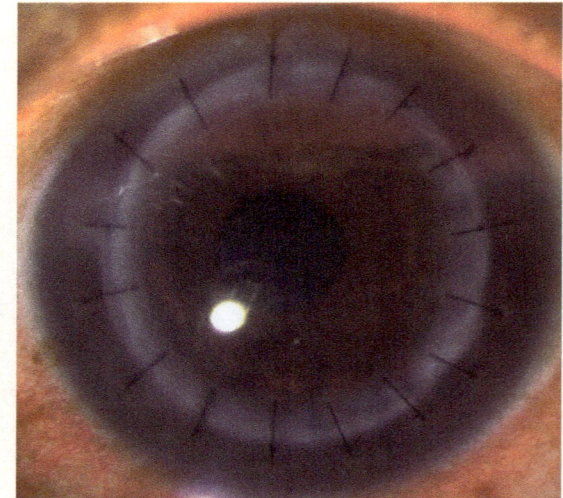

a. LASIK
b. Radial keratotomy
c. Keratoplasty
d. Photorefractive keratectomy

Answer Key: 13. c   14. a   15. c   16. c

Conjunctiva, Sclera and Cornea

17. A 10-year-old boy presented with history of cricket ball injury. He had complaints of pain, redness and watering since then. On examination, a large area of epithelial defect was seen on the cornea. It became clearly visible after staining and examination under cobalt blue filter as shown in the photograph above. What was the stain used?

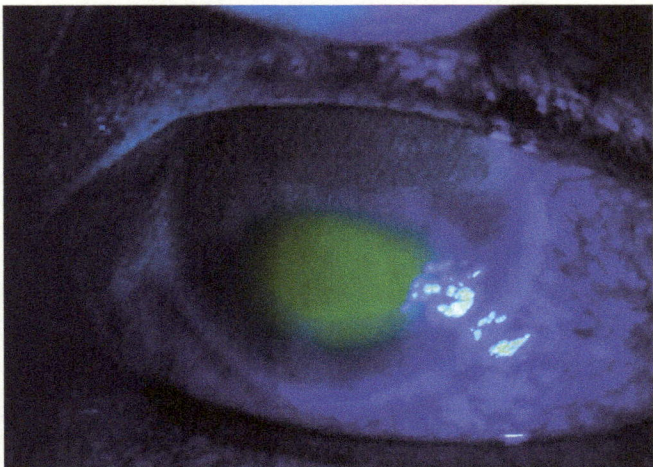

   a. Rose Bengal
   b. Sodium Fluorescein
   c. Masson's trichrome
   d. Trypan blue

18. A patient presents on first post-operative day after cataract surgery with severe decrease in vision. On examination, there is severe corneal oedema. Anterior segment OCT of the eye is given below. What is the diagnosis?

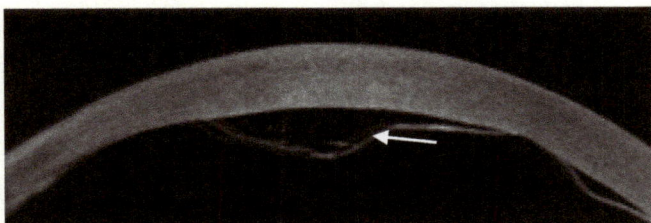

   a. Pseudophakic bullous keratopathy
   b. Striate keratopathy
   c. Descemet's membrane detachment
   d. Decompensated cornea

19. A 15-year-old boy complains of progressive increase in the power of his glasses. His refraction shows high astigmatism in both eyes. The corneal topography is given below. What is the possible diagnosis?

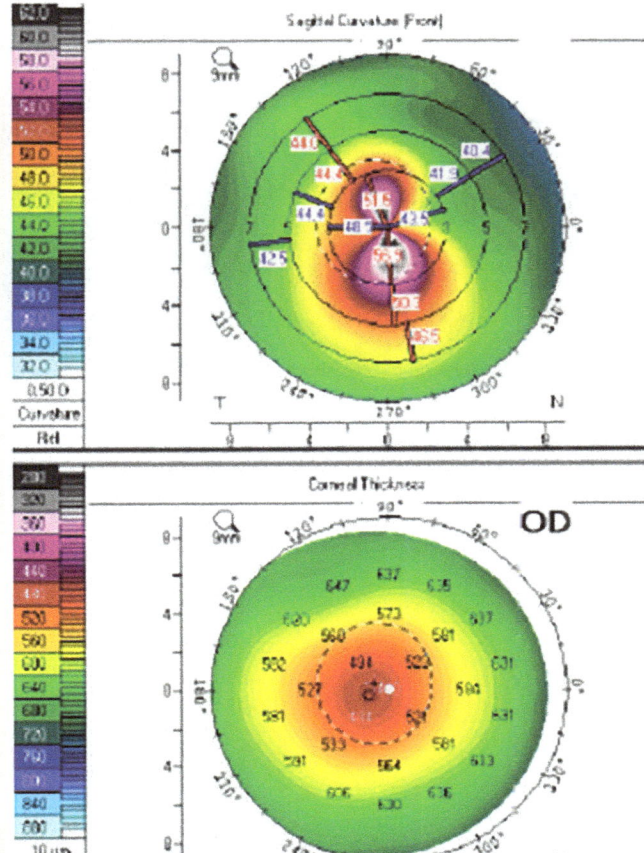

   a. Keratoconus
   b. Keratoglobus
   c. Refractive error
   d. Megalocornea

Answer Key: 17. b   18. c   19. a

20. From the photograph, what is the diagnosis?

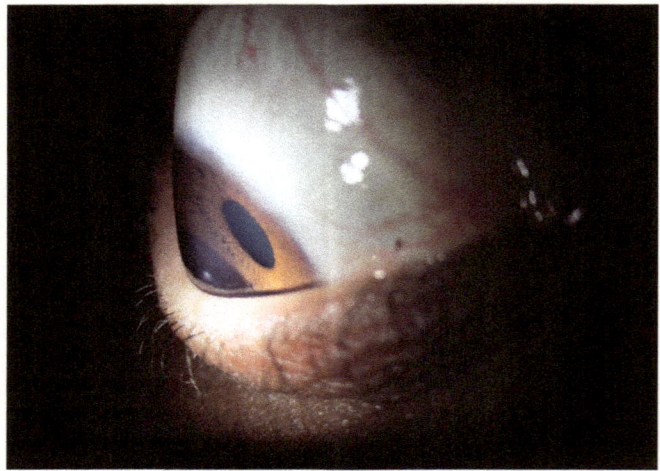

a. Keratoconus
b. Pellucid marginal degeneration
c. Terrien's marginal degeneration
d. Arcus juvenilis

21. From the photograph, what is the probable diagnosis?

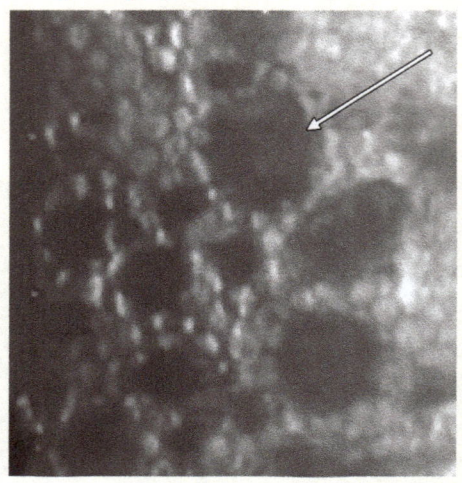

a. Granular dystrophy
b. Reis Buckler dystrophy
c. Macular dystrophy
d. Fuchs' dystrophy

22. A patient presents with history of alkali injury to the eye many years back resulting in severe loss of vision. From the clinical photograph, what would be the provisional diagnosis?

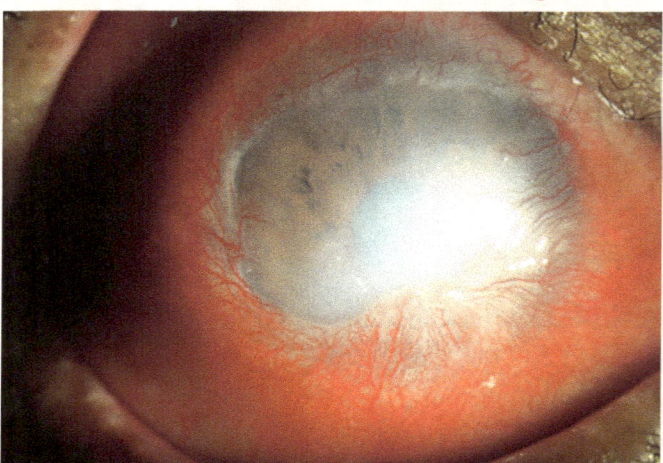

a. Pterygium
b. Peripheral ulcerative keratitis
c. Limbal stem cell deficiency
d. Adherent leucoma

Answer Key: 20. a   21. d   22. c

ANSWERS AND EXPLANATIONS

1. **Answer: c. With the rule astigmatism**
   (Ref: Yanoff & Duker 4th edition p 203-4)
   The clinical photograph shows **Pterygium**. The pterygium presses the cornea in the horizontal axis and tends to induce flattening. Thus the vertical axis of the cornea effectively becomes steeper than the horizontal axis. This is called '**with the rule astigmatism**'
   If the horizontal axis is steeper than the vertical axis, it would be called '**against the rule astigmatism**'

2. **Answer: c. Symblepharon**
   (Ref: Kanski 6th edition p 864-8)
   Symblepharon is a partial or complete adhesion of the palpebral conjunctiva to the bulbar conjunctiva resulting in the obliteration of the conjunctival fornix. Causes are
   - Chemical injuries
   - Thermal burns
   - Steven Johnson Syndrome
   - Trachoma
   - Herpes Zoster
   - Ocular cicatricial pemphigoid

3. **b. Vernal keratoconjunctivitis**
   (Ref: Yanoff & Duker 4th edition p 192-3)
   The photograph shows flat topped elevations on the conjunctiva which are known as papillae. The typical appearance is called cobblestone appearance.

4. **Answer: d: Phlyctenular conjunctivitis**
   (Peyman's Principles and Practice of Ophthalmology 2nd edition, p 405)
   Phlyctenular conjunctivitis is a unilateral allergic reaction to an antigen characterised by the formation of a circumscribed nodular lesion at the limbus. (as seen in the photograph)
   It is a type IV hypersensitivity reaction whose most common association in India is with **Mycobacterium tuberculosis.**

5. **Answer: a. Pterygium**
   (Ref: Kanski 8th edition p 162-3, 476-7)
   Pterygium is elastotic degeneration of the conjunctiva where a fold of conjunctiva grows on to the surface of the cornea. (Shown in the picture)

   The main differential diagnosis in case of recurrent or atypical looking pterygium is **ocular surface squamous neoplasia (OSSN)**. This includes a spectrum of pre-malignant and malignant epithelial lesions of conjunctiva and cornea. The lesions are gelatinous or fleshy in appearance with irregular surface. Superficial or feeder vessels may be present. Treatment is excision with 3–4 mm margins and assessment of edge clearance. Topical chemotherapy

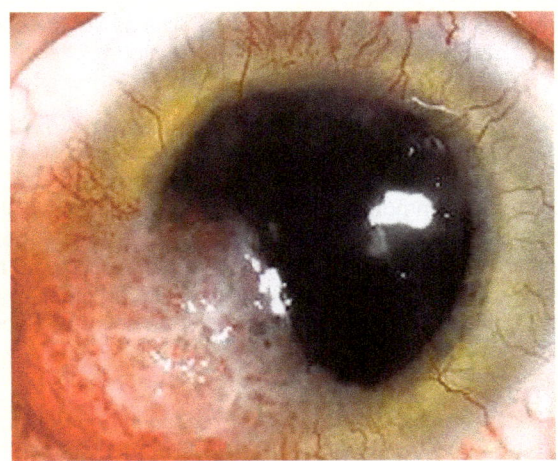
Ocular surface squamous neoplasia (OSSN)

with **Mitomycin C**^{Q}, **5-Fluorouracil**^{Q}, **Interferon alfa-2b**^{Q} are used as adjunct to avoid recurrence. However topical chemotherapy may be also used as a primary modality of management.

6. **Answer: c. Topical Natamycin only. No need to drain the Hypopyon.** *(Ref: Yanoff & Duker 4th edition p 225-7)*
   The clinical photograph shows a fungal ulcer with hyopyon. The ulcer has fuzzy margins with satellite lesions, hence clinically should be diagnosed as fungal. In India, most fungal ulcers are caused by filamentous fungi **Aspergillus**^{Q}, hence **Natamycin is the drug of choice**^{Q}. Drainage of Hypopyon is not done. **Steroids are absolutely contraindicated**^{Q}.

7. **Answer: b. Fungal keratitis**
   (Ref: Peyman's Principle and Practice of Ophthalmology, 2nd edition, p 476-480)
   The photograph shows a large central corneal lesion with smaller lesions surrounding it. These are satellite lesions, characteristic of fungal keratitis. Hence, the answer.

8. **Answer: b. *Acanthamoeba* keratitis**
   (Ref: Peyman's Principle and Practice of Ophthalmology, 2nd edition, p 488-91)
   The photograph shows a large ring ulcer, typically described in *Acanthamoeba* keratitis, associated with contact lens users. Hence, the answer

9. **Answer: b. Viral keratitis**
   (Ref: Peyman's Principle and Practice of Ophthalmology, 2nd edition, p 494-95)
   This photograph has been taken under cobalt blue filter of the slit-lamp after fluorescein staining. Fluorescein staining shows an irregular zig-zag, branching corneal ulcer with terminal bulbs. This is called a dendritic ulcer, typical of Herpes simplex virus.

10. **Answer: c. Therapeutic penetrating keratoplasty**
    (Ref: Peyman's Principle and Practice of Ophthalmology, 2nd edition, p 480-81)
    The photograph shows a perforated corneal ulcer with prolapse of iris tissue. The treatment is therapeutic penetrating keratoplasty where the entire cornea is replaced by cadaveric donor tissue. The aim of the surgery is to mainly restore the integrity of the globe.

11. **Answer: c. Mooren's ulcer**
    (Ref: Yanoff & Duker 4th edition p 244-5)
    The picture shows a corneal ulcer extending to the limbus. This is called as peripheral ulcerative keratitis (PUK). PUK is usually immunological and associated with systemic diseases like SLE, Rheumatoid arthritis etc. Mooren's ulcer is a type of PUK with no systemic association. It is a very painful condition and presents with an indolent ulcer with overhanging margins. Scraping is negative because it is non-infectious.

12. **Answer: b: Granular dystrophy**
    (Ref: Peyman's Principles and Practice of Ophthalmology, 2nd edition, p 181-82)
    The photograph shows multiple white opacities in the cornea **with clear intervening stroma**. These opacities are caused by deposition of hyaline in the corneal stroma and are characteristic of granular dystrophy.
    The patients maintain good visual acuity till middle age but complain of glare and photophobia

13. **Answer: c. Macular dystrophy**
    (Ref: Peyman's Principles and Practice of Ophthalmology, 2nd edition, pg 182-83)
    The photograph shows multiple white opacities in the cornea **with hazy intervening stroma.** These opacities are caused by deposition of Mucopolysaccharide in the corneal stroma and are characteristic of macular dystrophy. The patients presents with decreased visual acuity at a young age.
    The photograph looks similar to that of granular dystrophy given in question no 12. But the corneal opacities in macular dystrophy are denser and the intervening stroma is also hazy, which differentiates it clinically from granular dystrophy.

14. **Answer: a. Lattice dystrophy**
    (Ref: Peyman's Principles and Practice of Ophthalmology, 2nd edition, p 180-81)
    The photograph shows multiple criss-cross lines extending throughout the cornea suggestive of lattice dystrophy

15. **Answer: c. Leucomatous**
    The different types of corneal opacity are
    Nebular: This involves <1/3 rd of the corneal stroma. So the iris details can be seen quite clearly through the opacity
    Macular: This involves >1/3 rd to 1/2 of the corneal stroma. So iris details can be seen hazily through the opacity.
    Leucomatous: This involves >1/2 to full thickness of the stroma. Hence iris details are not visible through the opacity.
    Adherent leucoma: This is a leucomatous opacity with iris attached to it

16. **Answer: c. Keratoplasty** *(Ref: Yanoff & Duker 4th edition p 301)*
    Keratoplasty means cornea transplantation. The photograph shows a corneal graft sutured to the host bed by multiple sutures

17. **Answer: b. Sodium Fluorescein**
    Fluorescein stain is used to detect epithelial abrasion or epithelial defect in the cornea because it stains the areas where epithelium is absent. It is best examined under cobalt blue filter. The green area in the photograph is the epithelial defect.

18. **Answer: c. Descemet's membrane detachment**
    (Ref: Yanoff & Duker 4th edition p 455-6)
    Anterior segment OCT is an imaging technique which helps to evaluate the structures like cornea, angle, anterior chamber, iris and lens. The picture above shows an image of the cornea with detachment of the posterior layer which is the Descemet's membrane with endothelium

19. **Answer: a. Keratoconus**
    (Ref: Yanoff & Duker 4th edition p 168-172)
    The topography picture shown in the question contains two maps.
    The upper one is the **curvature map** showing the **keratometry** readings on the anterior corneal surface. The cool colours like green and yellow indicate normal values whereas high keratometry readings are depicted by the warmer colours like red, purple and black. So the curvature map shows increased curvature in the centre, slightly skewed to the inferior cornea
    The lower one is a **thickness map** showing the corneal thickness at various points in the cornea. The cool colours like yellow and green indicate normal thickness whereas the warmer colours indicate decreased thickness. So, the thickness map shows decreased thickness at almost the same place where the curvature map shows increased curvature
    Thus the question hints at a patient with **high astigmatism** with **increased corneal curvature** and **decreased thickness**. So the correct option is keratoconus.
    Keratoglobus shows increased curvature with decreased thickness throughout the cornea unlike keratoconus where the cone is in a localised area.

20. **Answer: a. Keratoconus**
    (Ref: Peyman's Principles and Practice of Ophthalmology, 2nd edition, p 515-9)
    The photograph shows corneal protrusion indenting the lower lid on downgaze. This is called **Munson's sign**, seen in keratoconus.

21. **Answer: d. Fuch's dystrophy**
    This is a picture of specular microscopy of cornea
    Specular microscopy
    - Specular microscope is a reflected light microscope
    - Light is projected on to the eye and the reflected light is captured by the instrument. The light reflected from the optical interface between the corneal endothelium and the aqueous humour is imaged and analyzed.

- The specular microscope is thus used to study the **corneal endothelium**[Q]
- It is useful to evaluate **corneal graft**[Q], endothelial dystrophies like **Fuch's dystrophy**[Q] and **donor corneal tissue**[Q] prior to keratoplasty.
- The endothelial cells are closely packed, **hexagonal in shape**[Q] with an average cell count of 2500–3000/mm². The cell density gradually decreases with age
- Cellular **pleomorphism**[Q], **polymegathism**[Q], decreased cell density with areas of cell loss or guttae are features of endothelial dysfunction

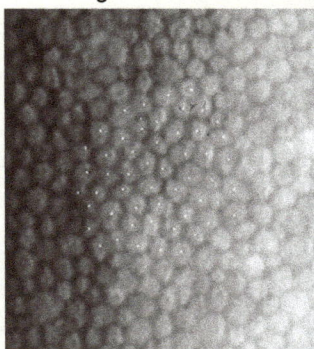
Normal corneal endothelium

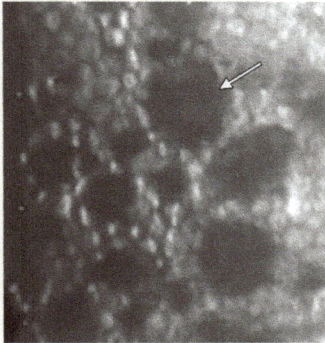
Fuchs' dystrophy

The picture in the question shows large areas of endothelial cell loss (indicated by arrow) with pleomorphism and polymegathism. This is suggestive of Fuchs' endothelial dystrophy

22. **Answer: c. Limbal stem cell deficiency**
    (Ref: Yanoff & Duker 4th edition p 296-8)

The photograph shows loss of corneal transparency. The inferior half of the cornea is conjunctivalised due to loss of the limbal stem cells.

Chemical injury to the eye is an ophthalmic emergency. **Alkali injury due to lime or chuna** is very common in children especially in the rural areas. If not treated properly it may have serious consequences. The features of alkali injury are

- Necrosis of the conjunctival and corneal epithelium.
- Loss of limbal stem cells leads to conjunctivalisation and vascularisation of the cornea with loss of corneal transparency[Q]
- Deep stromal necrosis may lead to perforation of the cornea
- Intraocular inflammation may also be seen

4
Lens

The lens is a biconvex, transparent crystalline structure which divides the eye into anterior and posterior segments. It is placed in a saucer shaped depression called **patellar fossa**[Q].

- Refractive index: 1.386[Q]
- Refractive power : 14–16 D[Q]
- Equatorial diameter: 10 mm
- It has two surfaces anterior and posterior. **The anterior surface is less convex than the posterior**[Q].
- Radius of curvature:
  - Anterior 10 mm
  - Posterior 6 mm

The lens is made up of
- *Lens capsule*: It is a transparent membrane covering the lens. It is **thickest in the pre-equatorial region**[Q] and **thinnest at the posterior pole**[Q]
- *Lens epithelium*: There is a single layer of epithelium on the anterior surface of the lens but no epithelium on the posterior surface
- *Lens fibres*: These are protein fibres arranged closely in concentric layers. Lens fibres are formed throughout life so that the oldest fibres are at the centre and the newest fibres are most superficial. Hence the lens fibres may be divided into
  - *Nucleus*: It is the central part of the lens containing the older fibres. It is again subdivided into embryonic nucleus (formed in first 3 months of gestation), foetal nucleus (formed till birth), infantile nucleus (formed from birth to puberty), adult nucleus (formed after puberty)
  - *Cortex*: It is the peripheral part containing the newly formed fibres

The lens is suspended from above and below by the ciliary zonules. The attachment of the vitreous to the posterior surface of the lens is called **Weigert's ligament**[Q]. The potential space between the lens and vitreous is called **retrolental space of Berger**[Q].

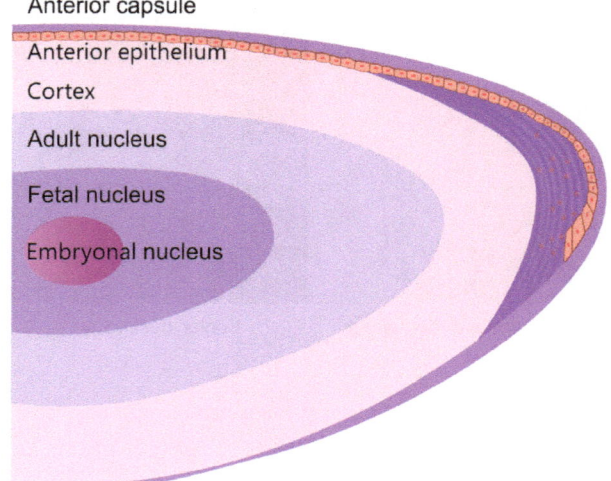

Fig. 1: Anatomy of the lens

Anti-oxidants present in lens
- **Glutathione**[Q]
- **Superoxide dismutase**[Q]
- **Catalase**[Q]
- **Vitamin C**[Q]
- **Vitamin E**[Q]

CONGENITAL AND DEVELOPMENTAL CATARACT

This is due to disturbance in the growth and development of the lens. Disturbance in development during the period of gestation leads to **congenital cataract** and usually affects the **embryonic or foetal nucleus. Developmental cataract** is due to disturbance in development after birth and hence affects the **infantile or adult nucleus and cortex.** The different morphological varieties are
- *Punctate cataract*: It consists of minute white dots throughout the lens but causes no visual disturbance. It is called **blue dot cataract**[Q]. **It is the most common type of congenital cataract**[Q]

- *Zonular or lamellar cataract*: **This is the most common type of congenital cataract associated with diminished vision**^{Q}. A zone in the foetal nucleus is usually affected. Hypocalcemia in pregnancy is an important cause^Q
- *Nuclear cataract*: This usually affects the **embryonic nucleus. Rubella in pregnancy is an important cause**^{Q}
- *Coronary cataract*: It usually occurs around puberty and is characterized by opacities in the periphery of the lens
- Anterior polar cataract
- Posterior polar cataract

Senile Cataract

It is the most common type of acquired cataract^Q. The different morphological types are

Nuclear cataract

- This is an age-related increase in the refractive index of the lens nucleus.
- It causes a myopic shift in refraction known as **index myopia**^{Q}
- Improvement of near vision occurs as a result of myopic shift in refraction. This is called second **sight of old age**^{Q}.
- The main mechanism of formation of nuclear cataract is **conversion of the soluble crystallins to insoluble crystalloids**^{Q}.

Cortical Cataract

- The main mechanism of formation of cortical cataract is decrease in concentration of proteins and amino acids and increase in sodium with associated hydration of the lens.
- In cuneiform cataract, there are wedge shaped cortical opacities in the peripheral portion of the lens. Hence it leads to **visual difficulty in dim light when the pupil is dilated**^{Q}.
- In cupuliform cataract, opacification is seen in the posterior cortex just below the capsule in the centre of the visual axis

Subcapsular Cataract

- It is usually seen beneath the posterior capsule at the posterior pole. As it lies just at the centre of the visual axis, it is the **most visually significant cataract**^{Q}.

- It causes **difficulty in vision in bright light**^{Q} and for **near work**^{Q}.
- **Glare is common**^{Q}

Mature Cataract

When the entire lens has become opacified, it is called mature cataract. **Pearly white**^{Q} **appearance with absence of iris shadow**^{Q} **is seen**. If not operated, it progresses to hypermature cataract.

Hypermature cataract

It has two varieties
- *Sclerotic cataract*: The lens becomes shrunken and small with calcification on the anterior capsule. There is wrinkling of the lens capsule. It predisposes to **subluxation of lens**^{Q}
- *Morgagnian cataract*: There is total liquefaction of the cortex as a result of which the nucleus sinks inferiorly. The liquefied cortex leaks through the intact capsule and blocks the trabecular meshwork. This leads to **phacolytic glaucoma**^{Q} **or lens protein glaucoma**. It also causes **phacoanaphylactic uveitis**^{Q}

Intumescent Cataract

This means a swollen cataract due to excessive hydration. The swollen lens pushes the iris forward leading to closure of the angle. This is called as **phacomorphic glaucoma**^{Q}.

Traumatic Cataract

It may be seen in different types of injury like:
- *Penetrating injuries as a result of direct injury to the lens*: It is usually **anterior subcapsular or anterior polar cataract**^{Q}.
- *Blunt trauma or concussion injuries*: Due to the impact of the trauma, the iris diaphragm moves backward and touches the lens capsule. As a result, the iris pigments form a ring on the anterior capsule called as **Vossius Ring**^{Q}. The typical cataract is called **rosette cataract**^{Q}
- Thermal injury
- Electrical and radiation injury

Metabolic Cataract

	Type of cataract	Cause	Associated features
Diabetes Mellitus	**Snowflake cataract**[Q]	Osmotic overhydration. Excess glucose is converted to **sorbitol** by the enzyme **aldose reductase**[Q]	**Fluctuation in refractive error is a sign of changing lens hydration**[Q]
Galactosemia	**Oil droplet cataract**[Q]	Accumulation of galactose due to deficiency of enzyme Galactose1-P-uridyl transferase	**Reversible cataract**[Q] Disappears when galactose is removed from the diet
Fabry's disease	Spoke –wheel like opacities		
Wilson's disease	**Sunflower cataract**[Q]	Deficiency of α-2 globulin ceruloplasmin leading to inadequate Cu binding and deposition of Cu in tissues	**Kayser –Fleischer ring (KF)**[Q] Sunflower cataract is also called **pseudo cataract** because it does not cause visual impairment
Lowe's (oculocerebrorenal) syndrome	Cataract with **posterior lenticonus**[Q]	Inborn error of metabolism	**Microspherophakia** Associated with mental retardation, renal dysfunction, osteomalacia, muscular hypotony, frontal prominence
Hypocalcemia	Spokes or riders in the lens		

Toxic Cataract

The drugs causing toxic cataract are:
- *Corticosteroids*: Steroids by systemic route of administration[Q] may lead to toxic cataract. The typical morphology is **posterior subcapsular cataract**[Q]
- Chloroquine
- *Chlorpromazine*: It causes **star shaped or stellate cataract**
- Miotics may cause **anterior subcapsular cataract**
- **Amiodarone**[Q] may cause **anterior subcapsular cataract**[Q]
- INH and Ethambutol
- Smoking

Complicated Cataract

This name is given to cataract arising due to inflammatory or degenerative diseases of the eye. It is usually **posterior subcapsular cataract**[Q]. It has a typical **bread crumb appearance**[Q] with **polychromatic lustre**[Q]. The causes are
- Anterior, intermediate or posterior uveitis
- Retinitis Pigmentosa[Q]
- High Myopia[Q]
- *Angle closure glaucoma*: This is typically **anterior subcapsular cataract**[Q] and is known as **glaucomflecken**[Q]
- Intraocular tumours

Presenile Cataract

The different conditions associated with presenile cataract are:
- *Myotonic Dystrophy*: The typical cataract is **Christmas Tree Cataract**[Q].
- *Syndermatotic cataract*: It is associated with skin disorders like atopic dermatitis, icthyosis and psoriasis
- **Down's syndrome**[Q]
- Werner's syndrome
- **Neurofibromatosis**

CLINICAL FEATURES OF CATARACT

- Gradually progressive decrease in vision
- *Glare and coloured haloes*: Coloured haloes are also seen in **mucopurulent conjunctivitis** and **acute angle closure glaucoma.** In conjunctivitis, the haloes disappear on washing the eye. For differentiating haloes of cataract and glaucoma, **Fincham's test**[Q] was used. On holding a stenopaeic slit in front of the eye, the haloes due to cataract will break but the haloes due to glaucoma will remain intact.
- *Monocular diplopia*: This is more common in intumescent cataract.

MANAGEMENT OF CATARACT

The treatment of cataract is cataract surgery. Cataract surgery has evolved over decades to the highest level of predictability and precision today. **The incision in modern day cataract surgery is very small with the benefit of no suture^Q, minimum postoperative astigmatism^Q and quick visual recovery. The intraocular lenses implanted today after cataract surgery are foldable, can be implanted through a very small incision and provide visual quality similar to the natural lens.**

Preoperative evaluation of cataract patient^Q

- *Systemic evaluation*: Diabetes, hypertension, heart disease, lung disease, infections
- *Visual acuity and refraction:* In case of advanced cataract where visual acuity is very poor, **perception of light and projection of rays^Q** should be assessed. This gives a rough idea about the retina and optic nerve function.
- *Colour vision*: To assess the optic nerve
- *Tests for macular function like* **Potential Acuity Meter (PAM):** This is used to predict postoperative visual acuity in patients with advanced cataract
- **IOP evaluation by Tonometry^Q**
- Gonioscopy is done if IOP is high
- **Pupillary reaction**
- Tests for stereoacuity
- Anterior segment evaluation on slit lamp
- *Fundus evaluation:* 90D lens, Direct and Indirect Ophthalmoscope
- **Syringing** to check for patency of the lacrimal drainage pathway
- **USG B-Scan** to assess the posterior segment in advanced cataract where fundus cannot be evaluated clinically.
- *Optical Coherence Tomography (OCT):* to assess the macula in case of any pathology
- **Keratometry and Axial length** to calculate IOL power. Axial length is measured by **A-Scan** biometry.

The different types of cataract surgery are:

- *Intracapsular cataract extraction (ICCE)*: In this technique, the lens along with the capsular bag is removed through a large incision. **The only indication of ICCE today would be subluxated lens^Q.** Intraocular lens has to be iris-fixated, sclera fixated or placed in the anterior chamber.
- *Extracapsular cataract extraction (ECCE)*: In this technique, the lens is removed in toto by making an opening in the anterior capsule. As a result a large limbal incision of 8-9 mm is needed. The capsular bag with an opening in the anterior capsule is left after removal of the lens. **The IOL is placed in the capsular bag^Q**
- *Small incision cataract surgery (SICS)*: The technique is almost similar to ECCE but a corneoscleral tunnel of 6-7 mm is made instead of a limbal incision
- *Phacoemulsification*: In this technique, the lens is emulsified and aspirated by an ultrasound probe after making a circular opening (capsulorrhexis) in the anterior capsule. So the incision is small, just enough to permit the entry of the probe **(2.8-3.2 mm)^Q. A foldable IOL is implanted in the capsular bag^Q**

The steps of Phacoemulsification surgery are

- Wound construction
- Entry into anterior chamber
- Anterior capsulorrhexis (a circular opening is made in the anterior capsule of the lens)
- Hydrodissection (This means injecting fluid beneath the capsule to separate the lens from the capsule. Hydrodelineation is a type of controlled hydrodissection done in posterior polar cataract)
- Phacoemulsification of the lens
- Cortical wash
- IOL implantation
- Wound closure by hydration

- *Micro incision cataract surgery (MICS)*: This is similar to conventional phacoemulsification but the incision is even smaller **(2.2-2.4 mm)**
- *Femtosecond laser assisted cataract surgery^Q*: This is the most recent advancement in the field of cataract surgery. Femtosecond laser is an **ultra short** pulse laser **(10^{-15} seconds)** which has a variety of application in ophthalmic practice. In cataract surgery, Femtosecond laser is used to create the **corneal incision^Q, capsulorrhexis^Q** and **fragmentation of lens nucleus^Q.** It may also be used to correct astigmatism by **astigmatic keratotomy^Q.**

IOL Power Calculation Formulae

- **SRK-II formula^Q**: This is used for emmetropic eyes (Axial length 22-25 mm). The formula states
- **P = A-2.5L-0.9K** (A = constant, L = Axial length, K = keratometry)
- **Hoffer^Q** formula: This is used for hypermetropic eyes. (Axial length < 22 mm)
- **SRK-T** formula: This is used for myopic eyes. (Axial length > 25 mm)
- **Haigis/Holladay II** formula: These are used in post-refractive surgery cases

Types of Intraocular Lenses

The different types of IOL are:

➢ *Non-foldable lenses*: These are usually made up of **Polymethylmethacrylate (PMMA)**^{Q}. They are posterior chamber IOLs, anterior chamber IOLs, iris-fixated IOLs and scleral fixated IOLs

➢ *Foldable lenses*: These are made up of **Acrylic**^{Q} **(hydrophobic or hydrophilic)** and hydrogels. They are all posterior chamber IOLs which are placed in the capsular bag.

Types of Foldable IOL

- *Monofocal IOL*: These provide good distance vision but glasses have to be used for near. (Since accommodation is lost after pseudophakia)
- *Multifocal IOL*: These IOLs have separate zones which focus for distance and near. So they provide good vision both for distance and near without glasses. **The main disadvantage is glare and haloes**^{Q}
- *Accommodative IOL*: These lenses can move in the capsular bag during accommodation to provide good vision for both distance and near without glasses.
- *Toric IOL*: These lenses have a cylindrical power incorporated in them and hence help to correct any associated **corneal astigmatism**^{Q}. They may be multifocal or monofocal.

Complications of Cataract Surgery

The complications related to surgery are

➢ **Posterior capsular tear with nucleus drop**^{Q}
➢ Vitreous loss
➢ **Retinal detachment**^{Q}
➢ Postoperative uveitis
➢ Toxic anterior segment syndrome (TASS)
➢ Cystoid macular oedema^Q
➢ Striate keratopathy
➢ Pseudophakic bullous keratopathy due to endothelial decompensation

Complications related to IOL

- *Malposition of IOL*: The IOL may be decentred, subluxated or dislocated leading to
  - *Sunset syndrome*^{Q}: Subluxated inferiorly
  - Sunrise syndrome: Subluxated superiorly
  - Windshield wiper syndrome: Lens keeps moving with movement of head
- *Posterior capsule opacification (PCO)*^{Q}: The posterior capsule behind the lens may opacify months or years after cataract surgery leading to visual impairment.
  - Morphological types are **Elschnig's pearls**^{Q} and **Sommering's ring**^{Q}.
  - Treatment is **Nd: YAG capsulotomy**

Endophthalmitis^Q

This is the most dreaded and worst possible complication of cataract surgery. **It is a suppurative inflammation starting from the vitreous which extends to all the parts of the eye except the sclera**^{Q}. If the sclera also becomes involved, the condition is then called as **panophthalmitis**^{Q}. Post-operative endophthalmitis has the following features

- *Early onset (within 7 days of surgery)*: The most common causative organism is **Staphylococcus epidermidis**
- *Late onset*: The most common causative organisms are **fungi and Propionibacterium acne**^{Q}
- Prevention is of utmost importance. The main source of infecting organisms is the patient's own flora. Hence prophylactic topical antibiotics are given 3 days prior to surgery. **Irrigation of the conjunctival cul-de-sac with povidone iodine prior to surgery is a must**^{Q}.
- Post operative topical antibiotics are given for 1-2 weeks
- The patient presents with sudden onset, pain, redness and decrease in vision. Exudates are seen in the vitreous on examination
- Treatment is **intravitreal tap and intravitreal antibiotics**. If the patient does not improve, **pars plana vitrectomy**^{Q} is done
- Treatment of panophthalmitis is **evisceration**^{Q}

MANAGEMENT OF CATARACT IN CHILDREN

➢ Cataract in children is an important cause for development of **stimulus deprivation amblyopia**^{Q}
➢ **Unilateral cataract is more dangerous than bilateral cataract because the risk of amblyopia is more**
➢ The ideal age for cataract surgery in children is **4–6 weeks**^{Q} because 6 weeks is the critical period for visual maturation in children. Thus early surgery decreases the possibility of amblyopia
➢ *IOL power selection in children*: In very small children, it is extremely difficult to calculate the IOL power as the axial length and keratometry values are not accurate. In older children, if IOL power is calculated according to the present axial length, there occurs a **myopic shift** as the child grows older. **Hence undercorrection of IOL power from the calculated value is needed.**
  - In children < 1yr of age, IOL is avoided. Patients are left aphakic and advised postoperative contact lenses. Secondary IOL implantation is planned at a later date when the child is older

- Between 1–8 years of age, IOL is implanted. The power of the IOL is undercorrected from the calculated value according to the age of the patient.
- Beyond 8 years, IOL power is the same as the calculated value from the formulae.

ANOMALIES OF LENS POSITION

The lens is located in a saucer shaped depression called the patellar fossa between the anterior and posterior chamber of the eye. A lens in abnormal position since birth is called **Ectopia lentis.** Acquired cases are called **subluxation and dislocation.** Subluxation means that a part of the lens still lies with the patellar fossa. Dislocation means that the lens is completely out of the patellar fossa.

Congenital causes
• Marfan's syndrome[Q] (associated with **superotemporal**[Q] subluxation)
• Homocystinuria[Q] (associated with **inferonasal**[Q] subluxation)
• Weil Marchesani (microspherophakia with anterior dislocation of lens)
• Ehler-Danlos syndrome
• Hyperlysinemia
• Stickler's disease

Contd…

• Sulphite oxidase deficiency
Acquired causes
• **Trauma (most common)**[Q]
• Buphthalmos
• Megalocornea
• High Myopia
• Pseudoexfoliation
• Hypermature sclerotic cataract
• Chronic uveitis
• Endophthalmitis
• Intraocular tumours

> **Must Remember**
> - *Snowflake cataract:* Diabetes mellitus
> - *Sunflower cataract:* Wilson's disease
> - *Rosette cataract:* Blunt trauma
> - *Oil droplet cataract:* Galactosemia
> - *Polychromatic lustre:* Complicated cataract
> - *Christmas tree cataract:* Myotonic dystrophy

QUESTIONS

Anatomy and Physiology of Lens

1. **The capsule of the crystalline lens is thinnest at:** *(UPPG)*
   a. Arterior pole
   b. Posterior pole
   c. Equator
   d. None

2. **Ascorbate and Alpha Tochopherol are maintained in the lens in reduced state by:** *(AIIMS 2014)*
   a. Glucose
   b. Glycoprotein
   c. Glutathione
   d. Fatty acids

3. **Which of the following does not handle free radicals in the lens?** *(AIPG)*
   a. Vitamin A
   b. Vitamin C
   c. Vitamin E
   d. Catalase

4. **The crystalline lens derives its nutrition from:** *(AIIMS)*
   a. Blood vessels
   b. Connective tissue
   c. Aqueous and vitreous
   d. Capsule of the lens

5. **Transport of ascorbic acid in the lens is done by:** *(AIPG)*
   a. Myoinositol
   b. Choline
   c. Taurine
   d. Na-K ATPase

6. **Ligament of Weigert is:** *(APPG)*
   a. Attachment of the vitreous to the posterior capsule of the lens
   b. Medial palpebral ligament
   c. Attachment of the superior oblique tendon
   d. Associated with the middle ear

7. **Zonules suspending the lens are attached to:** *(DNB 2015)*
   a. Root of iris
   b. Ciliary body
   c. Limbus
   d. Vitreous

Anomalies of Lens Position

8. **Position of the lens in Marfan's syndrome is:** *(COMEDK)*
   a. Superior
   b. Superotemporal
   c. Inferior
   d. Nasal

9. **Typical bilateral inferonasal subluxation of lens is seen in:** *(DNB)*
   a. Marfan's syndrome
   b. Homocystinuria
   c. Hyperlysinemia
   d. Trauma

10. **Ectopia lentis is seen in:** *(PGI)*
    a. Marfan's syndrome
    b. Congenital rubella
    c. Homocystinuria
    d. Sulphite oxidase deficiency
    e. Myotonic dystrophy

11. **Anterior lenticonus is seen in:** *(AIPG)*
    a. Alport's syndrome
    b. Lowe's syndrome
    c. Down's syndrome
    d. William's syndrome

12. **Spontaneous absorption of lens material is seen in:** *(COMEDK)*
    a. Marfan's syndrome
    b. Hallerman Streiff syndrome
    c. Aniridia
    d. Persistent hyperplastic primary vitreous (PHPV)

Cataract

13. **Phacodonesis is seen in all except:** *(NEET 2016)*
    a. Trauma
    b. Hypermature cataract
    c. Pseudoexfoliation
    d. Diabetes mellitus

14. **Gene commonly indicated in congenital cataract:** *(AIIMS 2014)*
    a. PAX-6
    b. CRYGS-3
    c. LMX-1B
    d. PITX-3

15. **Most common type of congenital cataract is:** *(AIIMS)*
    a. Capsular
    b. Zonular
    c. Cupuliform
    d. Blue dot

16. **Most common congenital cataract associated with decreased vision:** *(AIIMS)*
    a. Blue dot
    b. Cupuliform
    c. Zonular
    d. Coronary

17. **Rider's are seen in:** *(AIPG)*
    a. Blue dot cataract
    b. Zonular cataract
    c. Sutural cataract
    d. Coronary cataract

18. **Commonest type of cataract:** *(PGI)*
    a. Hereditary
    b. Trauma
    c. Diabetes
    d. Age related
    e. Radiation

19. **Which of the following is true regarding concentration of proteins in senile cataract?** *(AIIMS 2013)*
    a. More insoluble protein, less soluble protein
    b. More soluble protein, less insoluble protein
    c. Equal concentration of soluble and insoluble protein
    d. None of the above

20. **High molecular weight protein present in cataractous lens in humans:** *(AIIMS 2015)*
    a. HM 1 and HM 2
    b. HM 2 and HM 3
    c. HM 3 and HM 4
    d. HM 4 and HM 1

21. **Most visually significant cataract:** *(AIIMS)*
    a. Nuclear cataract
    b. Cortical cataract
    c. Posterior subcapsular cataract
    d. Zonular cataract

22. **Second sight phenomenon is seen in:** *(TNPG)*
    a. Nuclear cataract
    b. Cortical cataract
    c. Posterior subcapsular cataract
    d. Mature cataract

23. **Index myopia is seen in:** *(DNB)*
    a. Nuclear cataract
    b. Cortical cataract
    c. Mature cataract
    d. Posterior subcapsular cataract

24. True about posterior subcapsular cataract is:
    (DNB 2015)
    a. Visual loss is late
    b. It is a type of mature senile cataract
    c. Difficulty in bright light is a symptom
    d. Glare is uncommon
25. Which of the following is not seen in uncomplicated mature cataract? *(APPG)*
    a. Absence of iris shadow
    b. Pearly white colour
    c. Normal anterior chamber
    d. Absent light perception
26. The most common complication of hypermature sclerotic cataract: *(AIIMS)*
    a. Dislocation of lens
    b. Phacomorphic glaucoma
    c. Uveitis
    d. Neovascularisation of iris
27. Which type of cataract causes phacomorphic glaucoma? *(DNB)*
    a. Incipient cataract
    b. Intumescent cataract
    c. Morgagnian cataract
    d. Zonular cataract
28. Typical appearance of diabetic cataract is: *(AIIMS)*
    a. Sunflower cataract
    b. Breadcrumb cataract
    c. Polychromatic lustre
    d. Snowflake cataract
29. Cataract in diabetic patient is due to accumulation of sorbitol. The enzyme responsible is: *(AIIMS)*
    a. Hexokinase
    b. NADPH dependent aldose reductase
    c. Glucokinase
    d. Phosphofructokinase
30. Fluctuating refractive errors with cataract is seen in:
    (AIIMS)
    a. Morgagnian cataract
    b. Diabetic cataract
    c. Intumescent cataract
    d. Traumatic cataract
31. Sunflower cataract is seen in: *(AIPG)*
    a. Chalcosis
    b. Diabetes
    c. Syphilis
    d. Stargardt's disease
32. Polychromatic lustre is seen in: *(AIPG/ AIIMS)*
    a. Complicated cataract
    b. Diabetic cataract
    c. Post radiation cataract
    d. Congenital cataract
33. Prolonged use of corticosteroids results in which type of cataract? *(NEET 2016)*
    a. Posterior subcapsular
    b. Nuclear
    c. Anterior polar
    d. Posterior polar
34. Steroid induced cataract is: *(AIPG)*
    a. Posterior subcapsular
    b. Anterior subcapsular
    c. Nuclear cataract
    d. Cupuliform cataract
35. Rosette cataract is seen in: *(APPG)*
    a. Blunt trauma
    b. Diabetes
    c. Wilson's disease
    d. Myopia
36. Anterior polar cataract is seen in: *(PGI)*
    a. Diabetes
    b. Perforating injury
    c. Irradiation
    d. Chalcosis
37. Onion peel appearance is seen in: *(NEET 2016)*
    a. Posterior subcapsular cataract
    b. Posterior polar cataract
    c. Anterior polar cataract
    d. Nuclear cataract
38. Vossius ring is seen in: *(DNB)*
    a. Penetrating trauma
    b. Concussion injury
    c. Iridocyclitis
    d. Acute angle closure glaucoma
39. Christmas tree cataract is seen in: *(PGI)*
    a. Down's syndrome
    b. Rubella
    c. Myotonic dystrophy
    d. Diabetes
40. Which of the following does not cause complicated cataract? *(WBPG)*
    a. Pathological myopia
    b. Diabetes mellitus
    c. Retinitis pigmentosa
    d. Iridocyclitis
41. Select the correct match: *(PGI 2013)*
    a. Wilson's disease- Sunflower cataract
    b. Alport's syndrome-Posterior lenticonus
    c. Amiodarone-Anterior subcapsular cataract
    d. Myotonic dystrophy- Christmas tree cataract
    e. Down's syndrome- Cortical cataract
42. Specific pattern of cataract is not seen in: *(APPG)*
    a. Juvenile diabetes
    b. Leprosy
    c. Myotonic dystrophy
    d. Wilson's disease
43. Which of the following conditions is not associated with cataract? *(DNB 2015)*
    a. Diabetes mellitus
    b. Myotonic dystrophy
    c. Refsum's disease
    d. Wilson's disease

Cataract Surgery

44. The investigation to predict post-operative visual outcome after cataract surgery is: *(DNB 2016)*
    a. Pachymetry
    b. Topography
    c. Potential acuity meter
    d. Lensometry
45. Recovery after cataract surgery is fastest with: *(MPPG)*
    a. ICCE
    b. ECCE
    c. Phacoemulsification
    d. SICS
46. Advantages of ECCE over ICCE are: *(PGI)*
    a. Less chance of cystoid macular oedema
    b. Less chance of endophthalmitis
    c. Can be used in traumatic lens subluxation
    d. Less chance of vitreous haemorrhage and retinal detachment
    e. Minimal endothelial damage
47. In present scenario, only indication of ICCE is: *(DNB)*
    a. Mature cataract
    b. Paediatric cataract
    c. Subluxated cataract
    d. Immature cataract
48. The standard sutureless cataract surgery with phacoemulsification and foldable IOL implantation has an incision of: *(AIIMS)*
    a. 1–1.5 mm
    b. 2–2.5 mm
    c. 3–3.5 mm
    d. 4–4.5 mm
49. Phacoemulsification includes: *(PGI)*
    a. Hydrodissection
    b. Hydrodelineation
    c. Continuous curvilinear capsulorrhexis
    d. IOL implantation
    e. Lens aspiration

50. Which of the following steps is not done in phacoemulsification cataract surgery? *(NEET 2016)*
    a. Continuous curvilinear capsulorrhexis
    b. Sclerocorneal tunnel
    c. Irrigation and aspiration
    d. Foldable IOL implantation

51. Best irrigating fluid for cataract surgery is: *(AIIMS)*
    a. Normal saline
    b. Ringer lactate
    c. Balanced salt solution
    d. Balanced salt solution + glutathione

52. Power for nuclear fragmentation in cataract surgery is: *(DNB 2016)*
    a. Ultrasonic
    b. Thermal
    c. Electrical
    d. Magnetic

53. Treatment for congenital cataract is: *(DPG)*
    a. Pharmacotherapy
    b. Combined cataract surgery and goniotomy
    c. Cataract surgery with IOL implantation with posterior capsulotomy
    d. Pars plana lensectomy with no IOL implantation

54. A child has congenital cataract involving the visual axis which was detected by the parents right at birth. When should the child be operated? *(DPG)*
    a. Immediately
    b. At 2 months of age
    c. At 1 year of age when the globe attains normal size
    d. At 4 years when ocular and orbital growth is complete

55. Essential parameters for IOL power calculation are: *(TNPG)*
    a. Keratometry and corneal thickness
    b. Corneal thickness and axial length of the eyeball
    c. Keratometry and axial length of the eyeball
    d. Corneal thickness and anterior chamber depth

56. Axial length of the eye prior to cataract surgery is measured by: *(DNB 2015)*
    a. Keratometry
    b. A-Scan Biometry
    c. Specular microscopy
    d. Slit lamp Biomicroscopy

57. SRK formula is used for calculation of: *(NEET 2016)*
    a. IOL power
    b. Corneal endothelial count
    c. Corneal curvature
    d. Extent of retinal detachment

58. Which of the following is not needed for IOL power calculation prior to cataract surgery? *(DNB 2016)*
    a. Keratometry
    b. A-Scan biometry
    c. Corneal topography
    d. SRK formula

59. Best site for IOL implantation is: *(DPG)*
    a. Iris
    b. Anterior chamber
    c. Capsular bag
    d. Sulcus

60. Non-foldable IOLs are made up of: *(DNB 2015)*
    a. PMMA
    b. Silicon
    c. Acrylic
    d. Hydrogels

61. Modern IOLs are made up of: *(PGI)*
    a. PMMA
    b. Acrylic acid
    c. Glass
    d. Silicon
    e. Styrene

62. IOL which can correct astigmatism is: *(DNB 2015)*
    a. Toric IOL
    b. Multifocal IOL
    c. Monofocal IOL
    d. ACIOL

63. Most recent advance in the field of cataract surgery is the use of: *(NEET 2016)*
    a. Femtosecond laser
    b. Neodymium laser
    c. Picosecond laser
    d. Excimer laser

64. In which of the following conditions is IOL implantation after cataract surgery contraindicated? *(AIPG)*
    a. Fuch's heterochromic iridocyclitis
    b. Juvenile rheumatoid arthritis
    c. Psoriatic arthritis
    d. Reiter's syndrome

Complications of Cataract Surgery

65. Complications of cataract surgery are: *(PGI)*
    a. Endophthalmitis
    b. Optic neuropathy
    c. Retinal detachment
    d. Vitreous loss
    e. Lagophthalmos

66. Postoperative endophthalmitis in cataract surgery is decreased by all except: *(WBPG)*
    a. Antibiotic eye drops
    b. Intracameral antibiotic at the end of the surgery
    c. Post operative oral antibiotics
    d. Sterile operative preparation

67. Which is the most important factor in the prevention of postoperative endophthalmitis? *(AIPG)*
    a. Preoperative preparation with povidone iodine
    b. One week antibiotic therapy prior to surgery
    c. Trimming of eyelashes
    d. Use of intravitreal antibiotics

68. Late onset endophthalmitis after cataract surgery is caused by: *(AIPG)*
    a. Staphylococcus epidermidis
    b. Pseudomonas
    c. Streptococcus pyogenes
    d. Propionibacterium acne

69. A 56-year-old man presents after 3 days of cataract surgery with history of pain and decrease in vision after an initial improvement. The most likely diagnosis is: *(AIIMS)*
    a. Endophthalmitis
    b. After cataract
    c. Central retinal vein occlusion
    d. Retinal detachment

70. Endophthalmitis involves all the layers of the eyeball except: *(AIPG)*
    a. Cornea
    b. Choroid
    c. Sclera
    d. Retina

71. Most common late complication of cataract surgery: *(DNB)*
    a. Cystoid macular oedema
    b. Glaucoma
    c. Posterior capsule opacification
    d. Uveitis

72. **Ring of Sommering is seen in:** *(DNB)*
    a. Diabetes
    b. Galactosemia
    c. After cataract
    d. Wilson's disease
73. **Treatment of posterior capsule opacification is:**
    (AIIMS/ NEET 2016)
    a. Krypton laser
    b. Argon laser
    c. Nd- YAG laser
    d. CO_2 laser
74. **A 60-year-old patient operated 6 months back for cataract presents with floaters and decrease in vision. The likely diagnosis is:** *(AIIMS)*
    a. Vitreous haemorrhage
    b. Retinal detachment
    c. CRAO
    d. Cystoid macular oedema

Miscellaneous

75. **How many weeks after cataract surgery are spectacles prescribed?** *(AIPG)*
    a. 6 weeks
    b. 10 weeks
    c. 12 weeks
    d. 14 weeks
76. **Which of the following is the output indicator of NPCB?**
    (AIIMS 2014)
    a. Number of cataract surgeries leading to sight restoration
    b. Decrease in the prevalence of blindness
    c. Number of school children provided with glasses for refractive correction
    d. Number of eye surgeons trained

ANSWERS AND EXPLANATIONS

1. b. Posterior pole (Ref: Yanoff & Duker 4th edition p 329-30)
2. c. Glutathione (Ref: Yanoff & Duker 4th edition p 329-30)
3. a. Vitamin A (Ref: Yanoff & Duker 4th edition p 329-30)
4. c. Aqueous and vitreous (Ref: Yanoff & Duker 4th edition p 329-30)
5. d. Na-K ATPase (Ref: Yanoff & Duker 4th edition p 329-30)
6. a. Attachment of the vitreous to the posterior surface of the lens (Ref: Yanoff & Duker 4th edition p 431)
7. b. Ciliary body (Ref: Yanoff & Duker 4th edition p 329-30)
8. b. Superotemporal
9. b. Homocystinuria
10. a. Marfan's syndrome, c. Homocystinuria, d. Sulphite oxidase deficiency (Ref: Yanoff & Duker 4th edition p 418)
11. a. Alport's syndrome (Ref: Yanoff & Duker 4th edition p 418)
    Lenticonus is a congenital condition where the anterior or the posterior surface of the lens is protruded. It may be anterior or posterior.
    Anterior lenticonus is seen in Alport's syndrome[Q]
    Posterior lenticonus is seen in Lowe's syndrome[Q]
12. b. Hallerman Streiff syndrome
13. d. Diabetes mellitus
    Phacodonesis is seen in conditions where zonular weakness of the lens is seen. Hence causes of phacodonesis are the same as that of lens subluxation.
14. b. CRYGS-3
15. d. Blue dot cataract
16. c. Zonular cataract
17. b. Zonular cataract (Ref: Yanoff & Duker 4th edition p 415-16)
    Hypocalcemia or Vitamin D deficiency in pregnancy gives rise to spoke like opacities which are called riders. It is a type of zonular cataract.
18. d. Age related cataract (Ref: Yanoff & Duker 4th edition p 414-15)
19. a. More insoluble protein, less soluble protein (Ref: Yanoff & Duker 4th edition p 414)
20. c. HM 3 and HM 4
21. c. Posterior subcapsular cataract (Ref: Yanoff & Duker 4th edition p 416)
22. a. Nuclear cataract (Ref: Yanoff & Duker 4th edition p 416)
23. a. Nuclear cataract (Ref: Yanoff & Duker 4th edition p 416)
24. c. Difficulty in bright light is a symptom (Ref: Yanoff & Duker 4th edition p 415-16)
25. d. Absent light perception
    Mature cataract means that the lens is completely opacified. Iris shadow is absent. Unless complicated, the anterior chamber and IOP will be normal. Visual acuity is markedly diminished but light perception with accurate projection of rays will be present in the absence of any other pathology.
26. a. Dislocation of lens
27. b. Intumescent cataract
28. d. Snowflake cataract (Ref: Yanoff & Duker 4th edition p 415)
29. b. NADPH dependent aldose reductase (Ref: Yanoff & Duker 4th edition p 415)
30. b. Diabetic cataract
31. a. Chalcosis (Ref: Yanoff & Duker 4th edition p 415-16)
32. a. Complicated cataract (Ref: Yanoff & Duker 4th edition p 415-16)
33. a. Posterior subcapsular (Ref: Yanoff & Duker 4th edition p 415-16)
34. a. Posterior subcapsular cataract (Ref: Yanoff & Duker 4th edition p 415-16)
35. a. Blunt trauma (Ref: Yanoff & Duker 4th edition p 415-16)

Lens

36. b. **Perforating injury** *(Ref: Yanoff & Duker 4th edition p 415-16)*
    Anterior polar cataract occurs at the site of trauma to the lens capsule.
37. b. **Posterior polar cataract** *(Ref: Yanoff & Duker 4th edition p 415-16)*
38. b. **Concussion injury** *(Ref: Yanoff & Duker 4th edition p 415-16)*
39. c. **Myotonic dystrophy** *(Ref: Yanoff & Duker 4th edition p 415-16)*
40. b. **Diabetes mellitus** *(Ref: Yanoff & Duker 4th edition p 415-16)*
    Diabetes causes metabolic cataract not complicated cataract.
41. a. **Wilson's disease- Sunflower cataract, c. Amiodarone-anterior subcapsular cataract, d. Myotonic dystrophy- Christmas tree cataract** *(Ref: Yanoff & Duker 4th edition p 415-16)*
42. b. **Leprosy** *(Ref: Yanoff & Duker 4th edition p 415-16)*
43. c. **Refsum's disease** *(Ref: Yanoff & Duker 4th edition p 415-16)*
44. c. **Potential acuity meter**
45. c. **Phacoemulsification** *(Ref: Yanoff & Duker 4th edition p 345-48)*
46. a. **Less chance of cystoid macular oedema, b. Less chance of endophthalmitis, d. Less chance of vitreous haemorrhage and retinal detachment, e. Minimal endothelial damage** *(Ref: Yanoff & Duker 4th edition p 345-48)*
    All complications of cataract surgery are less with the techniques like ECCE, SICS and Phacoemulsification as compared to ICCE
    Also in ICCE, the capsular bag is removed; hence the IOL has to be iris fixated, scleral fixated or placed in the anterior chamber. In modern day cataract surgery, IOL is placed in the capsular bag.
    Thus the only indication of ICCE today would be markedly subluxated cataract where the capsular bag cannot be retained
47. c. **Subluxated cataract** *(Ref: Yanoff & Duker 4th edition p 345-48)*
48. c. **3–3.5 mm** *(Ref: Yanoff & Duker 4th edition p 371-73)*
49. a. **Hydrodissection, c. Continuous curvilinear capsulorrhexis, d. IOL implantation** *(Ref: Yanoff & Duker 4th edition p 371-73)*
50. b. **Sclerocorneal tunnel** *(Ref: Yanoff & Duker 4th edition p 371-73)*
    In phacoemulsification a corneal incision is usually made. Sclerocorneal tunnel is made in Small Incision Cataract Surgery (SICS)
51. d. **Balanced salt solution + Glutathione** *(Ref: Yanoff & Duker 4th edition p 353)*
52. a. **Ultrasonic** *(Ref: Yanoff & Duker 4th edition p 361)*
53. c. **Cataract surgery with IOL implantation with posterior capsulotomy** *(Ref: Yanoff & Duker 4th edition p 391)*
    In children it has been seen that after cataract surgery there is rapid opacification of the posterior capsule and anterior vitreous. Hence in children, two additional steps are added to the routine cataract surgery. They are
    - Primary posterior capsulotomy (Opening is made in the posterior capsule at the centre of the visual axis)
    - Anterior vitrectomy (removal of the anterior vitreous)
    - Needling, discision, lensectomy are old procedures which are not done now.
54. a. **Immediately** *(Ref: Yanoff & Duker 4th edition p 393)*
    The dictum for congenital cataract is 'operate as early as possible, best within 4-6 weeks of birth.
55. c. **Keratometry and axial length of the eye ball** *(Ref: Yanoff & Duker 4th edition p 337-40)*
56. b. **A-Scan biometry** *(Ref: Yanoff & Duker 4th edition p 337-40)*
57. a. **IOL Power** *(Ref: Yanoff & Duker 4th edition p 337-40)*
58. c. **Corneal topography** *(Ref: Yanoff & Duker 4th edition p 339)*
    Corneal topography is used to get accurate keratometry values in irregular corneas prior to cataract surgery. However it is not routinely needed in all cases prior to cataract surgery.
59. c. **Capsular bag** *(Ref: Yanoff & Duker 4th edition p 380)*
60. a. **PMMA** *(Ref: Yanoff & Duker 4th edition p 346)*
61. a. **PMMA, b. Acrylic, d. Silicon** *(Ref: Yanoff & Duker 4th edition p 346)*
62. a. **Toric IOL** *(Ref: Yanoff & Duker 4th edition p 368)*
63. a. **Femtosecond laser** *(Ref: Yanoff & Duker 4th edition p 371-73)*
    Femtosecond laser assisted cataract surgery (FLACS) is the most recent advancement in the field of cataract surgery. Femtosecond laser is used to improve precision in steps like incision making, capsulorrhexis and fragmentation of the nucleus.

Self Assessment and Review of Ophthalmology

64. b. **Juvenile rheumatoid arthritis.**
    Explained in chapter on uveitis
65. a. **Endophthalmitis, c. Retinal detachment, d. Vitreous loss** *(Ref: Yanoff & Duker 4th edition p 399-402)*
66. c. **Postoperative oral antibiotics** *(Ref: Yanoff & Duker 4th edition p 351-54)*

    Endophthalmitis is the most dreaded and vision threatening complication of cataract surgery. Hence prevention of infection is of paramount importance. The different steps to prevent endophthalmitis are
    - Preoperative antibiotic eye drops 3 days prior to surgery
    - Sterile operative preparation
    - Irrigation of conjunctival cul-de-sac with povidone iodine (most important) prior to surgery
    - Postoperative antibiotic eye drops

67. a. **Preoperative preparation with povidone iodine** *(Ref: Yanoff & Duker 4th edition p 352)*
68. d. **Propionibacterium acne** *(Ref: Yanoff & Duker 4th edition p 724)*
69. a. **Endophthalmitis** *(Ref: Yanoff & Duker 4th edition p 725)*
70. c. **Sclera** *(Ref: Yanoff & Duker 4th edition p 723)*
71. c. **Posterior capsular opacification** *(Ref: Yanoff & Duker 4th edition p 402-03)*
72. c. **After cataract** *(Ref: Yanoff & Duker 4th edition p 402-03)*

    After cataract is the old name for posterior capsule opacification. The more common variety is Elschnig's pearls. Sommering's ring is also a type of PCO.

73. c. **Nd:YAG laser** *(Ref: Yanoff & Duker 4th edition p 402-03)*
74. b. **Retinal detachment** *(Ref: Yanoff & Duker 4th edition p 403)*
75. a. **6 weeks** *(Ref: Yanoff & Duker 4th edition p 354)*

    After cataract surgery steroid eye drops are given in tapering doses over 4–6 weeks. Glasses are usually prescribed at the end of this period.

76. a. **Number of cataract surgeries leading to sight restoration**

IMAGE BASED QUESTIONS

1. The lens in the photograph shows a typical type of cataract. What history should be elicited from the patient?

   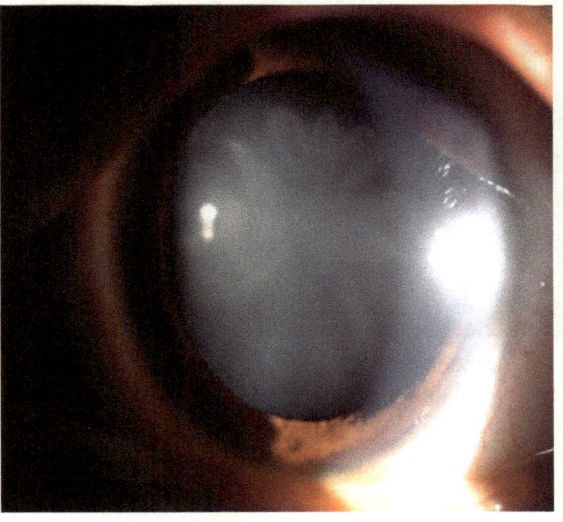

   a. Diabetes mellitus
   b. Trauma
   c. Steroid use
   d. History of using glasses

2. What is the most common complication associated with the condition shown in the clinical photograph?

   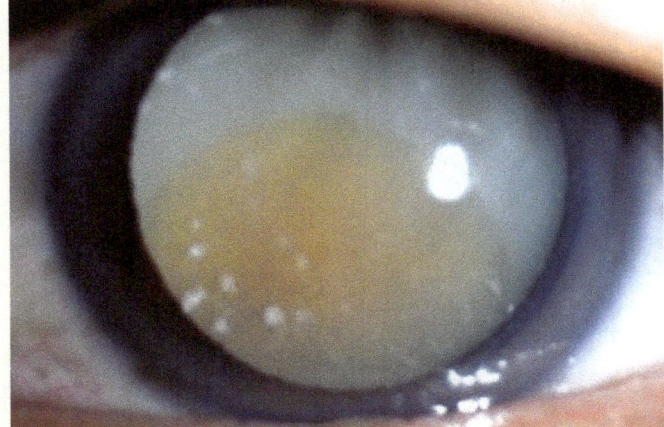

   a. Phacomorphic glaucoma
   b. Phacolytic glaucoma
   c. Endophthalmitis
   d. Angle closure glaucoma

3. What is the condition associated with the cataract shown in the photograph?

   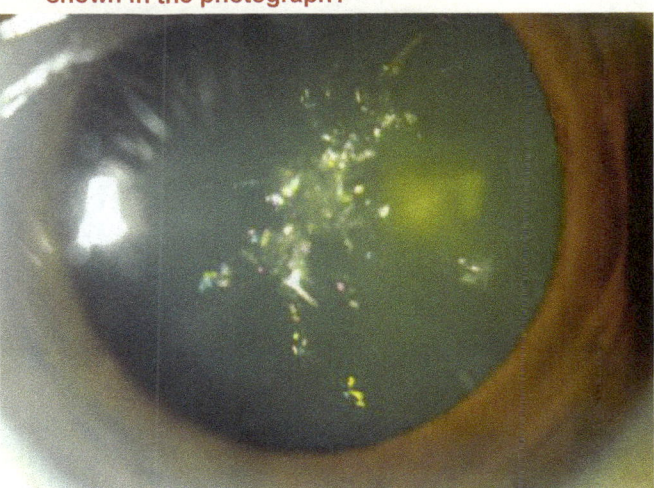

   a. Wilson's disease
   b. Galactosemia
   c. Myotonic dystrophy
   d. Down's syndrome

4. This is the anterior segment photograph of a patient who has history of cataract surgery with IOL done many years ago. He came with complaints of decrease in vision in the pseudophakic eye. What is the diagnosis?

   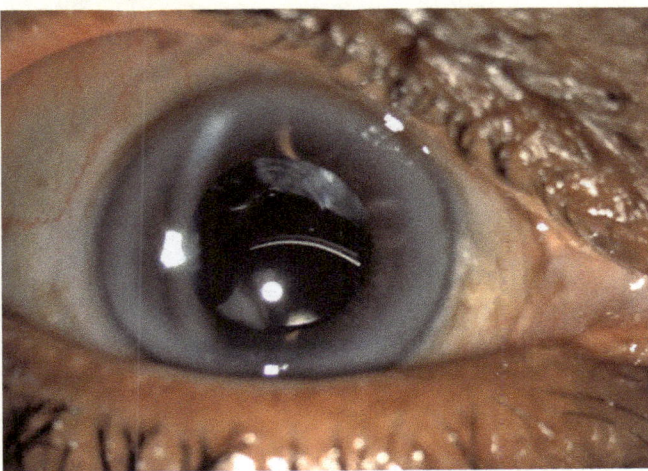

   a. Sunrise syndrome
   b. Sunset syndrome
   c. Dislocated IOL
   d. Windshield wiper syndrome

Answer Key: 1. b   2. b   3. c   4. b

5. The clinical photograph shows cataract with a certain associated condition. All of the following may be strongly associated with this patient except:

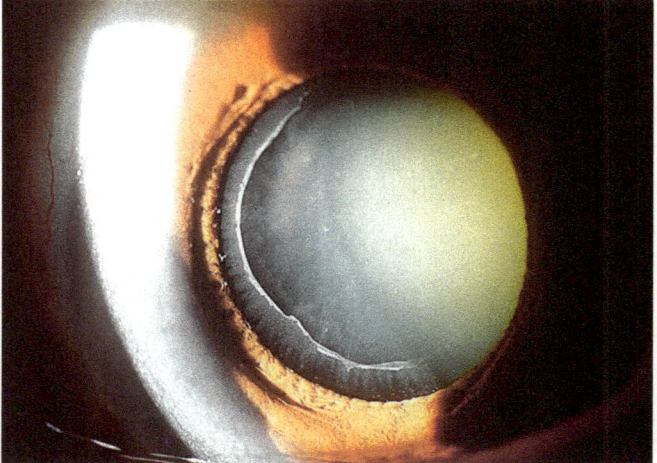

   a. Weak zonules
   b. Poorly dilating pupil
   c. Angle closure glaucoma
   d. Subluxation of the capsular bag

6. A patient presents with the cataract shown in the photograph. What is the most likely complain of the patient?

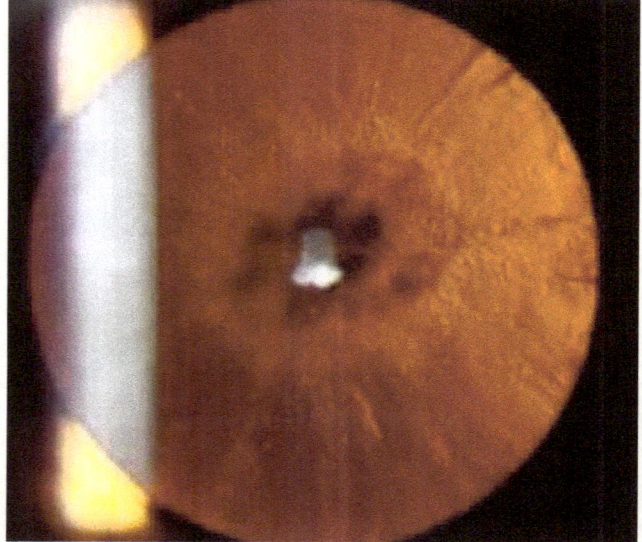

   a. Difficulty in vision in bright light
   b. Difficulty in vision in dim light
   c. Double vision
   d. Difficulty in vision in upgaze

7. A patients presents with severe pain, redness and decrease in vision within 3 days of uneventful cataract surgery. The clinical photograph is given. Fundal glow is not visible. What is the possible diagnosis?

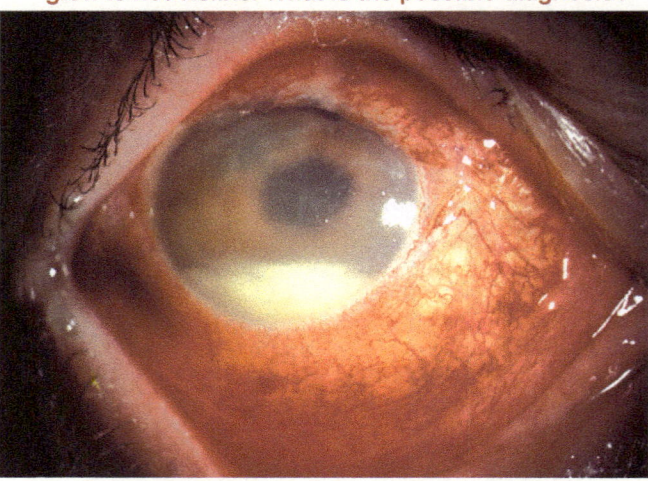

   a. Dislocated IOL
   b. Endophthalmitis
   c. Vitreous haemorrhage
   d. Retinal detachment

8. A patients presents with diminution of vision about 1 year after cataract surgery. From the clinical picture below, identify the diagnosis. *(May AIIMS 2017)*

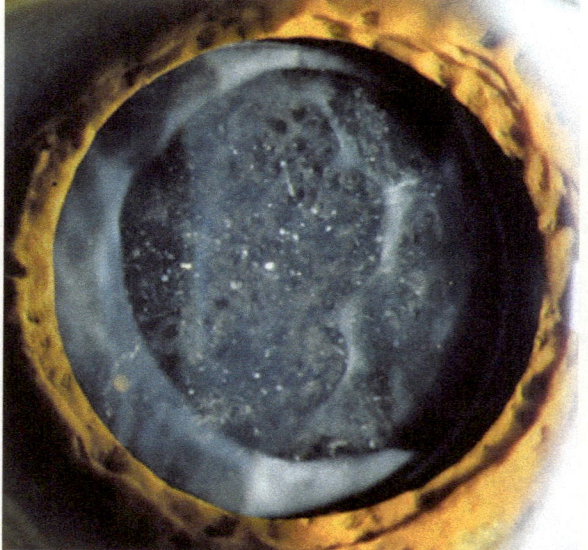

   a. Irvine Gass syndrome
   b. UGH syndrome
   c. After cataract
   d. Endophthalmitis

Answer Key: 5. c 6. a 7. b 8. c

9. Nowadays, cataract surgery is performed with the aid of lasers resulting in smaller incisions and fewer post-operative complications. What is the frequency of the laser shown below? *(Nov AIIMS 2016)*

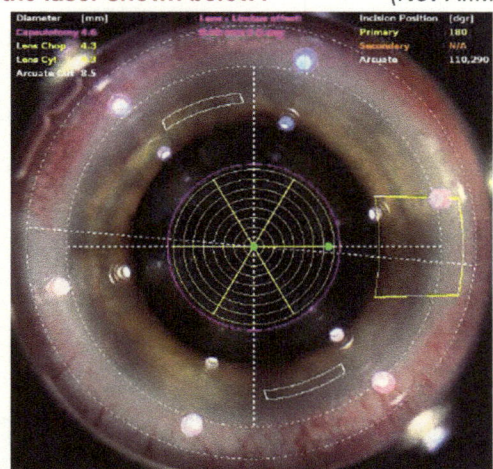

   a. 10^{-9}
   b. 10^{-15}
   c. 10^{-12}
   d. 10^{-6}

10. A patient post cataract surgery is implanted with the IOL shown in the picture. Which of the following statements regarding the patient is true?

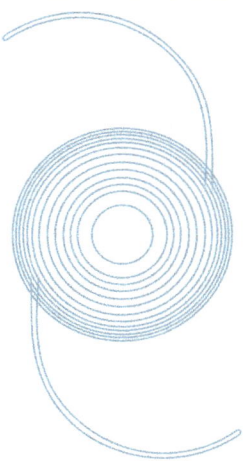

   a. He requires glasses only for reading
   b. He requires glasses only for distance
   c. He requires glasses for both distance and near
   d. He does not require glasses

11. What is the type of IOL shown in the picture?

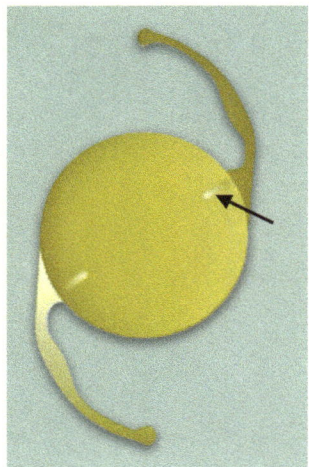

   a. Monofocal IOL
   b. Multifocal IOL
   c. Toric IOL
   d. Accommodative IOL

12. A patient post cataract surgery describes his visual experience as shown in the picture. What's the likely IOL implanted in the patient?

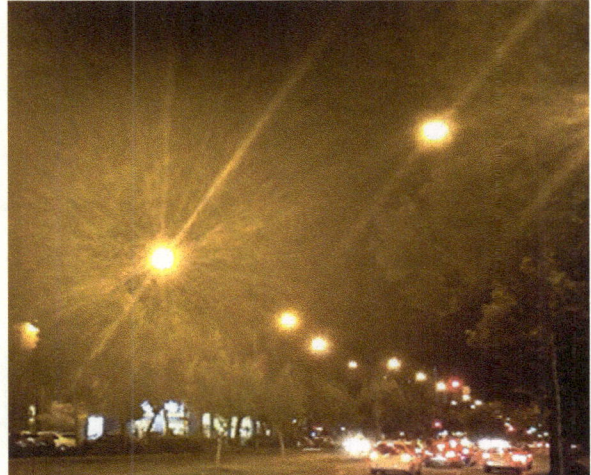

   a. Monofocal IOL
   b. Multifocal IOL
   c. Accommodative IOL
   d. There is no IOL

Answer Key: 9. b 10. d 11. c 12. b

13. The instrument shown in the photograph is used for

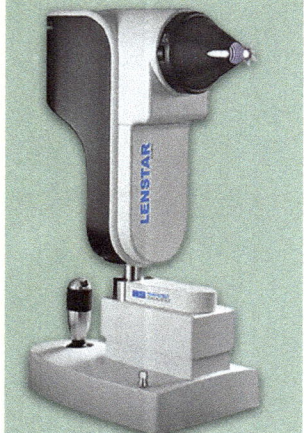

a. IOL power calculation
b. Keratometry
c. Pachymetry
d. USG B-Scan

14. The device shown in the photograph helps in the management of

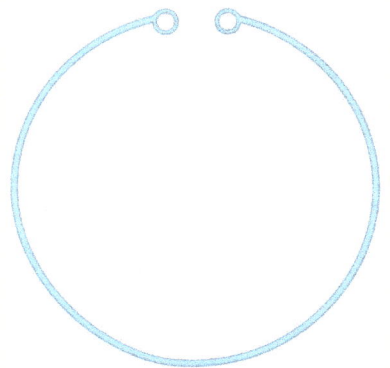

a. Posterior polar cataract
b. Subluxated cataract
c. Cortical cataract
d. Mature cataract

15. A 15-year-old patient with history of stroke is referred for ophthalmic evaluation. From the clinical photograph, what could be the possible diagnosis?

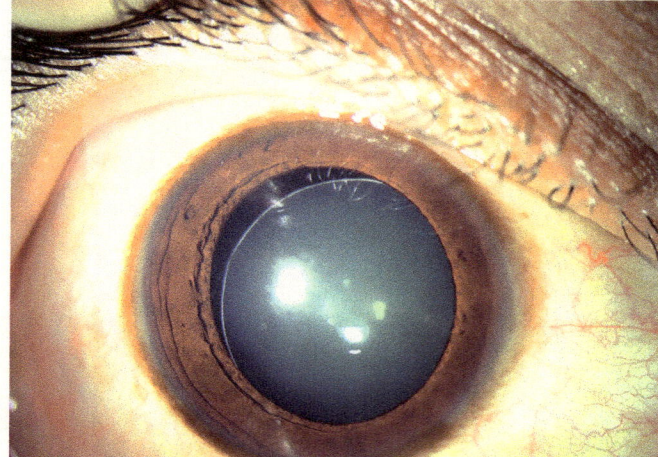

a. Galactosemia
b. Wilson's disease
c. Homocystinuria
d. Myotonic dystrophy

Answer Key: 13. a   14. b   15. c

ANSWERS AND EXPLANATIONS

1. **Answer: b. Trauma** *(Ref: Yanoff & Duker 4th edition p 415)*

   The typical cataract seen in the picture is rosette cataract (looks like petals of a flower). Hence the relevant history is that of blunt trauma.

2. **Answer: b. Phacolytic glaucoma**

   The photograph shows **hypermature morgagnian cataract** (sunken nucleus with liquefied cortex). The most common complication associated with this **is phacolytic glaucoma.**

3. **Answer: c. Myotonic dystrophy**
   (Ref: Peyman's Principles and Practice of Ophthalmology 2nd edition, p 184-85)

   This is a classical picture of Christmas tree cataract seen in Myotonic dystrophy.

4. **Answer: b. Sunset syndrome** *(Ref: Yanoff & Duker 4th edition p 401)*

   In the photograph it can be seen that the IOL is decentred inferiorly. This is called sunset syndrome.

5. **Answer: c. Angle closure glaucoma**
   (Ref: Peyman's Principles and Practice of Ophthalmology 2nd edition, p 714-15)

   The photograph shows cataract with a white ring on the anterior lens capsule. This white ring is caused by deposition of a fibrillar extracellular material. This condition is called **Pseudoexfoliation syndrome (PXF)^Q**
   The features of PXF syndrome are:
   - Deposition of white flaky fibrillar material in different anterior segment structures like lens capsule, zonules, pupillary margin, iris tissue, angle of anterior chamber
   - Weak zonules leading to subluxation of capsular bag during cataract surgery or in late postoperative period
   - Poorly dilating pupil
   - Secondary glaucoma due to deposition of PXF material in the angle. It is a type of secondary **open angle glaucoma.**

6. **Answer: a. Difficulty in vision in bright light**
   (Ref: Peyman's Principles and Practice of Ophthalmology 2nd edition, p 684-89)

   The picture shows central posterior subcapsular cataract which cause maximum visual disability when the pupil is constricted such as in bright light and near work.

7. **Answer: b. Endophthalmitis**
   (Ref: Peyman's Principles and Practice of Ophthalmology 2nd edition, p 1042-43)

   The clinical photograph shows congestion, corneal oedema with pus in the anterior chamber (hypopyon). This, with associated finding of absent fundal glow points to the possibility of exudates in the vitreous. Hence the diagnosis is endophthalmitis.
   The diagnosis is confirmed by USG B-Scan which shows dense vitreous echoes suggestive of vitreous exudates (indicated by arrow)

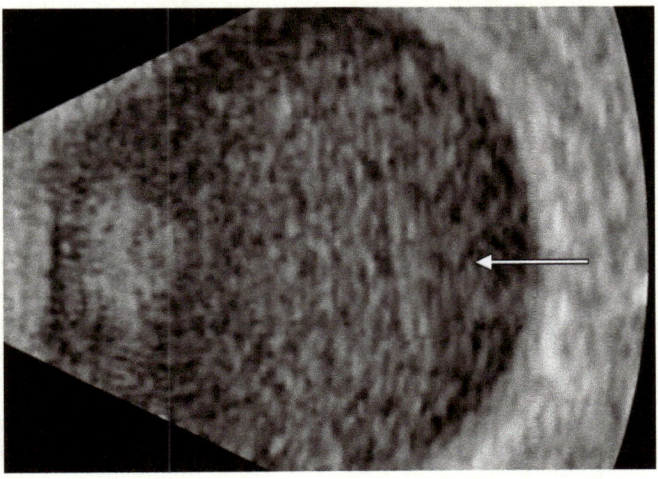

8. **Answer: c. After cataract** *(Ref: Kanski 8th edition p 293)*

   After cataract or posterior capsule opacification (PCO) is the **most common late complication of cataract surgery^Q.** It is caused by migration of the lens epithelial cells that have remained in the capsular bag after cataract extraction. Treatment is creation of an opening in the posterior capsule, known as **capsulotomy** with **Nd: YAG laser^Q**

9. **Answer: b. 10^{-15}** *(Ref: Yanoff & Duker 4th edition p 375-376)*

   Femtosecond laser is an infrared laser with a wavelength of **1053nm^Q** and an ultra-short pulse duration of **10^{-15} seconds (Femtosecond).** The main advantage of this ultra-short pulse is that the collateral damage to the tissues surrounding the target tissue is minimal. The applications of Femtosecond laser are
   - Femtosecond laser assisted cataract surgery where the laser is used for creating the incision, capsulorrhexis and fragmentation of the nucleus
   - Corneal refractive surgery: The important procedures are **Femtosecond Lenticule Extraction (FLEx), Small Incision Lenticule Extraction (SMILE),** Intrastromal corneal ring segment (ICRS) implantation.

Ophthalmic Lasers

Type of laser	Wavelength	Tissue effect	Procedure
Nd:YAG	1064 nm	Photodisruption	Iridotomy, capsulotomy
Double frequency Nd:YAG	532 nm	Photocoagulation	Selective laser trabeculoplasty (SLT)^Q, Panretinal photocoagulation (PRP)
Excimer	193 nm	Photoablation^Q	LASIK, Photorefractive keratectomy (PRK), Phototherapeutic keratectomy (PTK)
Argon	514 nm, 532 nm	Photocoagulation	Panretinal photocoagulation (PRP)
Femtosecond laser	1053 nm	Photodisruption	**FLEx, SMILE,** Femto assisted cataract surgery

10. Answer: d. He does not require glasses

The IOL shown in the picture is a multifocal IOL (it has multiple diffractive rings) which focuses for both distance and near. Hence the patient does not require glasses post cataract surgery.

In a monofocal IOL, these diffractive rings are absent. Hence it focuses only for distance and the patient requires glasses for reading.

11. Answer: c. Toric IOL

Toric IOL is used to correct **pre-existing corneal astigmatism** at the time of cataract surgery. The line on IOL (as indicated by the arrow) shows the axis of toricity or cylinder incorporated in the IOL.

12. Answer: b. Multifocal IOL

The picture is typical of glare and haloes around light at night. This problem is commonly experienced with multifocal IOL.

13. Answer: a. IOL power calculation

The photograph shows an optical biometer which is used for IOL power calculation prior to cataract surgery.

14. Answer: b. Subluxated cataract

(Ref: Peyman's Principles and Practice of Ophthalmology 2nd edition, p 713)

The device shown in the photograph is a **capsule tension ring.** It is used intra-operatively in cases where the capsular bag is weak as in subluxated cataract, weak zonules etc.

15. Answer: c. Homocystinuria

(Ref: Peyman's Principles and Practice of Ophthalmology 2nd edition, p 185)

The photograph shows inferonasal subluxation of the crystalline lens which is classically described in Homocystinuria. This, along with history of thrombotic disorder (stroke) suggests the answer.

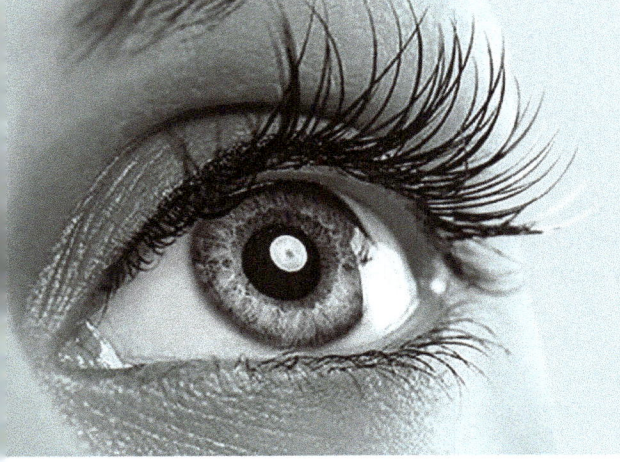

5

Retina

ANATOMY OF RETINA

The retina is the innermost neural coat of the eyeball. It consists of ten layers. From outside inwards, the layers are Figure 1:

1. *Retinal pigment epithelium (RPE)*: This is the outermost layer of the retina which is separated from the choroid by a layer called the Bruch membrane. It has no role in the neural transmission. Hence, the remaining layers of the retina which are involved in neural activity are collectively called as **neurosensory retina**. The functions of RPE are:
    * It acts as metabolic pump to prevent the accujmulation of debris in the subretinal space
    * It provides nutrition to the photoreceptors
2. *Layer of Photoreceptors*: This contains the outer segments of the photoreceptors namely the rods and the cones
    * The rods are responsible for vision in dim light or scotopic vision. About 120 million rod cells are present in the retina with maximum concentration in the mid periphery. Rods are absent at the foveola. They contain a pigment called **rhodopsin**^{Q}
    * The cones are responsible for colour vision and vision in bright light or scotopic vision. About 6.5 million cones are present in the retina with maximum concentration in the fovea. They contain a pigment called **iodopsin**
3. External limiting membrane
4. *Outer nuclear layer*: It contains the cell bodies of the photoreceptor cells
5. *Outer plexiform layer*: It contains the synapses between the photoreceptors and bipolar cells^Q
6. *Inner nuclear layer*: It contains the cell bodies of the bipolar cells. It also contains the cells bodies of the horizontal cells, amacrine cells and Müller's cells

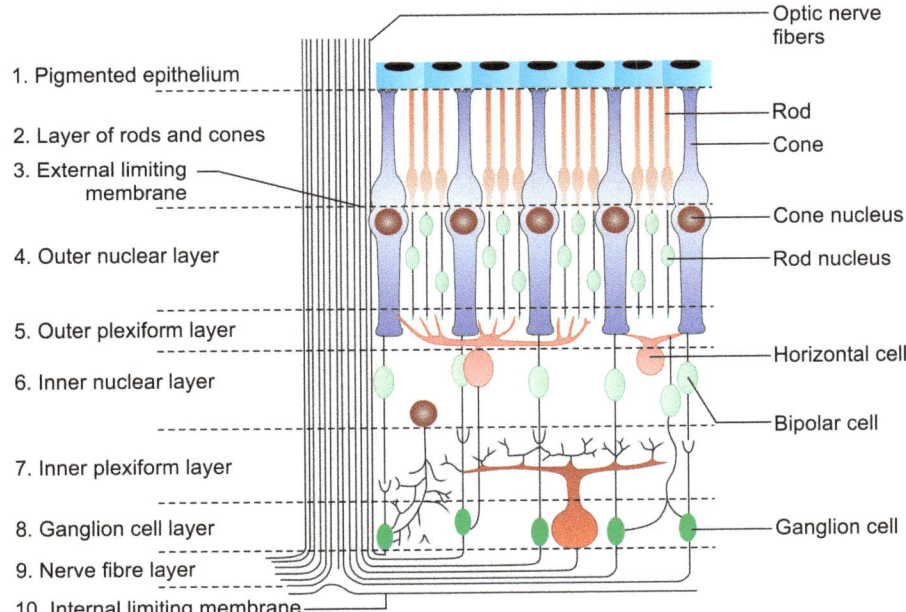

Fig. 1: Layers of the retina

Function of Horizontal cells: Lateral inhibition^Q
Function of Amacrine cells: Negative feedback inhibition^Q

7. *Inner plexiform layer*: It contains the synapses between the bipolar cells and ganglion cells
8. *Ganglion cell layer*: It contains the cell bodies of the ganglion cells
9. *Retinal nerve fibre layer (RNFL)*: **It is constituted by the axons of the ganglion cells**[Q]
10. *Internal limiting membrane*: It separates the retina from the vitreous and is formed by the foot processes of the Müller's cells

IMPORTANT REGIONS OF THE RETINA

➢ *Optic disc*: It is also known as the optic nerve head and signifies the point of origin of the optic nerve. It is **1.5 mm**[Q] in diameter and consists of only the nerve fibre layer of the retina. Due to the absence of photoreceptors, no visual response is seen if light falls in this area of the retina. Hence it also called as the blind spot (Fig. 2)
➢ *Macula*: The oval area on the posterior pole of the eye is the macula. It has an overall diameter of **5.5 mm**[Q].

The centre of the macula is the fovea (**1.5 mm in diameter**). The centre of the fovea is called the foveola (**0.35 mm**). It has the highest concentration of cones. Rods are absent in this region. The centre of the macula is about **2 disc diameters (3 mm)**[Q] from the margin of the optic disc (Fig. 3)
➢ *Ora Serrata*: Junction of retina and ciliary body.

TRANSMISSION OF VISUAL IMPULSE

Phototransduction (Fig. 4)

EXAMINATION OF RETINA

➢ *Indirect ophthalmoscope*: It is used to visualize Peripheral Retina.
➢ *Direct ophthalmoscope, 90D lens*: Used to visualize the posterior pole
• Goldmann three mirror lens
  ◆ *Central part*: Used to visualize the posterior pole
  ◆ *Equatorial mirror*: Used to visualize the area surrounding the equator
  ◆ *Peripheral mirror*: Used to visualize the peripheral retina up to the ora serrata.

	Direct Ophthalmoscope	Indirect Ophthalmoscope
Magnification	15 times[Q]	2-5 times[Q]
Field of view	Limited: About 2 disc diameter	Large: Up to ora serrata
Hazy media	Not much useful	Useful because of bright illumination
Type of image	Virtual and erect[Q]	Real and inverted[Q]
Stereopsis	No stereopsis	Stereopsis is present as examination is done binocularly by the examiner
Condensing lens	Not needed	Needed. A converging lens of usually **20D**[Q] is used

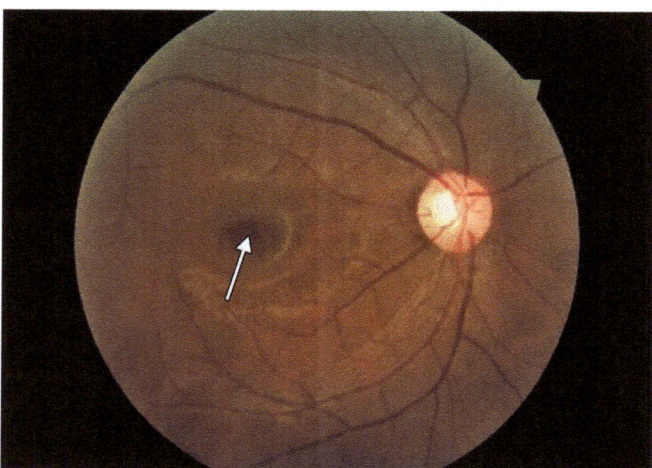

Fig. 2: Normal fundus (arrow points to the fovea)

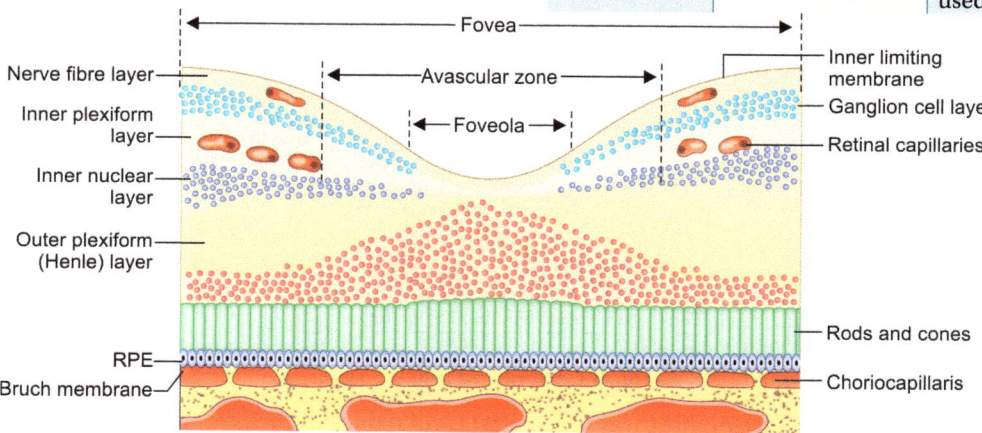

Fig. 3: Layers at the fovea

Retina

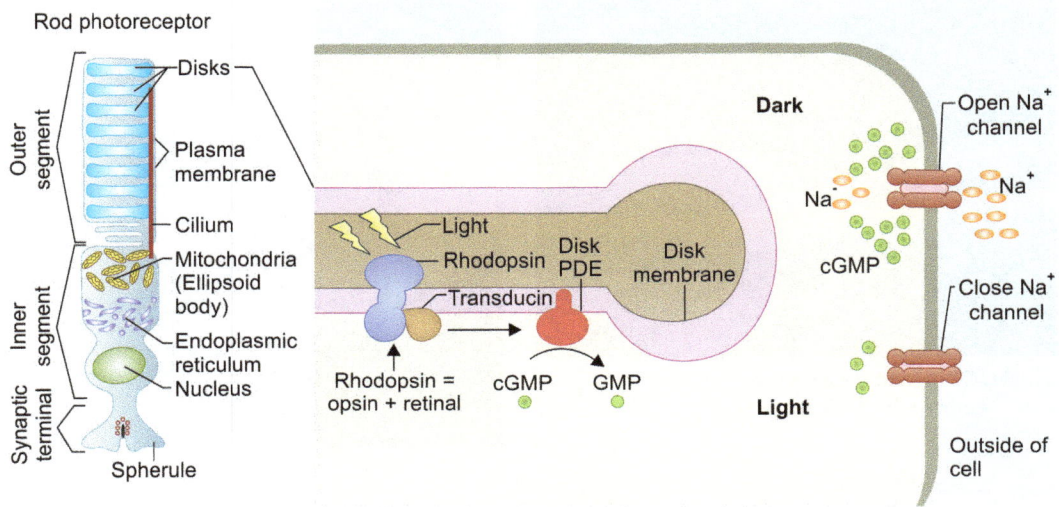

Fig.4: Phototransduction

Blood Supply of Retina

- The **inner six layers** of the retina are supplied by the **central retinal artery (CRA)**[Q]
- The **outer four layers** of the retina are supplied by the chorcapillaris which are derived from the **short posterior ciliary arteries**[Q]
- These two systems of blood vessels form an anasmotic circle around the margin of the optic disc. This is called the **circle of Zinn-Haler**[Q]

INVESTIGATIONS RELATED TO RETINA

➢ *Fundus fluorescein angiography (FFA)*: It is used to study the normal physiology of retinal and choroidal circulation. 5 mL of 10% solution of sodium fluorescein dye is injected in the **antecubital vein**[Q]. Serial fundus photographs are taken. There are typically four phases in FFA:
1. *Pre-arterial phase*: Dye is seen in the choroidal vessels
2. *Arterial phase*: Dye is seen in the retinal arteries
3. *Arteriovenous phase*: There is complete filling of retinal arteries and capillaries. Lamellar blood flow appears in the veins
4. *Venous phase*: Dye is seen in the retinal veins only

FFA helps to identify areas of retinal hypoperfusion, abnormal blood vessels and neovascularization, leakage due to disruption of the blood retinal barrier (Fig. 5)

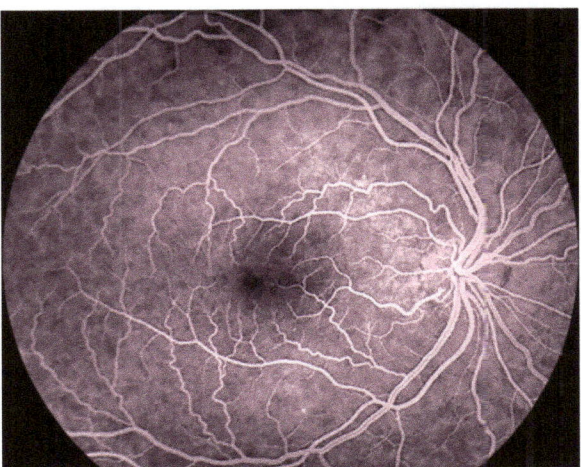

Fig. 5: Normal FFA showing fluorescein dye inside the blood vessels

➢ *Indocyanine green angiography (ICGA)*: This is a type of angiography done with Indocyanine green dye. It helps to study the **choroidal vasculature**[Q]
➢ *Optical coherence tomography (OCT)*: This is an optical scan of the retinal **layers using infra-red light**[Q]. It is useful in evaluating retinal thickness, especially in macular oedema (Fig. 6)
➢ *Ocular electrophysiology*: The different tests are
  • Electroretinogram (ERG): This is a mass response of the retina to flash light. It helps to identify gross retinal pathologies like **retinal dystrophies**. ERG has three waves (Fig. 7), namely
    1. *a wave*: It arises from the photoreceptors[Q]
    2. *b wave*: It arises from the bipolar cells
    3. *c wave*: It arises from the RPE.

57

Self Assessment and Review of Ophthalmology

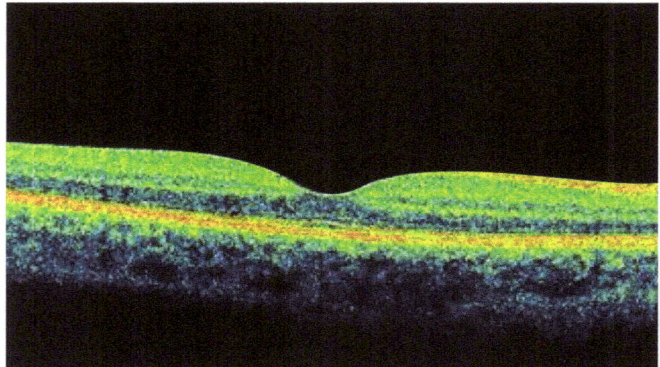

Fig. 6: Normal OCT of macula showing depression at the centre which is the fovea

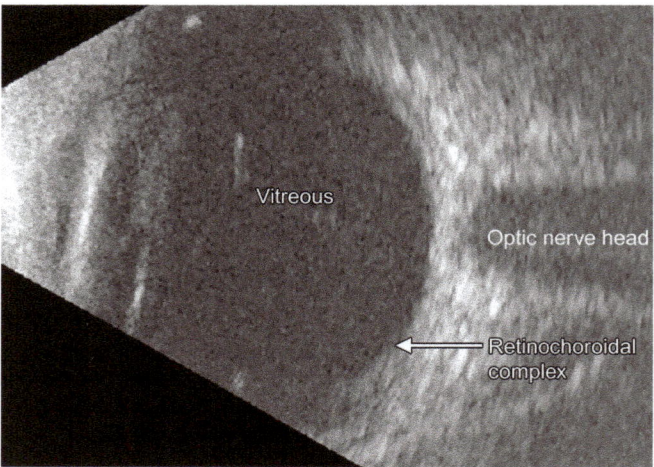

Fig. 8: Normal USG B-Scan

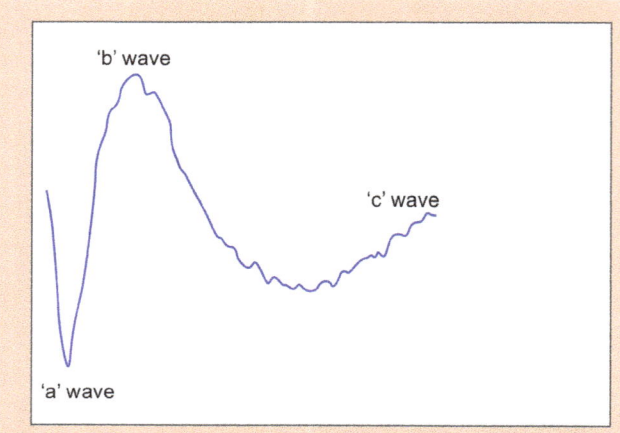

Fig. 7: Waves of electroretinogram

- Pattern ERG: Special ERG which is used for macular diseases.
- Multifocal ERG: Special ERG used for localized retinal diseases.
- Electroculogram: This test is used to evaluate the function of RPE. It is measured in terms of a ratio called **Arden's ratio**[Q]. (Normal value > 1.5[Q])
- Visual evoked potential (VEP): This test is used to evaluate the visual pathway, mainly the optic nerve. The main wave is P100 wave. Increase in latency and decrease in amplitude of this wave indicates dysfunction of the visual pathway, mainly the optic nerve
- USG B-Scan: USG B-Scan is an important imaging modality used to evaluate the posterior segment of the eye in conditions where dense media opacities do not allow direct visualization of the fundus as in dense cataract, corneal opacity or vitreous haemorrhage. The frequency of the probe is **8–10 MHz.** Common conditions diagnosed on USG are retinal **detachment, choroidal detachment and vitreous hemorrhage (Fig. 8)**.

RETINAL DETACHMENT

Separation of the **Neurosensory Retina**[Q] from retinal pigment epithelium (RPE).

Types

- Rhegmatogenous retinal detachment
- Tractional retinal detachment
- Exudative retinal detachment

Rhegmatogenous RD

Pathophysiology

The essential lesion is a **rhegma** (retinal break) through which the liquefied vitreous gains access to the retina. This liquefied vitreous accumulates beneath the neurosensory retina leading to RD. This is commonly seen in:

- *High myopes*: Peripheral retinal degenerations like **lattice degeneration**[Q], holes and breaks with liquefaction of overlying vitreous predispose to RD
- *Retinoschisis*: This is a condition where there is splitting of the neurosensory retina and vitreous degeneration. It is of two types:
  1. *Typical retinoschisis*: Split at the level of Outer Plexiform Layer[Q]
  2. *Reticular retinoschisis*: Split at the level of Nerve Fibre Layer[Q]. Seen more commonly in hypermetropes in the inferotemporal periphery of retina
- Trauma
- Aphakia[Q]
- Pseudophakia[Q]

Retina

- Most dangerous type of retinal break: **Horse shoe tear**[Q]
- Most dangerous location of retinal break: **Supero-temporal retina**[Q]

Symptoms

- Premonitory features:
  - *Photopsia*[Q]: Flashes of light due to vitreo-retinal traction at site of break
  - *Floaters*: Due to associated vitreous haemorrhage
- Visual field defect which is described by the patient as a black curtain or veil[Q] in front of the eye
- Loss of vision when the detachment involves the macula.

Signs

- Decrease in visual acuity
- *Hypotony*: The liquefied vitreous in the subretinal space is absorbed through the RPE leading to hypotony
- *Shafer's sign*[Q]: Pigments in anterior vitreous (tobacco dusting) is a feature of **fresh RD**[Q]
- Detached retina is **convex** in configuration. Surface is corrugated with free undulation. Break is identified at the periphery.

Treatment

- *Prophylactic laser barrage*: It is done in
  - Symptomatic break (associated with photopsia and floaters)
  - Horse shoe tear[Q]
  - Superior, especially supero-temporal tears
  - Aphakia[Q]
  - One eyed patient
- *Surgery for retinal detachment*
  - *Scleral buckling*: In this procedure, the sclera is indented by attaching an explant known as a buckle. This pushes the RPE inwards towards the neurosensory retina. Subretinal fluid is drained and the break is closed by laser or cryotherapy[Q]
  - *Pneumatic retinopexy*[Q]: In this procedure, the neurosensory retina is pushed towards the RPE by injecting an expansile gas in the vitreous cavity. The break is then sealed with laser. The gases commonly used are **Sulphur Hexafluoride (SF6**[Q] and **Perfluoropropane (C3F8)**
  - *Pars plana vitrectomy*

Tractional RD

Pathophysiology

Fibrovascular membranes[Q] in the vitreous due to long standing vitreous hemorrhage exert traction on the retina. This pulls the retina forward leading to retinal detachment.

Causes

- Proliferative diabetic retinopathy(PDR)[Q]
- Central retinal vein occlusion
- Eales' disease
- Retinopathy of prematurity (ROP).

Signs

- Detached retina is **concave** in configuration with highest elevation at the site of the tractional band. No breaks are seen
- Minimal mobility

Treatment

Pars plana vitrectomy and **endophotocoagulation**[Q].

Exudative RD

Pathophysiology

Exudative fluid, mainly from choroid, collects in the sub retinal space leading to retinal detachment.

Causes

- Inflammatory conditions like choroiditis, choroidal vasculitis, posterior scleritis[Q]
- Choroidal tumours like melanoma, hemangioma, metastasis[Q]
- Toxemia pregnancy[Q]
- Malignant hypertension[Q]
- Coat's disease[Q].

Symptoms

- Floaters due to vitritis but no photopsia
- Visual field defect
- Loss of vision due to involvement of macula.

Signs

- Detached retina has a **convex** configuration. Surface is **smooth**. No break is seen
- **Shifting fluid is seen.**[Q]

Treatment

- Systemic steroids
- Treatment of the cause.

To summarise:

	Rhegmatogenous RD	**Tractional RD**	**Exudative RD**
Causes	Retinal breaks seen in: • High myopia • Retinoschisis • Trauma • Aphakia, pseudophakia	• Proliferative diabetic retinopathy • CRVO • Eales' dieases • ROP • Sickle cell disease	• Choroiditis • Posterior scleritis • Malignant HTN • Choroidal tumours • Coat's disease
Premonitory symptoms	**Photopsia** **Floaters**	None	None
Symptoms	Curtain or veil in front of eye	Decrease in vision	Decrease in vision
Signs	Detached retina is **convex** **Surface is corrugated**	Detached retina is **concave**	Detached retina is **convex** **Surface is smooth** **Shifting fluid is** seen
Treatment	Scleral buckling surgery	Pars plana vitrectomy	Systemic steroids

RETINAL VASCULAR DISORDERS

Diabetic Retinopathy

Risk Factors

- **Duration of the diabetes (most important risk factor)**^{Q}
- Poor glycemic control
- Hypertension
- Hyperlipidemia
- Pregnancy
- Nephropathy

Pathophysiology

- The hallmark of diabetic retinopathy is the alteration in the structure and cellular composition of the microvasculature
- Hyperglycemia leads to the formation of advanced glycation end products (AGE) which are deposited in the walls of the retinal blood vessels. AGE cause **loss of pericytes**^{Q} and damage to the endothelial cells. This in turn leads to **microaneurysm**^{Q} formation due to weakening of the vessel walls
- Endothelial cells are responsible for maintenance of the blood retinal barrier. Hence endothelial cell damage leads to abnormal capillary permeability and leakage
- Retinal leucostasis is another important factor in the development of diabetic retinopathy. Increase in inflammatory cytokines causes influx of leucocytes which adhere to the vascular endothelium and cause a decrease in capillary perfusion
- Retinal hypoperfusion leads to increase in angiogenic mediators like **Vascular Endothelial Growth Factor (VEGF)** which stimulate **neovascularization**.

Classification

- Non-proliferative diabetic retinopathy (NPDR)
- Proliferative diabetic retinopathy (PDR)
- Diabetic maculopathy

Non-Proliferative Diabetic Retinopathy

- *Microaneurysms*: They are the **first detectable lesions of DR**^{Q}. They are dilated capillaries present at level of **Inner Nuclear Layer**^{Q} of the retina due to **loss of pericytes**^{Q} in the capillary walls
- *Intraretinal hemorrhages*: Rupture of the weakened capillaries leads to intraretinal hemorrhages. They are of two types: Superficial flame-shaped hemorrhages and dot blot hemorrhages. **Flame-shaped hemorrhages are located in the Nerve Fibre Layer**^{Q}. **Dot blot hemorrhages are located in the Inner Nuclear Layer**^{Q}
- *Hard exudates*: These are **lipoproteins**^{Q} leaking from the damaged retinal blood vessels. They are mainly located in the **Outer Plexiform Layer**^{Q}
- *Cotton wool spots*: Occlusion of the small retinal blood vessels leads to infarcts mainly in the retinal nerve fibre layer. These are called cotton wool spots or soft exudates
- *Intraretinal microvascular abnormalities (IRMA)*: Bending, looping, beading and dilatation of the veins.

Proliferative Diabetic Retinopathy

- Widespread retinal ischaemia leads to increase in a mediator called **Vascular Endothelial Growth Factor (VEGF)**^{Q} which causes neovascularization
- Neovascularization may occur at the disc (**NVD**) or along the arcades, in which case it is called Neovascularization elsewhere (**NVE**)
- The new blood vessels are friable and may rupture leading to **vitreous hemorrhage (VH)**
- Long standing vitreous hemorrhage leads to fibrous organization. The fibrous bands in the vitreous exert traction on the retina leading to **Tractional Retinal Detachment (TRD)**^{Q}

- Effect of VEGF in the anterior segment is neovascularisation of the iris called **rubeosis iridis**
- New vessels at the angle of anterior chamber lead to **neovascular glaucoma**.

Diabetic Maculopathy

Maculopathy includes microaneurysm, hemorrhages and hard exudates at the macula leading to macular thickening or oedema. This may due to **focal leakage or diffuse leakage from the capillary bed**. But maculopathy needs to be treated only when it becomes **Clinically Significant Macular Edema (CSME)**[Q].

The criteria for CSME are:
- Retinal oedema or thickening within 500 microns of the centre of the macula
- Hard exudates within 500 microns of the centre of the macula
- One or more disc diameters of retinal thickening, part of which is within one disc diameter of the centre of the macula

Investigations

- Systemic investigations like blood sugar and lipid profile
- *Fundus fluorescein angiography (FFA)*: It helps to identify vascular leakage, nonperfusion and abnormal new vessels
- *Optical coherence tomography (OCT)*: It helps to evaluate the macular thickness.
- Most common cause of severe vision loss in diabetes: **Vitreous Haemorrhage**[Q]
- Most common cause of moderate vision loss in diabetes: **Diabetic Maculopathy**[Q]

RETINAL VEIN OCCLUSION

Predisposing factors:
- Systemic hypertension
- Atherosclerosis
- Hypercoagulative conditions
- Venous stasis, periphlebitis
- Raised IOP

Retinal vein occlusion can either be **Central Retinal Vein Occlusion (CRVO)** or **Branch Retinal Vein Occlusion (BRVO)**.

Central Retinal Vein Occlusion (CRVO)

Symptoms

Sudden painless loss of vision.

Signs
- *Visual acuity*: Decrease in visual acuity, usually less than 6/60
- Relative afferent pupillary defect (RAPD)
- Anterior segment is normal

Treatment of Diabetic Retinopathy

- Control of systemic parameters like hypertension, hyperglycemia and hyperlipidemia.
- **Panretinal Photocoagulation (PRP)**[Q]: This is done in **Proliferative Diabetic Retinopathy (PDR)**[Q]. The lasers used are Double Frequency **Nd:YAG and Argon**

  (*Note*: The mechanism of action of laser is described as **conversion of hypoxia to anoxia**[Q]. This means that the laser converts a hypoxic dying peripheral retinal tissue to an anoxic dead tissue. This decreases the level of VEGF and helps the remaining central retinal tissue to survive)
- For diabetic maculopathy
  - In focal leakage: Focal laser
  - **In diffuse leakage: Macular grid laser**[Q]
- Intravitreal Injections
- **Steroids:** Triamcinolone, Dexamethasone

  (*Note*: Intravitreal Dexamethasone is available in the form of an implant containing **700 micrograms**[Q] of the drug which is slowly released over a period of **6 months**)
- **Anti-VEGF:** Bevacizumab, Ranibizumab
  Aflibercept is a new drug in this group.
- Surgery-**Pars plana vitrectomy**[Q]. Indications for surgery are:
  - **Tractional Retinal Detachment**[Q]
  - Non-resolving vitreous haemorrhage
  - Patients not responding to laser

- Fundus changes
  - Marked tortuosity and dilatation of the veins
  - Extensive hemorrhages in both the central and peripheral retina. This is called **Splashed Tomato Appearance**[Q] **or Blood and Thunder Appearance**
  - Cotton wool spots
  - Disc oedema
  - Macular oedema.

Branch Retinal Vein Occlusion (BRVO)

Features are similar to CRVO but fundus changes are localised along the involved blood vessel only.

Complications

- Occlusion of the vein results in decrease in forward blood flow through the retinal arteries leading to widespread ischaemia. This, in turn, causes increase in the level of vascular endothelial growth factor (VEGF) which leads to neovascularisation. Thus the complications of venous occlusion are **NVD, NVE, Vitreous haemorrhage, Tractional RD** and **Neovascular Glaucoma.**

Treatment

- Panretinal photocoagulation
- Intravitreal injection: Steroids and anti-VEGF
- Pars plana vitrectomy

  - Most common complication of BRVO: **Vitreous haemorrhage**[Q]
  - Most common complication of CRVO: **Neovascular Glaucoma**[Q]
  - Neovascular Glaucoma in CRVO is also called **100 Day Glaucoma**[Q]

CENTRAL RETINAL ARTERY OCCLUSION

Predisposing Factors

- Hypertension, Atherosclerosis, Hypercoagulative conditions
- Atrial fibrillation
- Emboli

Symptoms and Signs

- Marked decrease in visual acuity
- Relative afferent pupillary defect (RAPD)
- Anterior segment is normal
- Fundus
  - White opaque retina due to ischaemia of the inner retinal layers mainly the nerve fibre layer
  - *Cherry red spot*[Q]: The fovea which is devoid of the inner retinal layers receives blood supply from the choriocapillaries. Hence it appears bright red in contrast to the surrounding ischaemic retina
  - Marked narrowing of the retinal arterioles
  - **Sludging & segmentation of blood column (Cattle Track Sign)**[Q].

Treatment

- CRAO is an **ocular emergency** whose window period of treatment is **3 hours**
- Ocular massage for 15 min—This leads to lowering of IOP which in turn increases the blood flow and may dislodge the thrombus
- IV Mannitol
- Inhalation of 5% CO_2 + 95% O_2
- Paracentesis.

HYPERTENSIVE RETINOPATHY

In chronic hypertension, the changes that are seen in the retinal vasculature can be grouped as:

- **Arteriolar narrowing** which may be diffuse or focal: Severe narrowing leads to the development of infarcts or **cotton wool spots**[Q]
- *Vascular leakage*: Damage to microvasculature leads to intraretinal hemorrhages and **hard exudates**[Q]
- *Arteriosclerosis*: Thickening of the vessel wall characterized by hypertrophy and hyalinization of the vessel wall. Arteriosclerotic changes are classified as:
  - *Grade I*: Broadening of the arteriolar light reflex
  - *Grade II*: Deflection at the AV crossing junction (Salu's sign)
  - *Grade III*: Copper wiring of arterioles
  - *Grade IV*: Silver wiring of the arterioles.

Keith–Wagener-Barker Classification

- *Grade I*: Mild generalized arteriolar attenuation
- *Grade II*: Severe grade I + Focal arteriolar attenuation
- *Grade III*: Flame-shaped hemorrhages and cotton wool spots
- *Grade IV*: Papilloedema

> Changes in acute hypertension or **malignant hypertension** are:
> - Extensive flame-shaped hemorrhages
> - Hard exudates in a ring around the macula also called as **macular star**[Q]
> - Cotton wool spots
> - Choroidal infarcts which are called **Elschnig's spots**[Q]
> - Papilloedema
> - **Exudative Retinal detachment**[Q]

Retina

RETINOPATHY OF PREMATURITY

- Retinopathy of prematurity (ROP) is a proliferative retinopathy seen in premature infants of low birth weight, especially those who have been exposed to ambient oxygen
- The important risk factors which predispose to development of ROP include
    - **Prematurity**[Q]
    - Low birth weight[Q]
    - Oxygen therapy
    - Anemia needing blood transfusion
    - Sepsis.

Screening for ROP

- Neonates born **at ≤32 week of gestation or birth weight< 1500 g must be screened for ROP**[Q]
- Neonates born at ≥**32 weeks weighing between 1500 and 2000 g** who have been exposed to oxygen are also screened.
- Screening is done within 4 weeks of birth

Pathogenesis of ROP

- The retinal vasculature starts developing at around the fourth month of gestation. At about the eighth month, the vessels have reached the nasal retina but they do not reach the temporal periphery till the tenth month (1 month after delivery of a term baby)
- Premature infants, thus, have an incompletely vascularised retina which is dependent on an optimum level of VEGF for their vessel migration
- With oxygen therapy, there is suppression of the basal VEGF which causes halting of the vessel migration.
- Thus the normal development of the retinal vasculature is disturbed. Later on, this incompletely vascularised hypoxic retina starts generating excess VEGF which leads to proliferative retinopathy or ROP

Classification of Retinopathy of Prematurity

1. Location (Fig. 9)	Zone I	Circle with optic nerve at centre and a radius of twice the distance from optic nerve to macula
	Zone II	From edge of Zone I to the nasal ora serrata nasally and equator temporally
	Zone III	Lateral most crescent shaped area from Zone II to ora-serrata temporally
2. Severity (Figs 10A to D)	Stage 1	Presence of thin **white demarcation line**[Q] separating the vascular from avascular retina
	Stage 2	The line becomes prominent because of lifting of retina to form **a ridge**[Q]
	Stage 3	Presence of **extra-retinal fibrovascular proliferation**[Q] with abnormal vessels and fibrous tissue arising from the ridge and extending into vitreous
	Stage 4	**Partial retinal detachment**[Q]; not involving macula (4A) or involving macula (4B)
	Stage 5	Total retinal detachment[Q]
3. **Plus disease**[Q]		Presence of **dilatation and tortuosity of posterior retinal vessels**[Q]

International Classification of Retinopathy of Prematurity (ICROP) Zones

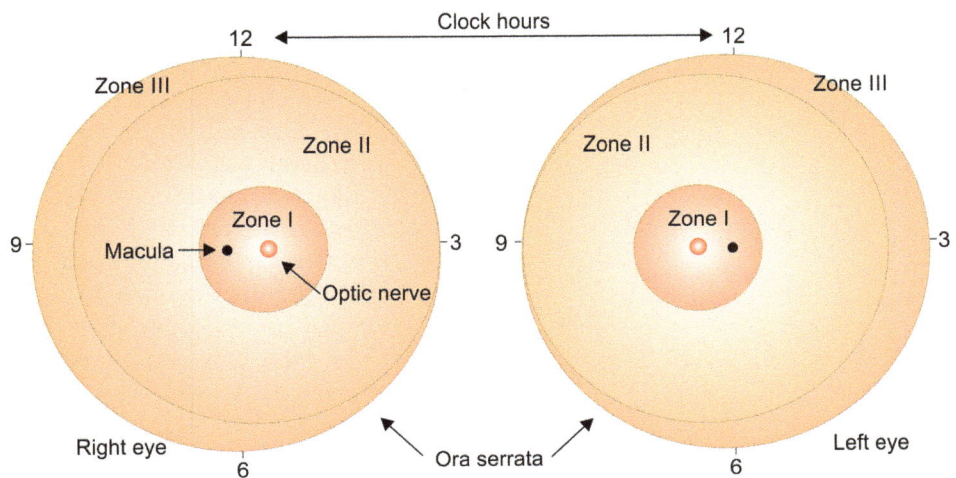

Fig. 9: Zones of ROP

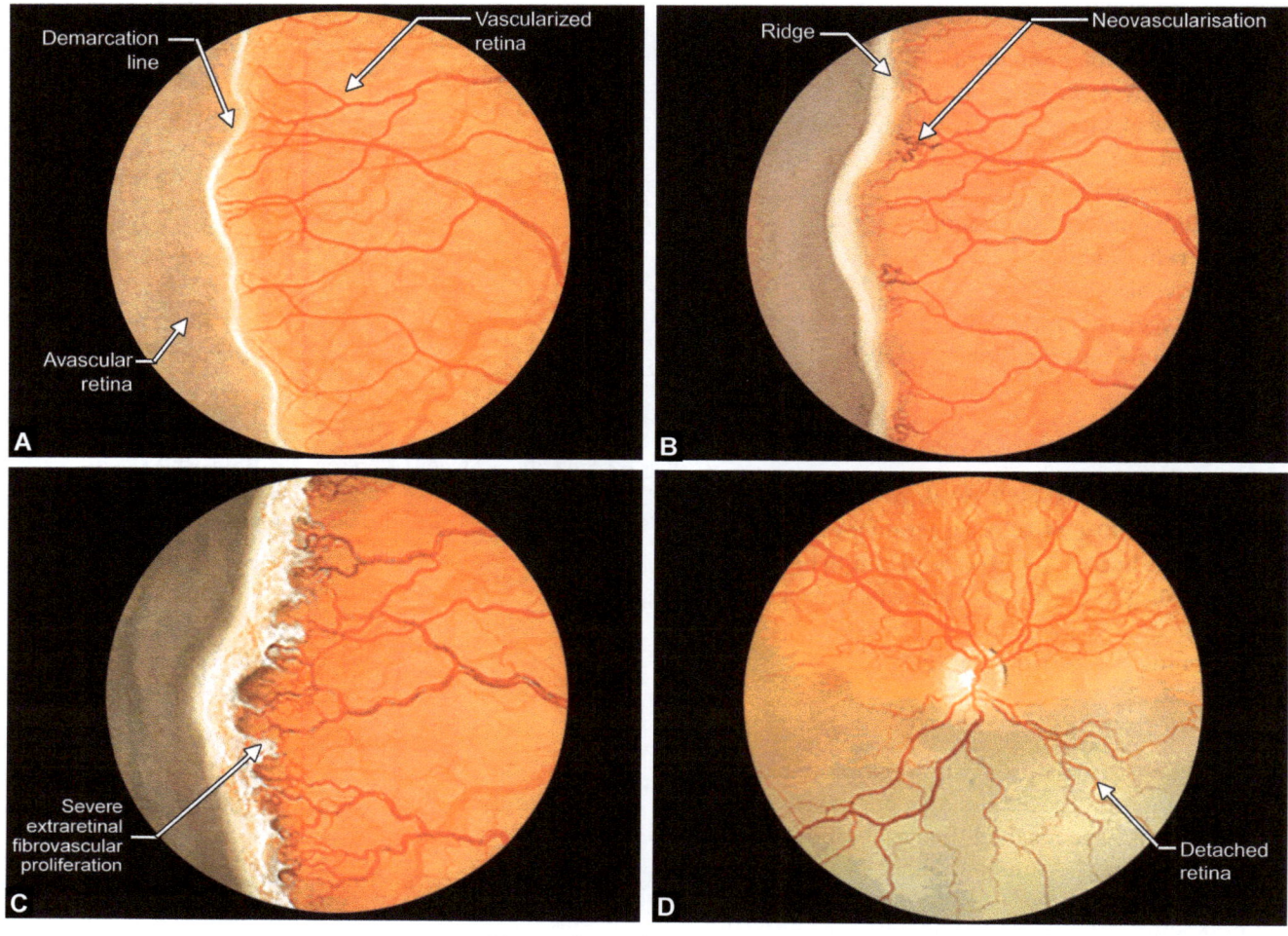

Figs. 10 (A to D): Stages of ROP

Based on results of ETROP (**Early Treatment of Retinopathy of Prematurity**) study, the treatment of ROP is described as:

Type	Treatment
Type 1 ROP or Threshold ROP:[Q] Zone I, any stage ROP with plus disease Zone I, stage 3 ROP with or without plus disease Zone II, stage 2 or 3 ROP with plus disease.	**Peripheral retinal ablation should be carried out**[Q]
Type II ROP: ROP not meeting the criteria for threshold ROP	Follow up

Prevention

- Judicious oxygen therapy : PaO_2 should be maintained between 50 and 80 mm Hg. SaO_2 should be maintained between 89 and 95%
- Judicious use of blood transfusions
- Prenatal steroids prevent respiratory distress and intraventricular hemorrhage which are two important risk factors of ROP.

Eales Disease

- Bilateral idiopathic, occlusive, **peripheral retinal periphlebitis**[Q] with neovascularisation
- Commonly seen in young males
- Strong association with **Tuberculosis**[Q]
- The disease is characterized by the occlusion of peripheral retinal veins associated with vasculitis. Retinal hypoperfusion leads to increase in VEGF which causes retinal neovascularisation.
- As the disease is mainly localized to the peripheral retinal veins, presentation is usually late. Presentation is usually with **vitreous hemorrhage**[Q]. This is the **most common cause of spontaneous vitreous hemorrhage in young adult**[Q]
- Retinal photocoagulation is the treatment. Anti-VEGF injection, Pars plana vitrectomy are other options

> Most common cause of vitreous hemorrhage in adult: **Diabetes**[Q]
> Most common cause of vitreous hemorrhage in young adults: **Trauma**[Q]

ACQUIRED MACULOPATHIES

The main symptoms of macular disease: Blurring of central vision associated with **metamorphopsia**[Q] **and micropsia** (image distortion).

Examination of Macula
- Direct slit-lamp biomicroscopy with 90D lens
- **Amsler Grid**[Q]
- Photostress Test
- Two light discrimination test
- Laser interferometry (LI)
- **Potential Acuity Meter (PAM)**[Q]

AGE-RELATED MACULAR DEGENERATION (ARMD)

ARMD is an age-related atrophy of the RPE and the photoreceptors associated with choroidal neovascularization. It is of two types:
1. Non-exudative/Dry ARMD
   - Accumulation of debris between the retinal pigment epithelium and Bruch's membrane of the choroid. These are called as **Drusens**
   - Progressive atrophy of the RPE, photoreceptors and choroid which is called **Geographic Atrophy**
2. Exudative/Wet ARMD
   - RPE Detachment
   - Breaks in the Bruch membrane allow the choriocapillaries to grow into the retina. This is called **Choroidal Neovascular Membrane (CNVM)**[Q]
   - Disciform Scar

Investigation

Indocyanine green angiography (ICGA)[Q]

(*Note*: ICGA is useful for evaluation of the choroidal vasculature whereas FFA is useful for the study of the retinal vasculature).

Treatment
- Dry ARMD: Anti-oxidants like **Vitamin C**, **Vitamin E**, zinc along with **Lutein, Zeaxanthin** and **Omega 3 fatty acids** have been shown to be beneficial in preventing progression of Dry AMD. A new drug **Lampalizumab** is under trial for treatment of geographic atrophy
- Wet ARMD:
  - Anti-VEGF injection[Q]
  - *Photodynamic therapy (PDT)*[Q]: This is a combination therapy using laser along with a photosensitizer **Verteporfin** which is taken up by the target tissue and enhances the effect of laser. It is less effective than Anti-VEGF
  - Transpupillary thermotherapy (TTT)
- Low vision aids: For advanced burnt out disease.

CENTRAL SEROUS RETINOPATHY (CSR)

Central serous retinopathy is an idiopathic detachment of the neurosensory retina in the region of the macula due to the accumulation of serous fluid
- More common in males aged between 20 and 40 years
- *Risk factors*: **Stress**[Q], **smoking**[Q] **and steroids**[Q]
- Seen in **Type A personalities**[Q]
- Sudden onset decrease in vision associated with micropsia and metamorphopsia
- Localized detachment of neurosensory retina at the posterior pole leading to **acquired hypermetropia** (effective shortening of the globe)
- *Fundus fluorescein angiography*: The classical patterns are
  - **Smoke Stack Pattern**[Q] or Mushroom/Umbrella pattern
  - **Ink Blot Pattern**[Q] (Enlarging Dot Sign)
- *Treatment*:
  - Wait and watch[Q] (as spontaneous resolution occurs in about **12 weeks**)
  - Photocoagulation, anti-VEGF injections are options where resolution does not occur in three month.

CYSTOID MACULAR OEDEMA (CME)

- CME is defined as accumulation of fluid in the **Outer Plexiform Layer**[Q] of the retina in the area of the macula due to defect in the **inner blood retinal barrier**[Q]
- Cause of CME is intraocular inflammation like **pars planitis**, anterior uveitis, intraocular surgery, etc
- Fundus fluorescein angiography: The typical pattern is called **flower petal appearance**[Q]
- Treatment is **steroids**, nonsteroidal anti-inflammatory drugs, anti-VEGF.

RETINAL DYSTROPHIES

Retinitis Pigmentosa

Retinitis pigmentosa (RP) is a type of retinal dystrophy predominantly affecting the rod photoreceptor cells of the retina with subsequent degeneration of the cones
- *Sporadic*: **Most common**[Q]
- Inheritance may be **Autosomal Dominant (AD)**, Autosomal Recessive (AR) or X-Linked Recessive (least common)

Symptoms

Night blindness or Nyctalopia^Q.

Signs

The fundus picture of RP is described as triad
- Arteriolar attenuation^Q
- Waxy disc pallor^Q
- Mid peripheral pigmentary changes described as **bony spicules**^{Q}

Other features are Myopia, Keratoconus, Glaucoma, **Posterior Subcapsular Cataract**^{Q}, Cystoid Macular Oedema.

Investigations

- **Scotopic flash ERG: Decrease in the amplitude of the 'a' wave**^{Q}
- Visual field assessment shows mid peripheral **Ring Scotoma**^{Q} **or Annular Scotoma**^{Q}. There is gradual constriction of the visual field from the periphery with a **central tubular vision** remaining in the advanced stages of the disease.

Atypical RP

- *RP sine pigmento*: Inconspicuous pigmentary change.
- *Retinitis punctata albescens*: Scattered white dots are seen in the fundus

Syndromes Associated with Atypical RP

- *Refsum's disease*^{Q}: Peripheral neuropathy, cerebellar ataxia, deafness
- *Usher's Syndrome*^{Q}: Non progressive sensorineural **deafness**
- *Cockayne's syndrome*: Dwarfism, bird-like facies, deafness, nystagmus, ataxia, mental retardation
- *Kearns-Sayre syndrome*^{Q}: Chronic progressive external ophthalmoplegia, heart block
- *Laurence moon biedl syndrome*^{Q}: Mental retardation, polydactyly, obesity, hypogonadism.
- *Bassen-Kornzweig syndrome*
- *Friedrich's ataxia*
- *NARP* (Neuropathy, Ataxia, Retinitis Pigmentosa)

Best's Disease (Juvenile Vitelliform Dystrophy)

- **Autosomal dominant (AD)**^{Q}
- Dystrophy of **RPE layer**^{Q} at the macula
- **Deposition of lipofuscin**^{Q} **pigment at the macula**
- Typically has the following stages
  - Vitelliform Stage: **Egg yolk appearance of macula**
  - Pseudohypopyon Stage
  - Vitelloruptive Stage: **Scrambled eggs appearance of macula**
- Investigation: **EOG**^{Q}

Stargardt's Disease and Fundus Flavimaculatus

- **Autosomal Recessive (AR) inheritance**
- Stargardt's disease is a retinal dystrophy with predominant macular involvement, hence also called **Juvenile Macular Dystrophy**
- Presents in first-second decade with decreased central vision
- Mottled appearance of the macula is seen. It is typically described as **beaten bronze appearance**^{Q}
- Adult variant is Fundus Flavimaculatus where involvement is predominantly in the peripheral retina. Hence patients may be asymptomatic
- **Pattern ERG** is affected. Routine flash ERG and EOG are normal.

Leber's Congenital Amaurosis

- This condition is associated with very poor vision since birth or very early childhood
- Fundus shows **salt and pepper retinopathy**^{Q}
- Characteristic feature is **oculodigital syndrome** where constant rubbing of the eyes by the child due to poor vision leads to **enophthalmos**

Congenital Stationary Night Blindness

- Group of retinal disorders characterized by infantile onset nyctalopia which is non-progressive
- It may have autosomal dominant, autosomal recessive or X-linked recessive inheritance
- The fundus may be normal or abnormal in appearance. Two characteristic types are
  1. Fundus albipunctatus
  2. **Oguchi's disease** ^{Q}: The fundus has an unusual golden-yellow colour in light adapted condition which becomes normal after prolonged dark adaptation. This is called **Mizuo phenomenon**^{Q}

RETINOBLASTOMA

Most common primary malignant intraocular tumor of childhood^Q

- Seen in 1:17000 live births and accounts for 3% of all childhood cancers
- Familial cases: 6%
- Sporadic cases: 94%

Genetics
- Gene for retinoblastoma is Rb gene (oncosuppressor gene), the locus of which is **13q14**^{Q}
- **Knudson's two hit hypothesis**^{Q} is used to explain the genetic pattern of retinoblastoma

Clinical Features
The common age of presentation is **18–24 months**^{Q}. The presenting features are:
- **Leukocoria (Amaurotic cat's eye reflex): Most common presenting feature**^{Q}
- *Strabismus*^{Q}: Second most common presenting feature
- Proptosis
- Keratitis/Perforated ulcer
- Hyphaema/Hypopyon
- Rubeosis iridis
- Complicated cataract
- Endophthalmitis
- Retinal detachment
- Orbital cellulitis
- Phthisis bulbi

Types
- **Exophytic:** Grows outwards into the subretinal space resulting in total retinal detachment
- **Endophytic:** Projects from the retina into the vitreous cavity. It is associated with **secondary calcification** which gives **cottage cheese appearance.**

Mode of Spread
- Intraocular extension
- Extraocular extension: **Most common mode of spread is via the Optic Nerve**^{Q}. It spreads to the brain via the optic nerve and to the orbit via emissary veins
- Metastasis.

Associated Tumours
- **Osteosarcoma**^{Q} **(most common)**
- Malignant melanoma
- Testicular Ca
- Ewing's tumour
- Wilm's tumour

Trilateral retinoblastoma: Bilateral retinoblastoma + pinealoblastoma^Q

Investigations
- *USG B-Scan*: **Presence of intraocular mass with calcification**^{Q}
- CT Scan
- MRI: Investigation of choice. It confirms the diagnosis and detects the extent of the disease
- *Aqueous humour paracentesis*: **Aqueous: Plasma LDH > 1**^{Q}.

Treatment
- *Cryotherapy*: Small tumor anterior to the equator
- *Photocoagulation*: Small tumors posterior to the equator
- *Brachytherapy*: Small tumors anterior to the equator
- *Enucleation*: **Tumours involving more than 50% of the globe** have to be enucleated with **a minimum optic nerve stump of 10 mm**^{Q}
- *External beam radiotherapy*: Adjuvant therapy after enucleation in tumours with orbital and intracranial extension.
- *Chemotherapy*: Metastatic disease is treated with palliative chemotherapy. Extraocular disease is treated with neo-adjuvant chemotherapy prior to enucleation to downstage the disease. **Carboplatin, Etoposide, Vincristine**^{Q} are the drugs used in chemotherapy
- Other modalities
    - Thermochemotherapy
    - Photodynamic therapy (PDT)

Leucocoria^Q
- Retinoblastoma
- Cataract
- Coloboma
- Persistent hyperplastic primary vitreous (PHPV)
- Toxocariasis
- Metastatic endophthalmitis
- Retinal astrocytoma
- Coat's disease
- ROP
- Retinal detachment

Coat's Disease
- This is a vascular disorder of the retina associated with **intraretinal telengiectasia**
- It is a **unilateral** condition seen in **boys** between **4 and 10 years** of age
- In this condition, abnormal telengiectatic and leaky blood vessels are seen most commonly in the **infero-temporal quadrant**^{Q} of the retina. These blood vessels cause severe intraretinal and subretinal exudation leading to **exudative retinal detachment**^{C}
- Presentation is with **leucocoria** and **strabismus**^{Q} associated with **vision loss**

Self Assessment and Review of Ophthalmology

- On examination exudation with retinal detachment is seen.
- Treatment is laser photocoagulation of the telengiectatic vessels
- A variant of Coat's disease is called **Idiopathic Juxtafoveal Telengiectasia**[Q].

Persistent Hyperplastic Primary Vitreous (PHPV)

- It is a congenital condition where the primary vitreous fails to regress. It is of two types, anterior and posterior. **Anterior PHPV is more common**
- In anterior PHPV, the persistent primary vitreous presents as a retrolental mass into which elongated ciliary processes are inserted. The contraction of the ciliary body pulls these processes and tears the capsule of the lens. Complications are cataract and glaucoma.
- Presents with **leucocoria in a microphthalmic eye**[Q]. It is always **unilateral**[Q].
- The features of anterior PHPV are summarized as ABC
  - Decreased **axial length** or microphthalmos
  - **Bands** in the vitreous
  - Elongated **ciliary body**
- Posterior PHPV is a rare condition where a dense white membrane is seen to extend from the disc to the peripheral retina. **It presents with retinal detachment**

> **Must Remember**
> - *Cattle track sign:* Central retinal artery occlusion (CRAO)
> - *Splashed tomato appearance:* Central retinal vein occlusion (CRVO)
> - *Mizuo phenomenon:* Oguchi's disease
> - *Oculodigital syndrome:* Leber's congenital amaurosis
> - *First detectable lesion in diabetic retinopathy:* Microaneurysm
> - *Most common type of retinal detachment:* Rhegmatogenous retinal detachment

QUESTIONS

Ophthalmoscopy/Investigations Related to Retina

1. Which of the following is not true about direct ophthalmoscopy? *(AIIMS 2015)*
   a. 2 disc diameters field
   b. Image is virtual and erect
   c. Magnification is 5 times
   d. Self-illuminated device

2. Which of the following is false about indirect ophthalmoscopy? *(AIIMS 2013)*
   a. Convex lens is used
   b. Image is virtual and erect
   c. Magnification is 4-5 times
   d. It is so bright that regular haziness is penetrated

3. Which of the following is false about indirect ophthalmoscopy? *(DNB 2016)*
   a. Condensing lens is required
   b. Examination through hazy media is possible
   c. Image is virtual and erect
   d. Stereopsis is present

4. There is a retained intraocular foreign body in the eye. Which is the most important test for monitoring vision? *(AIIMS 2014)*
   a. Dark adaptometry
   b. Visual evoked potential
   c. ERG
   d. EOG

5. Normal value of Arden index is *(AIIMS 2014)*
   a. 1
   b. 1.5
   c. Less than 185%
   d. More than 185%

6. 'b' wave in ERG arises from: *(APPG 2014)*
   a. Rods and cones
   b. Bipolar cells
   c. Ganglion cells
   d. Retinal pigment epithelium

7. In fluorescein angiography of retina, the dye is injected in *(AIPG 2009)*
   a. Femoral artery
   b. Antecubital vein
   c. Ophthalmic artery
   d. Internal carotid artery

Anatomy of Retina

8. The retina receives its blood supply from all except *(AIPG 2006)*
   a. Posterior ciliary arteries
   b. Central retinal artery
   c. Retinal arteries
   d. Circle of Zinn haler

9. The distance of the fovea from the temporal margin of the optic disc is *(AIPG)*
   a. 1 disc diameter
   b. 2 disc diameters
   c. 3 disc diameters
   d. 4 disc diameters

10. Regarding the fovea, which of the following is true: *(PGI)*
    a. Has the lowest threshold for light
    b. Contains only rods
    c. Contains only cones
    d. Maximum visual acuity
    e. Located on the optic nerve

11. Which area of the retina has the highest concentration of rods? *(Bihar PG 2014)*
    a. Parafoveal region
    b. Optic disc
    c. Fovea
    d. Ora serrata

12. Ratio of diameter of retinal arteriole to venule is: *(DNB 2016)*
    a. 1:2
    b. 2:3
    c. 3:4
    d. 3:2

13. The retina develops from: *(COMEDK 2013)*
    a. Neuroectoderm
    b. Surface ectoderm
    c. Endoderm
    d. Mesoderm

14. The layer between retina and choroid is: *(NEET 2016)*
    a. Descemet's membrane
    b. Bruch's membrane
    c. Ganglion cell layer
    d. Retinal pigment epithelium

Retinal Detachment

15. The risk of rhegmatogenous retinal detachment is increased in all of the following except *(AIIMS 2013)*
    a. Pseudophakia
    b. Trauma
    c. Hyperopia
    d. Lattice degeneration

16. Which of the following is not true about rhegmatogenous retinal detachment? *(AIIMS 2014)*
    a. It is caused due to fibrous bands in the vitreous
    b. It presents with floaters and photopsia
    c. It may extend up to ora serrata
    d. Surgery is the primary treatment

17. Shafer's sign is seen in: *(DNB 2015)*
    a. Retinal detachment
    b. Congenital glaucoma
    c. Stargardt's disease
    d. Retinopathy of prematurity

18. Subretinal demarcation line or watershed line is seen in *(AIIMS 2014)*
    a. Fresh rhegmatogenous retinal detachment
    b. Old rhegmatogenous retinal detachment
    c. Retinopathy of prematurity
    d. Retinitis pigmentosa

19. Pneumatic retinopexy is an outpatient procedure where retinal detachment is sealed with air insufflation. Which is the gas used in the process? *(AIIMS 2014)*
    a. Carbon dioxide
    b. Sulphur hexafluoride
    c. Nitrous oxide
    d. Oxygen

20. A young patient with history of using glasses for the past 10 years comes with complains of photopsia and sudden loss of vision in the right eye. Which of the following tests should be done.
    (AIIMS 2014, AIPG 2000)
    a. Cycloplegic refraction
    b. Gonioscopy
    c. Direct ophthalmoscopy
    d. Indirect ophthalmoscopy

21. A patient presents with sudden onset floaters and perception of a curtain or veil in front of his right eye. What is the most probable diagnosis? *(AIIMS 2011)*
    a. Vitreous haemorrhage   b. Retinal detachment
    c. Eales' disease   d. Glaucoma

22. Causes of exudative retinal detachment are
    (AIPG 2008)
    a. Scleritis   b. Toxemia pregnancy
    c. Dysthyroid eye disease   d. Sickle cell retinopathy

23. Causes of exudative retinal detachment are   *(PGI)*
    a. Central retinal artery occlusion
    b. Harada's disease
    c. Hypertensive retinopathy
    d. Coat's disease

24. Retinal detachment may be treated by: *(Bihar PG 2014)*
    a. Cryosurgery   b. Enucleation
    c. Evisceration   d. Ranibizumab

25. All of the following are used in the treatment of retinal detachment except: *(NEET 2016)*
    a. Scleral buckling
    b. Drainage of subretinal fluid
    c. Vitrectomy
    d. Transpupillary thermotherapy

Diabetic Retinopathy

26. A person is diagnosed to have diabetes on his 45th birthday. When will you recommend a dilated fundus examination for him? *(AIIMS 2014)*
    a. Immediately
    b. Before his 50th birthday
    c. After his 50th birthday
    d. When he complains of decrease in vision

27. Microaneurysms are the earliest feature of diabetic retinopathy. In which layer of retina are they seen
    (AIIMS 2014)
    a. Outer plexiform layer
    b. Inner nuclear layer
    c. Layer of rods and cones
    d. Retinal pigment epithelium

28. Which of the following is not a feature of diabetic retinopathy? *(DPG 2014)*
    a. Microaneurysm   b. Cotton wool spots
    c. Hard exudates
    d. Choroidal neovascularisation

29. Features of non-proliferative diabetic retinopathy are all except *(DNB 2013)*
    a. Neovascularisation   b. Hard exudates
    c. Soft exudates   d. Microaneurysm

30. Classical feature of Proliferative Diabetic Retinopathy (PDR) is: *(NEET 2016)*
    a. Hard exudates   b. Soft exudates
    c. Neovascularization   d. Retinal hemorrhages

31. Diabetic retinopathy can lead to   *(PGI)*
    a. Vitreous haemorrhage
    b. Retinal detachment
    c. IIIrd, IVth and VIth cranial nerve palsies
    d. Rubeosis iridis
    e. Hypermetropia

32. Grid photocoagulation is indicated in *(COMEDK 2009)*
    a. Ischaemic maculopathy
    b. Clinically significant macular edema
    c. Macular hole
    d. Proliferative diabetic retinopathy

33. Panretinal photocoagulation is indicated in
    (DNB 2014)
    a. Clinically significant macular edema
    b. Retinal break
    c. Proliferative diabetic retinopathy
    d. Tractional retinal detachment

34. A patient with Clinically Significant Macular Edema (CSME) was treated with macular grid photocoagulation. After 3 months the OCT showed persistent vitreo-retinal traction. What is the next line of management? *(AIIMS 2011)*
    a. Wait and watch
    b. Intravitreal bevacizumab
    c. Pars plana vitrectomy
    d. Repeat macular grid photocoagulation

35. All of the following are involved in the pathogenesis of diabetic macular oedema except *(AIIMS 2008)*
    a. Retinal pigment epithelium dysfunction
    b. Oxidative stress
    c. Increase in VEGF
    d. Increase in protein kinase C

36. ETDRS chart is used for vision evaluation in diabetic patients. What does ETDRS stand for? *(AIIMS)*
    a. Extended treatment for diabetic retinopathy study
    b. Early treatment for diabetic retinopathy study
    c. Emergency treatment for diabetic retinopathy study
    d. Emerging treatment for diabetic retinopathy study

37. Treatment of advanced diabetic retinopathy with vitreo-retinal fibrosis and tractional retinal detachment include all the following except *(AIPG 2009)*
    a. Removal of epiretinal membrane
    b. Pars plana vitrectomy
    c. Reattachment of retina
    d. Exophotocoagulation

38. A 35-year-old patient of Insulin Dependent Diabetes Mellitus (IDDM) on insulin for the past 10 years complains of gradual progressive, painless loss of vision. What is the possible diagnosis? *(AIIMS)*
    a. Cataract   b. Vitreous haemorrhage
    c. Rhegmatogenous retinal detachment
    d. Tractional retinal detachment not involving the macula

Retinal Vascular Occlusion

39. A young patient presents with sudden, painless loss of vision in one eye. Ocular examination reveals visual acuity of perception of light and cherry red spot on the fundus. A systolic murmur is heard on the chest. The probable diagnosis is: *(AIIMS 2002)*
    a. Central retinal artery occlusion
    b. Central retinal vein occlusion
    c. Multifocal choroiditis with infective endocarditis
    d. Central serous retinopathy

40. Cherry red spot is seen in all except: *(AIPG 2010)*
    a. Niemann-Pick disease   b. CRAO
    c. Tay-Sach's disease   d. CRVO

41. A 20-year-old presents with history of tennis ball injury to the right eye. On examination a red spot is seen on the macula. The most likely diagnosis is: *(AIIMS)*
    a. Macular hole   b. Berlin's oedema
    c. Macular tear   d. Macular haemorrhage

42. Cherry red spot in children after trauma is seen in: *(AIIMS 2015)*
    a. CRAO   b. CRVO
    c. Berlin's oedema   d. Niemann-Pick disease

43. Splashed tomato appearance of retina is seen in: *(DNB 2016)*
    a. CRAO   b. CRVO
    c. Eales' disease   d. Sickle cell retinopathy

Retinopathy of Prematurity

44. Premature baby weighing 1000 gms or less is most likely to suffer from: *(AIIMS 2013)*
    a. Cataract   b. Glaucoma
    c. Retinopathy of prematurity
    d. Retinal detachment

45. A 28-week-old baby suffered from respiratory distress syndrome at birth. On day 14, he developed sepsis. At what postnatal age should the baby undergo retinal evaluation for ROP? *(AIIMS 2014)*
    a. 2 weeks   b. 4 weeks
    c. 6 weeks   d. 8 weeks

46. A premature baby on examination shows bilateral ROP (Zone 1, Stage II with plus disease). How will you manage the patient? *(AIIM 2011)*
    a. Examine the patient again after 1 week
    b. Laser photocoagulation of both eyes
    c. Laser photocoagulation of worse eye
    d. Vitreoretinal surgery

47. Retinopathy of prematurity: True statement is: *(DNB 2015)*
    a. It is classified into 4 stages depending on severity
    b. It resolves spontaneously without any treatment
    c. Zone III involves the nasal retina
    d. Polyhydramnios is a risk factor

48. Retrolental fibroplasia: Which of the following statements is false: *(NEET 2016)*
    a. Total retinal detachment is seen in Stage V
    b. Treatment of threshold disease is laser photocoagulation
    c. Demarcation line is seen in Stage II
    d. It is seen in premature infants with high oxygen exposure

Retinal Vascular Disorders—Miscellaneous

49. A 25-year-old male presents with sudden painless loss of vision in one eye. There is no history of trauma. On examination, the anterior segment is normal but there is no fundal glow. Which of the following is the most likely cause? *(AIIMS 2010)*
    a. Vitreous haemorrhage
    b. Developmental cataract
    c. Optic atrophy
    d. Acute angle closure glaucoma

50. Which of the following is not a feature of vitreous haemorrhage? *(Jipmer 2015)*
    a. Sudden loss of vision   b. Floaters
    c. Metamorphopsia   d. Absence of fundal glow

51. A young male patient presents with recurrent vitreous haemorrhage. Probable diagnosis is: *(PGI)*
    a. Eales' disease
    b. CRVO
    c. Coat's disease
    d. Proliferative vitreoretinopathy
    e. Episcleritis

52. Eales disease is: *(DNB 2015)*
    a. Periphlebitis retinae
    b. Intraretinal cyst
    c. Posterior vitreous detachment
    d. Exudative retinal detachment

53. Which of the following is not true about Eales' disease? *(DNB 2015)*
    a. Retinal detachment may occur
    b. Associated with optic neuritis
    c. AKT is given
    d. Vitreous hemorrhage is seen

54. Investigation of choice in vitreous hemorrhage is: *(DNB 2016)*
    a. Ultrasound biomicroscopy
    b. USG A-Scan
    c. USG B-Scan
    d. Optical coherence tomography

55. A 30-year-old male with history of headache is sent for fundus evaluation. On examination he was found to have generalised arterial attenuation with multiple cotton wool spots and flame-shaped hemorrhages in both eyes. The probable diagnosis is: *(AIIMS)*
    a. Diabetic retinopathy
    b. Hypertensive retinopathy
    c. Central retinal artery occlusion
    d. Temporal arteritis

56. Hard exudates are seen in all except: *(PGI 2014)*
    a. Diabetic retinopathy
    b. Retinitis pigmentosa
    c. Eales' disease
    d. Retinal artery macroaneurysm
    e. Choroidal neovascular membrane

Self Assessment and Review of Ophthalmology

57. Cotton wool spots are seen in: *(PGI 2013)*
    a. Diabetic retinopathy
    b. Hypertensive retinopathy
    c. AIDS
    d. Retinoblastoma
    e. Toxemia pregnancy

58. Soft exudates are seen in all except: *(NEET 2016)*
    a. Diabetic retinopathy
    b. Hypertensive retinopathy
    c. CMV retinitis
    d. Retinopathy of prematurity

59. Which of the following is not associated with rubeosis iridis? *(DNB 2013)*
    a. Proliferative diabetic retinopathy
    b. Retinopathy of prematurity
    c. Central serous retinopathy
    d. Eales' disease

60. Ocriplasmin is a recombinant protease used to treat: *(AIIMS 2013)*
    a. Retinal break
    b. Diabetic macular oedema
    c. Uveovitreal membrane
    d. Submacular bleeding

Retinal Dystrophies

61. Retinitis pigmentosa is not associated with: *(AIIMS 2008)*
    a. Usher syndrome
    b. Barren-Kornzweig syndrome
    c. Kearns Sayre syndrome
    d. Marfan syndrome

62. Retinitis pigmentosa is a feature of all except: *(AIIMS 2010)*
    a. Refsum's disease
    b. Hallervorden-Spatz disease
    c. NARP
    d. Abetalipoproteinemia

63. Features of Usher syndrome include all except: *(DNB 2015)*
    a. Night blindness
    b. Visual impairment
    c. Multiple neurofibromas
    d. Hearing deficit

64. All are true about Retinitis pigmentosa except: *(AIIMS)*
    a. It may have X-linked inheritance
    b. Early diagnosis and treatment prevent progression of the disease
    c. Visual acuity is preserved even in advanced stage of the disease
    d. Associated with systemic abnormalities

65. Most common type of cataract seen in Retinitis pigmentosa is: *(DNB 2012)*
    a. Nuclear cataract
    b. Posterior subcapsular cataract
    c. Cortical cataract
    d. Anterior polar cataract

66. Ring scotoma is a feature of: *(AIIMS 2000)*
    a. Blue dot cataract
    b. Nuclear cataract
    c. Retinitis pigmentosa
    d. Diabetic retinopathy

67. All of the following are true about Retinitis pigmentosa except: *(DNB 2012)*
    a. Presence of pigments in the retina
    b. Narrowing of the arterioles
    c. Pale waxy disc
    d. Normal ERG

68. Confirmatory investigation in Retinitis pigmentosa is: *(DNB 2015)*
    a. Optical coherence tomography
    b. Pachymetry
    c. Electroretinogram
    d. Visual acuity assessment

69. Retinitis Pigmentosa—all of the following are true except: *(CET JUNE2017)*
    a. Night blindness and defective dark adaptation are seen
    b. It is associated with Usher's syndrome and Refsum's disease
    c. Annular scotomas may be seen
    d. The readings of electroretinogram are very highly elevated

70. A retinal disease is characterised by progressive rod-cone dystrophy. It presents with pale disc and retinal vessel attenuation. What is the third feature of the triad? *(COMEDK 2015)*
    a. Macular degeneration
    b. Bony spicule pigmentary changes
    c. Pre-retinal hemorrhages
    d. Cotton wool spots

71. Idiopathic nyctalopia is due to hereditary: *(AIIMS)*
    a. Absence of rod function
    b. Absence of cone function
    c. Absence of both rod and cone function
    d. Decrease in function of bipolar cells

72. Night blindness is seen in all except: *(WBPG 2013)*
    a. Retinitis pigmentosa
    b. Cone dystrophy
    c. Oguchi's disease
    d. Vitamin A deficiency

73. Mizuo phenomenon is seen in: *(AIIMS 2011)*
    a. Oguchi's disease
    b. Fundus albipunctatus
    c. Fundus flavimaculatus
    d. Retinitis pigmentosa

74. A young patient presents with loss of central vision. There is no significant family history. Both ERG and EOG are normal. Which is the most likely diagnosis? *(AIPG 2010)*
    a. Retinitis pigmentosa
    b. Rod-cone dystrophy
    c. Stargardt's disease
    d. Best's disease

75. A young patient presents with loss of central vision. ERG is normal but EOG is abnormal. What is the likely diagnosis? *(AIPG 2010)*
    a. Retinitis pigmentosa
    b. Rod-cone dystrophy
    c. Stargardt's disease
    d. Best's disease

76. Ideal diagnostic test for Best's disease is:
    (Jipmer 2000, CMC 2001)
    a. Dark adaptometry   b. ERG
    c. EOG   d. Perimetry
77. Which of the following has Autosomal Dominant inheritance pattern? (AIIMS 2010)
    a. Best's disease
    b. Gyrate atrophy
    c. Laurence-Moon-Biedl syndrome
    d. Barren-Kornzweig syndrome
78. Pigmentary changes between the posterior pole and equator known as ' salt and pepper retinopathy' is seen in all except:
    (AIIMS 2013)
    a. Resolving retinal detachment
    b. Phenothiazine toxicity
    c. Congenital rubella
    d. Fundus flavimaculatus

Macular Disorders

79. A young male presents with central scotoma in the left eye. His right eye showed 6/6 vision. On examination there is focal foveal detachment in the left eye. What should be the next step? (AIIMS 2014)
    a. Examine retrolental cells
    b. Inquire about use of steroids
    c. Inquire about trauma to the other eye
    d. Examination on slit lamp
80. A 25-year-old executive presents with metamorphopsia in his right eye. On examination, there is a shallow detachment at the macula. FFA shows smoke-stack appearance. Which of the following should be the line of management?
    (AIIMS 2013)
    a. Topical antibiotic steroid
    b. Systemic steroids
    c. Pulse methylprednisolone
    d. Wait and watch for spontaneous recovery
81. Enlarging dot sign on FFA is seen in: (PGI)
    a. Cystoid macular edema
    b. Central serous retinopathy
    c. Clinically significant macular edema (CSME)
    d. Coat's disease
82. ICGA is primarily indicated in: (AIPG 2010)
    a. Minimal classic CNVM
    b. Occult CNVM
    c. Angioid streaks
    d. Polypoidal choroidal vasculopathy
83. Choroidal neovascular membrane (CNVM) is seen in all except: (AIIMS)
    a. Hypermetropia
    b. Myopia
    c. Traumatic choroidal rupture
    d. Angioid streaks
84. Photodynamic therapy is used for the treatment of:
    (AIPG 2004)
    a. Cataract   b. Glaucoma
    c. Wet ARMD   d. Uveitis
85. Which of the following is not used in the treatment of neovascular ARMD? (COMEDK 2015)
    a. Alemtuzumab   b. Bevacizumab
    c. Ranibizumab   d. Pegaptanib sodium
86. Ring scotoma is seen in all except: (NEET 2016)
    a. High myopia   b. Aphakic glasses
    c. Retinitis pigmentosa d. ARMD
87. Angioid streaks are seen in (AIIMS 2005)
    a. Pseudoxanthoma elasticum
    b. Tendinous xanthoma
    c. Xanthelasma
    d. Eruptive xanthoma
88. Angioid streaks are seen in all except: (NEET 2016)
    a. Ehler Danlos
    b. Pseudoxanthema elasticum
    c. Paget's disease
    d. Hypertensive retinopathy

Retinoblastoma

89. Most common clinical presentation of retinoblastoma is: (AIIMS 2013)
    a. Leucocoria+ Heterochromia iridis
    b. Leucocoria+ Pseudohypopyon
    c. Leucocoria+ Hyphaema
    d. Leucocoria + Strabismus
90. Hereditary retinoblastoma is associated with which chromosomal segment: (AIPG)
    a. 13q14   b. 13p14
    c. 14q13   d. 14p13
91. Knudson's two hit hypothesis describes the occurrence of: (PGI 2000)
    a. Glaucoma   b. Retinoblastoma
    c. Optic nerve glioma d. Meningioma
92. Familial retinoblastoma: (PGI 2001)
    a. Has autosomal recessive inheritance
    b. Usually bilateral
    c. Occurs due to mutation of Rb gene
    d. More common than sporadic retinoblastoma
    e. Poorer prognosis than sporadic retinoblastoma
93. The most common second malignancy in survivors of retinoblastoma is: (AIPG 2006)
    a. Thyroid cancer   b. Osteosarcoma
    c. Chondrosarcoma   d. Pinealoblastoma
94. Increased LDH in aqueous humour suggests a diagnosis of: (AIPG 2009)
    a. Galactosemia   b. Glaucoma
    c. Retinoblastoma   d. Gyrate atrophy
95. Most common route of spread of retinoblastoma:
    (AIIMS 2015)
    a. Lymphatics   b. Optic nerve
    c. Direct spread   d. Vascular

96. As regards to retinoblastoma, which of the following statements is false? *(AIIMS)*
    a. 94% of the cases are sporadic
    b. Patients with sporadic disease do not pass the genes to their offspring
    c. Calcification in the tumour is detected on USG B-scan
    d. Reese-Ellsworth classification is useful for predicting prognosis after radiotherapy

97. A 2-year-old child presents with leucocoria in the right eye since 2 months. On examination total retinal detachment is seen. USG B-scan reveals the presence of a subretinal mass with calcification. What is the most probable diagnosis? *(AIIMS 2001)*
    a. Coat's disease   b. Retinoblastoma
    c. Toxocariasis   d. Retinal tuberculoma

98. A one-year-old child having leucocoria was diagnosed to have large unilateral retinoblastoma filling half the globe. What is the management of the patient? *(AIPG 2003)*
    a. Enucleation
    b. Chemotherapy followed by local therapy
    c. Photodynamic therapy
    d. Radiotherapy followed by chemotherapy

99. A 5-year-old boy is diagnosed to have bilateral retinoblastoma. In the right eye there is advanced retinoblastoma almost filling the globe whereas in the left eye, a few small lesions are seen in the periphery. What is the management? *(AIPG 2011)*
    a. Enucleation of both eyes
    b. Enucleation of right eye and focal therapy of left eye
    c. Radiotherapy
    d. Six cycles of chemotherapy

100. Ideal treatment of bilateral advanced retinoblastoma: *(PGI 2004/ Jipmer 2002)*
    a. Enucleation   b. Chemotherapy
    c. Radiotherapy   d. Photocoagulation

101. Pseudo-rosettes are seen in *(PGI/ DNB 2013)*
    a. Ophthalmia nodosum b. Retinoblastoma
    c. Trachoma   d. Phacolytic glaucoma

102. Poor prognostic factors for retinoblastoma are: *(PGI 2015)*
    a. Size >4 mm   b. Size >2 mm
    c. Associated glaucoma
    d. Undifferentiated tumour cells
    e. Scleral involvement

103. Enucleation means: *(PGI)*
    a. Removal of the contents of the globe
    b. Removal of the entire globe with portion of the optic nerve
    c. Removal of the contents of the orbit
    d. Removal of the globe leaving a frill of sclera around the optic nerve

104. Evisceration is contraindicated in: *(AIIMS 2015)*
    a. Malignancy
    b. Panophthalmitis
    c. Severe ocular trauma
    d. Expulsive choroidal haemorrhage

105. Leucocoria is seen in all except: *(AIIMS 2002)*
    a. Persistent hyperplastic primary vitreous
    b. Congenital glaucoma
    c. Endophthalmitis   d. Retinoblastoma

Miscellaneous

106. A 7-year-old male presents with 6/6 vision in the right eye and hand movements close to face vision in the left eye. On fundoscopy, the right eye was normal. The left eye showed retinal detachment, subretinal yellowish exudates and telangiectatic vessels. What is the most probable diagnosis? *(AIIMS 2014)*
    a. Coat's disease
    b. Sympathetic ophthalmitis
    c. Familial exudative vitreoretinopathy
    d. Retinopathy of prematurity

107. All of the following are true about Idiopathic Juxtafoveal Telangiectasia except: *(AIIMS 2013)*
    a. It is a variant of Coat's disease
    b. It is associated with macular telangiectasia
    c. It is associated with structural abnormalities of the retinal blood vessels
    d. It is associated with peripheral retinal telangiectasia

108. Which of the following is associated with Persistent hyperplastic primary vitreous: (PHPV)? *(AIPG 2008)*
    a. Patau syndrome   b. Edward syndrome
    c. Trisomy 14   d. Down's syndrome

109. Which of the following does not show calcification? *(AIIMS 2014)*
    a. Persistent hyperplastic primary vitreous
    b. Choroidal osteoma
    c. Optic nerve head drusen
    d. Retinoblastoma

110. Acute loss of vision in a case of alcoholic pancreatitis: *(AIPG 2010)*
    a. Purtscher's retinopathy
    b. Acute congestive glaucoma
    c. Central retinal artery obstruction
    d. Optic neuritis

111. Purtscher's retinopathy is associated with: *(DNB 2015)*
    a. Diabetes   b. Head trauma
    c. Rheumatoid arthritis d. Wilson's disease

112. Roth's spots are seen in: *(PGI/COMEDK 2009)*
    a. Hypertension
    b. Diabetes
    c. Bacterial endocarditis
    d. Central retinal artery occlusion

113. Retinal hemorrhage with a white centre is known as: *(DNB 2015)*
    a. Cotton wool spot   b. Roth spot
    c. Drusen
    d. Flame-shaped haemorrhage

114. Bull's eye maculopathy is seen in toxicity of: *(PGI/AIIMS)*
    a. Chloroquine   b. Dapsone
    c. Rifampicin   d. Ethambutol

115. **Mucopolysaccharide hyaluronic acid is present in :**
 (AIIMS 2010, 2007)
 a. Vitreous humour
 b. Cornea
 c. Lens
 d. Blood vessels

116. **Strongest attachment of the vitreous is at:**
 (DNB 2016)
 a. Vitreous base at ora serrata
 b. Optic disc
 c. Macula
 d. Blood vessels

117. **A vitreous sample has been collected at 9pm. What advice would you like to give to the staff on duty regarding the overnight storage of the sample?**
 (AIPG)
 a. The sample should be stored at 4 degrees Celsius
 b. The sample should be incubated at 37 degrees Celsius
 c. The sample should be kept in the deep freezer
 d. The sample should be refrigerated for the initial 3 hours and then incubated

118. **When compared to blood, vitreous humour has higher concentration of:** *(AIIMS 2015)*
 a. Glucose
 b. Sodium
 c. Potassium
 d. Ascorbate

119. **Which of the following is not an ocular emergency?**
 (PGI 2015)
 a. Ocular trauma
 b. Sympathetic ophthalmitis
 c. CRAO
 d. CRVO
 e. Endophthalmitis

120. **What is reverse hypopyon?** *(DNB 2015)*
 a. Collection of pus in the vitreous
 b. Collection of emulsified silicon oil in the anterior chamber
 c. Abscess in the orbit
 d. Perforated corneal ulcer

121. **Shape of subhyaloid hemorrhage is:** *(DNB 2015)*
 a. Boat shaped
 b. Crescent shaped
 c. Round
 d. Flame shaped

122. **Most common age-related change seen in the vitreous:** *(DNB 2013)*
 a. Anterior vitreous detachment
 b. Posterior vitreous detachment
 c. Vitreous haemorrhage
 d. Vitritis

123. **Which of the following will not cause hypotonic maculopathy?** *(May AIIMS 2017)*
 a. Suprachoroidal haemorrhage
 b. Cyclodialysis
 c. Corneal perforation
 d. Filtration site leak

ANSWERS AND EXPLANATIONS

1. c. **Magnification is 5 times** *(Ref: Kanski 7th edition, p 692)*
2. b. **Image is virtual and erect** *(Ref: Kanski 7th edition, p 692)*
3. c. **Image is virtual and erect** *(Ref: Kanski 7th edition, p 692)*
4. c. **ERG** *(Ref: Yanoff & Duker 4th edition, p 460)*

    Electroretinogram is an important prognostic tool for intraocular metal foreign body especially iron. In siderosis bulbi, the early change in ERG is increase in the amplitude of the negative a wave with a normal b wave. Later the amplitude of the b wave also decreases. In the end stage disease, ERG becomes completely extinguished.

5. d. **More than 185%** *(Ref: Yanoff & Duker 4th edition, p 460)*

    The value should exceed 1.5 or 150%, hence the answer.

6. b. **Bipolar cells** *(Ref: Yanoff & Duker 4th edition, p 458)*
7. b. **Antecubital vein** *(Ref: Yanoff & Duker 4th edition, p 441)*
8. a. **Posterior ciliary arteries** *(Ref: Yanoff & Duker 4th edition, p 426)*

    This is a slightly controversial question because all the mentioned vessels are involved in the blood supply to the retina. I would choose posterior ciliary artery as the answer because the short posterior ciliary arteries do not directly supply the retina. They form the choriocapillaries from where the outer layers of retina are supplied.

9. b. **2 disc diameters** *(Ref: Yanoff & Duker 4th edition, p 420)*
10. a. **It has the lowest threshold for light, c. Contains only cones, d. Maximum visual acuity**

    (Ref: Yanoff & Duker 4th edition, p 420–21)

11. a. **Parafoveal region**

    The highest concentration of rods is in the mid periphery of the retina. But among the options here the most appropriate is parafoveal

12. b. **2:3** *(Ref: Yanoff & Duker 4th edition, p 426)*
13. a. **Neuroectoderm**

    Explained in the chapter on Ocular Embryology

14. b. **Bruch's membrane** *(Ref: Yanoff & Duker 4th edition, p 420–21)*
15. c. **Hyperopia** *(Ref: Yanoff & Duker 4th edition, p 648)*

    Rhegmatogenous RD is associated with high myopia and not hypermetropia

16. a. **It is caused due to fibrous bands in the vitreous** *(Ref: Yanoff & Duker 4th edition, p 649)*

    Fibrous bands in the vitreous are responsible for causing tractional RD, not rhegmatogenous

17. a. **Retinal detachment** *(Ref: Yanoff & Duker 4th edition, p 649)*
18. b. **Old rhegmatogenous retinal detachment** *(Ref: Yanoff & Duker 4th edition, p 649)*
19. b. **Sulphur hexafluoride** *(Ref: Yanoff & Duker 4th edition, p 651)*
20. d. **Indirect ophthalmoscopy** *(Ref: Yanoff & Duker 4th edition, p 642–43)*

    The question hints at a possible myopic patient presenting with complaints of flashes and floaters. This may be due to a peripheral retinal break and has the potential to progress to Rhegmatogenous RD. Hence, this patient should undergo a peripheral retinal screening with indirect ophthalmoscopy and scleral indentation. If a break is identified, laser barrage of the break should be done to prevent RD.

21. b. **Retinal detachment** *(Ref: Yanoff & Duker 4th edition, p 649)*
22. a. **Scleritis, b. Toxemia of pregnancy** *(Ref: Yanoff & Duker 4th edition, p 653–58)*
23. b. **Harada's disease, c. Hypertensive retinopathy, d. Coat's disease** *(Ref: Yanoff & Duker 4th edition, p 653–58)*

    Causes of exudative RD:
    - Inflammatory disorders like choroiditis, choroidal vasculitis, posterior scleritis
    - Choroidal tumours
    - Vogt Koyanagi Harada's disease (This is a panuveitis with multifocal choroiditis leading to exudative RD)
    - Malignant hypertension/ Toxemia pregnancy
    - Coat's disease (Retinal telengiectasia with leaking retinal blood vessels leading to exudative RD)

Retina

24. **a. Cryosurgery** *(Ref: Yanoff & Duker 4th edition, p 468)*
    Rhegmatogenous retinal detachment is treated by Scleral Buckling surgery. The important steps of the surgery are:
    - Application of the buckle
    - Drainage of the subretinal fluid
    - Cryotherapy to the breaks
    - Hence we choose the answer cryosurgery (though the term is not completely appropriate)

25. **d. Transpupillary thermotherapy** *Ref: Yanoff & Duker 4th edition, p 468)*
    Scleral buckling with drainage of subretinal fluid is done in rhegmatogenous retinal detachment. Vitrectomy is done in tractional retinal detachment

26. **a. Immediately** *(Ref: Kanski 7th edition, p 534)*
    Screening for diabetic retinopathy:
    - For Insulin Dependent Diabetes Mellitus (IDDM) or juvenile-onset DM: Screening should be started 5 years after diagnosis^Q
    - For Non-insulin Dependent Diabetes Mellitus (NIDDM) or late-onset diabetes: Screening should be started at the time of diagnosis^Q

    The patient in the question belongs to the NIDDM group

27. **b. Inner nuclear layer** *(Ref: Yanoff & Duker 4th edition, p 542)*
28. **d. Choroidal neovascularisation** *(Ref: Yanoff & Duker 4th edition, p 543–44)*
    Proliferative diabetic retinopathy is associated with retinal neovascularisation
29. **a. Neovascularisation** *(Ref: Yanoff & Duker 4th edition, p 543–44)*
    Neovascularisation is a feature of PDR not NPDR
30. **c. Neovascularisation** *(Ref: Yanoff & Duker 4th edition, p 543–44)*
31. **a. Vitreous haemorrhage, b. Retinal detachment, c. IIIrd, IVth, VIth cranial nerve palsies, d. Rubeosis iridis**
    (Ref: Yanoff & Duker 4th edition, p 544–45)
    Diabetes may lead to myopic shift and frequent changes in refraction due to fluctuation in blood sugar levels but hypermetropia is not seen
32. **b. Clinically significant macular oedema** *(Ref: Yanoff & Duker 4th edition, p 548)*
33. **c. Proliferative diabetic retinopathy** *(Ref: Yanoff & Duker 4th edition, p 547)*
34. **c. Pars plana vitrectomy** *(Ref: Yanoff & Duker 4th edition, p 548–49)*
    This question is an example of a case where the macular oedema is caused by a tractional band at the macula. Hence the treatment is pars plana vitrectomy
35. **d. Increase in protein kinase C** *(Ref: Yanoff & Duker 4th edition, p 542)*
36. **b. Early treatment for diabetic retinopathy study** *(Ref: Kanski 7th edition, p 536)*
37. **d. Exophotocoagulation** *(Ref: Yanoff & Duker 4th edition, p 548–49)*
    The different procedures that are done in diabetic vitrectomy are
    - Pars plana vitrectomy
    - Release of vitreous membranes
    - Removal of epiretinal membranes
      (The removal of the tractional bands will cause the retina to settle)
    - **Endophotocoagulation**
    - Silicon oil injection (This is a vitreous substitute used to reform the vitreous cavity)
38. **a. Cataract**
    Diabetes is associated with snow flake cataract. It may also lead to rapid progression of senile cataract
39. **a. Central retinal artery occlusion** *(Ref: Yanoff & Duker 4th edition, p 519)*
40. **d. CRVO** *(Ref: Yanoff & Duker 4th edition, p 519)*

Important causes of Cherry Red Spot	
CRAO/BRAO^Q	Hurler's syndrome
Berlin's oedema (blunt trauma)^Q	Sialodosis
Gaucher's disease^Q	Multiple sulfatase deficiency
Niemann Pick's disease^Q	Hallervorden-Spatz
Tay-Sach disease^Q	Farber's disease
Metachromatic leukodystrophy^Q	

41. b. **Berlin's oedema** *(Ref: Yanoff & Duker 4th edition, p 670)*
42. c. **Berlin's oedema** *(Ref: Yanoff & Duker 4th edition, p 671)*
    Berlin's oedema is seen after blunt trauma or concussion injury. This gives the appearance of cherry red spot.
43. b. **CRVO** *(Ref: Yanoff & Duker 4th edition, p 526–27)*
44. c. **Retinopathy of prematurity** *(Ref: Yanoff & Duker 4th edition, p 534)*
45. b. **4 weeks** *(Ref: Yanoff & Duker 4th edition, p 538)*
46. b. **Laser photocoagulation** *(Ref: Yanoff & Duker 4th edition, p 536–38)*
    The question describes a case of Threshold ROP in both eyes. Hence the treatment is laser photocoagulation of both eyes
47. d. **Polyhydramnios is a risk factor**
    Any antenatal condition leading to perinatal complication or premature delivery is an indirect risk factor
48. c. **Demarcation line is seen in Stage II** *(Ref: Yanoff & Duker 4th edition, p 536–38)*
    Retrolental fibroplasia is the old term for ROP
49. a. **Vitreous haemorrhage** *(Ref: Kanski 7th edition, p 585)*
    The question describes a young male with sudden painless vision loss. Absence of fundal glow means dense media opacity. So this is a case of Eales' disease presenting with vitreous haemorrhage
50. c. **Metamorphopsia** *(Ref: Kanski 7th edition, p 595)*
    Metamorphopsia is a feature of macular disease, not vitreous haemorrhage
51. a. **Eales' disease** *(Ref: Yanoff & Duker 4th edition, p 572)*
52. a. **Periphlebitis retinae** *(Ref: Kanski 7th edition, p 583, 585)*
53. b. **Associated with optic neuritis** *(Ref: Yanoff & Duker 4th edition, p 572)*
54. c. **USG B-Scan** *(Ref: Yanoff & Duker 4th edition, p 438–39)*
    Vitreous hemorrhage causes media haziness as a result of which direct visualization of retina by ophthalmoscopy becomes difficult. Also optical scans cannot be done in hazy media. Hence, in order to evaluate the retina, USG B-Scan is done. The main use of USG A-Scan is to determine axial length of the eye prior to cataract surgery.
55. b. **Hypertensive retinopathy** *(Ref: Yanoff & Duker 4th edition, p 514)*
56. b. **Retinitis pigmentosa** *(Ref: Kanski 7th edition, p 651–54)*
    Hard exudates are lipoproteins leaking from the retinal blood vessels due to damage to the endothelium.

Causes of hard exudates
♦ Diabetes Mellitus^Q
♦ Hypertension (macular star)^Q
♦ Retinal artery macroaneurysm^Q
♦ Capillary haemangioma of the retina (Von-Hippel-Lindau disease)^Q
♦ Retinal vascular occlusions like CRVO, BRVO^Q
♦ Coat's disease
♦ Choroidal neovascular membrane
♦ Radiation retinopathy
♦ Neuroretinitis (macular star)

57. a. **Diabetic retinopathy, b. Hypertensive retinopathy, c. AIDS, e. Toxemia pregnancy**
    (Ref: Kanski 7th edition, p 536, 442, 567, 586, 589, 553)
    Cotton wool spots are infarcts in the retinal nerve fibre layer due to microvascular occlusion. They were previously called soft exudates.

Causes of Cotton wool spots
♦ Diabetes Mellitus^Q
♦ Hypertension/Toxemia pregnancy^Q
♦ Retinal ischaemic disorders like CRVO, BRVO, ocular ischaemic syndrome^Q
♦ Embolic disorders
♦ Infections like **HIV**^{Q}, CMV, leptospirosis, fungal infections
♦ Collagen vascular disorders like SLE
♦ Neoplastic disorders like lymphoma, leukaemia
♦ Radiation retinopathy^Q

Retina

58. **d. Retinopathy of prematurity**
    See explanation of Question No 54

59. **c. Central serous retinopathy** *(Ref: Kanski 7th edition, p 632–33)*
    Causes of rubeosis iridis
    - Proliferative diabetic retinopathy
    - CRVO
    - Eales' disease
    - Retinopathy of prematurity
    - Sickle cell retinopathy
    - Chronic iritis
    - Iris tumours

60. **c. Uveovitreal membrane**

61. **d. Marfan's syndrome**

62. **b. Hallervorden- Spatz disease** *(Ref: Yanoff & Duker 4th edition, p 485)*

63. **c. Multiple neurofibromas** *(Ref: Yanoff & Duker 4th edition, p 482–85)*

64. **b. Early diagnosis and treatment prevents progression of the disease** *(Ref: Yanoff & Duker 4th edition, p486)*
    Progression is the natural course of the disease and cannot be prevented. However visual acuity in bright light in good till advanced stage of the disease.

65. **b. Posterior subcapsular cataract** *(Ref: Yanoff & Duker 4th edition, p483)*

66. **c. Retinitis pigmentosa** *(Ref: Yanoff & Duker 4th edition, p482)*

67. **d. Normal ERG** *(Ref: Yanoff & Duker 4th edition, p 482–83)*

68. **c. Electroretinogram** *(Ref: Yanoff & Duker 4th edition, p 1102–03)*

69. **d. The readings on electroretinogram are highly elevated** *(Ref: Yanoff & Duker 4th edition, p 1102–03)*
    The readings on ERG are low or extinguished

70. **b. Bony spicule pigmentary changes** *(Ref: Yanoff & Duker 4th edition, p 483)*
    The classical triad of Retinitis pigmentosa is
    - Waxy disc pallor
    - Arteriolar attenuation
    - Bony spicules or retinal pigmentary changes

71. **a. Absence of rod function** *(Ref: Yanoff & Duker 4th edition, p 480)*

72. **b. Cone dystrophy** *(Ref: Kanski 7th edition, p 656)*

Causes of Night blindness
• Vitamin A deficiency^Q
• Retinitis pigmentosa^Q
• Congenital stationary night blindness (Oguchi's disease, Fundus albipunctatus)
• Choroideremia
• Advanced glaucoma
• Pathological Myopia

73. **a. Oguchi's disease** *(Ref: Yanoff & Duker 4th edition, p 486)*

74. **c. Stargardt's disease** *(Ref: Yanoff & Duker 4th edition, p 492)*
    Stargardt's disease being localised to the macula does not produce any appreciable change in the routine Flash ERG. It shows decrease in the amplitude of Pattern ERG.

75. **d. Best's disease** *(Ref: Yanoff & Duker 4th edition, p 494)*

76. **c. EOG** *(Ref: Yanoff & Duker 4th edition, p 494)*

77. **a. Best's disease** *(Ref: Yanoff & Duker 4th edition, p 494)*

78. **a. Resolving retinal detachment**
    Salt and pepper retinopathy refers to areas of pigmentation along with areas of hypopigmentation in large areas of retina.

Important causes of Salt and Pepper Retinopathy
• Congenital syphilis^Q
• Congenital rubella^Q
• Retinitis pigmentosa
• Leber's congenital amaurosis^Q
• Fundus flavimaculatus^Q
• Albinism
• Cystinosis
• Phenothiazine toxicity^Q

79. b. **Inquire about the use of steroids** (Ref: Yanoff & Duker 4th edition, p 653, 605)
    The question describes features suggestive of Central Serous Retinopathy (CSR). Steroids are one of the risk factors for CSR and hence the answer.

80. d. **Wait and watch for spontaneous recovery** (Ref: Yanoff & Duker 4th edition, p 654, 608)
    The question describes a case of CSR. Treatment for CSR is to wait for spontaneous resolution for 3 months. Hence the answer.

81. b. **Central serous retinopathy** (Ref: Yanoff & Duker 4th edition, p 653)

82. b. **Occult CNVM** (Ref: Yanoff & Duker 4th edition, p 585)
    Indocyanine Green Angiography (ICGA) is used to visualise the choroidal vasculature. One of its main uses is to differentiate an Occult CNVM from a Classic CNVM when the clinical picture is not completely clear. The regimen of Anti-VEGF injection is different for the two types. Prognosis is worse for Occult CNVM.
    Idiopathic Polypoidal Choroidal Vasculopathy (IPCV) is a relatively uncommon condition where the clinical picture is similar to CNVM but the prognosis is poor. Diagnosis of IPCV is also confirmed by ICGA.

83. a. **Hypermetropia** (Ref: Yanoff & Duker 4th edition, p 600–04)
    Causes of CNVM are:
    • Age-related macular degeneration (ARMD) ^Q
    • High myopia ^Q
    • Traumatic choroidal rupture ^Q
    • Angioid streaks ^Q

84. c. **Wet ARMD** (Ref: Yanoff & Duker 4th edition, p 589)

85. a. **Alemtuzumab** (Ref: Yanoff & Duker 4th edition, p 589–92)
    The drugs used for Wet/ Exudative/Neovascular AMD are Bevacizumab and Ranibizumab. Aflibercept is a new drug in this group.

86. d. **ARMD** (Ref: Yanoff & Duker 4th edition, p 589–92)
    Ring scotoma is caused by degeneration in the peripheral retina as in high myopia or Retinitis pigmentosa. Aphakic glasses cause peripheral scotoma due to edge effect.
    ARMD affects the central retina and hence causes central scotoma

87. a. **Pseudoxanthema elasticum** (Ref: Yanoff & Duker 4th edition, p 601)
    Angioid Streaks are idiopathic breaks in the Bruch membrane. (Membrane separating choroid from the RPE). Conditions associated with angioid streaks are
    • Pseudoxanthema elasticum^Q
    • Ehler-Danlos^Q
    • Paget's disease
    • Sickle cell disease

88. d. **Hypertensive retinopathy** (Ref: Yanoff & Duker 4th edition, p 601)

89. d. **Leucocoria + strabismus** (Ref: Yanoff & Duker 4th edition, p 794)
    The most common presentation of Rb is leucocoria followed by strabismus
    The common age of presentation is 18–24 months

90. a. **13q14** (Ref: Yanoff & Duker 4th edition, p 793)

91. b. **Retinoblastoma** (Ref: Yanoff & Duker 4th edition, p 793)

92. b. **Usually bilateral, c. Occurs due to mutation of Rb gene, e. Poorer prognosis then compared to sporadic retinoblastoma** (Ref: Yanoff & Duker 4th edition, p 793)

Retina

93. b. Osteosarcoma (Ref: Kanski 7th edition, p 510)
94. c. Retinoblastoma (Ref: Yanoff & Duker 4th edition, p 794)
95. b. Optic nerve (Ref: Yanoff & Duker 4th edition, p 795)
96. b. Patients with sporadic disease do not pass the gene to their offsprings (Ref: Yanoff & Duker 4th edition, p 793)

    Sporadic retinoblastoma accounts for 94% cases and only 6% cases are familial. But even patients with sporadic disease can transmit the defective gene to the offspring. However, the prognosis is better than the familial variety.

97. b. Retinoblastoma (Ref: Yanoff & Duker 4th edition, p 794-95)

    2-year-old child, leucocoria, intraocular mass with calcification- Diagnosis of Retinoblastoma

98. a. Enucleation (Ref: Yanoff & Duker 4th edition, p 796-99)

    In the section on Retinoblastoma we have discussed the different treatment modalities available for the disease. Indications for different treatment modalities are:

    A. Enucleation
    - Intraocular retinoblastoma involving more than 50% of the globe
    - Intraocular retinoblastoma extending to anterior segment
    - Retinoblastoma with orbital extension (after chemoreduction)

    B. Focal therapy: Photocoagulation, Cryotherapy, Brachytherapy
    - Small intraocular tumours
    - Larger tumours may be treated with focal therapy after chemoreduction (to avoid enucleation)

    C. Chemotherapy
    - Palliative therapy for retinoblastoma with metastasis
    - Bilateral advanced retinoblastoma (to avoid bilateral enucleation)
    - Chemoreduction

    D. Radiotherapy
    - Advanced cases with intracranial extension
    - Orbital radiotherapy for cases with extension to orbital wall

99. b. Enucleation of the right eye and focal therapy of the left eye (Ref: Yanoff & Duker 4th edition, p 796–99)
100. b. Chemotherapy (Ref: Yanoff & Duker 4th edition, p 796)
101. b. Retinoblastoma (Ref: Yanoff & Duker 4th edition, p 796)

    Retinoblastoma arises as a malignant proliferation of the primitive retinal cells called retinoblasts. Histopathological examination shows typical arrangement of tumour cells called rosettes. The different types are
    - **Flexner-Wintersteiner rosettes (highly specific to Rb)**[Q]
    - **Homer-Wright rosettes**[Q]
    - **Pseudo-rosettes**[Q]
    - **Fleurettes**[Q]

102. a. Size> 4 mm, c. Associated glaucoma, d. Undifferentiated tumour cells, e. Scleral involvement (Ref: Yanoff & Duker 4th edition, p 799)

103. b. Removal of the entire globe with portion of the optic nerve (Ref: Yanoff & Duker 4th edition, p 796)

    There are three types of destructive ocular procedures
    1. Enucleation: Removal of the entire globe with a portion of the optic nerve. Absolute indication is **intraocular malignancy**[Q] (retinoblastoma, malignant melanoma). Relative indications are painful blind eye, anterior staphyloma, microphthalmos, and phthisis bulbi. Absolute contraindication is **panophthalmitis**[Q]
    2. Evisceration: Removal of the contents of the globe leaving behind the sclera and the extraocular muscles. Absolute indication is **panophthalmitis**[Q]. Absolute contraindication is **intraocular malignancy**[Q]
    3. Exanteration: It is a radical procedure involving removal of the globe, extraocular muscles, adnexa and a portion of the bony orbit. It is rarely done today

104. a. Malignancy (Ref: Kanski 7th edition, p 116)
105. b. Congenital glaucoma (Ref: Yanoff & Duker 4th edition, p 795)
106. a. Coat's disease (Ref: Yanoff & Duker 4th edition, p 560–61)

    The question describes a male child between 4-10 years of age with telangiectatic retinal vessels and exudative retinal detachment only in one eye. The other eye is normal. Hence the answer is Coat's disease.

107. d. It is associated with peripheral retinal telangiectasia (Ref: Yanoff & Duker 4th edition, p 562)

    Idiopathic Juxtafoveal Telangiectasia is a variant of Coat's disease. In Coat's disease, the telangiectatic vessels are peripherally located along the inferotemporal arcade. In juxtafoveal telengiectasia, the abnormal vessels are macular

108. a. Patau syndrome (Ref: Koole FD et al. Ocular abnormalities in Patau syndrome. Ophthalmic Paediatr Genet; 1990:11:15–21)

109. a. Persistent hyperplastic primary vitreous
(Ref: Kachewar et al. An imaging review of intraocular calcification. J Clin Diagn Res 2014;8:203–05)

Causes of intraocular calcification
• Optic nerve head drusen^Q
• Retinoblastoma^Q
• Choroidal osteoma^Q (Tuberous sclerosis)
• Choroidal angioma
• Coat's disease^Q
• Retinopathy of prematurity^Q
• Healed chorioretinitis^Q (mainly toxoplasmosis)
• Dystrophic calcification: Phthisis bulbi
• Metastatic calcification: Systemic hypercalcemia

110. a. Purtscher's retinopathy
(Ref: Yanoff & Duker 4th edition, p 679)

It is a blockage of the retinal capillaries by emboli leading to multiple hemorrhages and cotton wool spots throughout the retina

Causes are
- **Acute pancreatitis^Q**
- Head and chest trauma
- SLE
- Scleroderma
- Chronic renal failure
- Thrombotic thrombocytopenic purpura
- Fat embolism
- Amniotic fluid embolism

111. b. Head trauma
(Ref: Yanoff & Duker 4th edition, p 679)

112. c. Bacterial endocarditis
(Ref: Kanski 7th edition, p 589)

Roth's spots are retinal hemorrhages with pale or white centres. The important causes are
- Bacterial endocarditis
- Diabetes, hypertension
- Leukaemia
- Pernicious anaemia
- HIV (rarely)

113. b. Roth spot
(Ref: Kanski 7th edition, p 589)

114. a. Chloroquine
(Ref: Yanoff & Duker 4th edition, p 685)

Bull's eye maculopathy is a term given to a condition where the macula shows a central area of hyperpigmentation surrounded by a zone of hypopigmentation. Chloroquine and less commonly Hydroxychloroquine are associated with this type of maculopathy when given for long periods of type as in rheumatoid arthritis

Dose of chloroquine causing maculopathy: 250mg/day for 3 years, cumulative dose of 300 gm ^{Q}

Other causes of Bull's eye maculopathy
• Cone dystrophy
• Cone-rod dystrophy
• Stargardt's disease
• Atypical retinitis pigmentosa (Bardet-Biedl syndrome)
• Benign concentric annular macular dystrophy
• Fenestrated sheen macular dystrophy
• Central areolar choroidal atrophy
• Lipofuscinosis
• Chronic macular hole, ARMD

115. a. Vitreous humour
(Ref: Yanoff & Duker 4th edition, p 430)

Retina

116. a. **Vitreous base at ora serrata** *(Ref: Yanoff & Duker 4th edition, p 431)*

    The attachments of the vitreous are:
    - **Vitreous base (strongest)**[Q]
    - Posterior lens capsule
    - Margins of the optic disc
    - **Macula**
    - Along the blood vessels (weakest)

117. a. **The sample should be stored at 4 degrees Celsius**
118. d. **Ascorbate** *(Ref: Kanski 7th edition, p 730)*
119. d. **CRVO** *(Ref: Kanski 7th edition, p 551–59)*
120. b. **Collection of emulsified silicon oil in the anterior chamber** *(Ref: Yanoff & Duker 4th edition, p 474)*

    Silicon oil is a **vitreous substitute** which is injected into the vitreous cavity after vitrectomy. When the silicon oil gets emulsified, it comes to the anterior chamber and collects in the upper part. It looks like a hypopyon in the upper part of anterior chamber, hence the name. Complications of emulsified silicon oil in anterior chamber are
    - Glaucoma
    - **Band Shaped Keratopathy (BSK)**[Q]

    Vitreous substitutes are
    - Air
    - Expansile gases like **Sulphur hexafluoride (SF6)**[Q], **Perfluoropropane (C3F8)**[Q]
    - Silicon oil
    - Perfluorocarbon liquids (PFCL)
    - Polymeric hydrogels

121. a. **Boat shaped**

    Subhyaloid hemorrhage is collection of blood in the potential space between the posterior vitreous and the internal limiting membrane of retina. It is classically boat-shaped

122. b. **Posterior vitreous detachment** *(Ref: Yanoff & Duker 4th edition, p 433)*
123. a. **Suprachoroidal haemorrhage**

    (Ref: Hypotonic maculopathy: Clinical presentation and therapeutic methods: Thomas M et al; Ophthalmol Ther. 2015 Dec; 4(2): 79–88.)

    Suprachoroidal hemorrhage causes increase in IOP, not hypotony

IMAGE BASED QUESTIONS

1. This is the fundus picture of a 60-year-old male patient who presented with sudden loss of vision in the right eye. He is a known hypertensive and diabetic. What is the possible diagnosis?

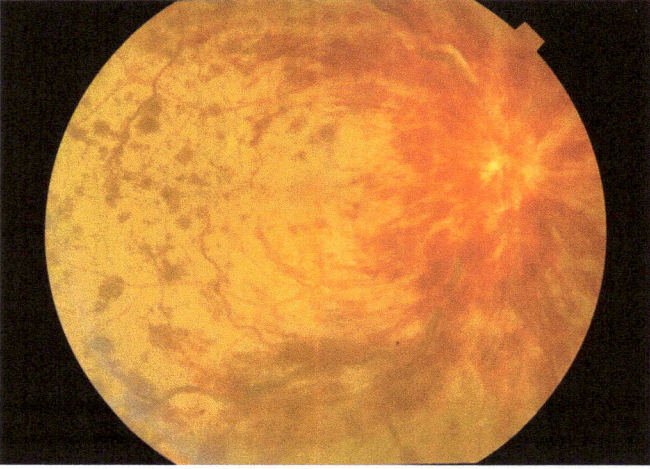

   a. Central retinal artery obstruction
   b. Central retinal vein obstruction
   c. Hypertensive retinopathy
   d. Diabetic retinopathy

2. This is the fundus picture of a 60-year-old patient with history of heart disease who presents with sudden onset loss of vision in the right eye. What is the likely diagnosis?

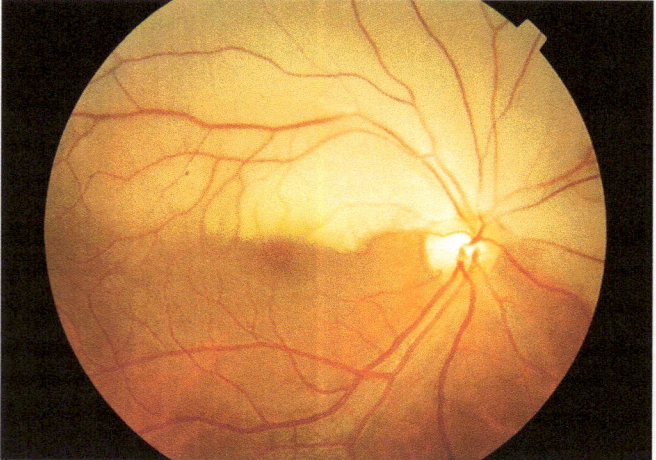

   a. Central retinal artery occlusion
   b. Branch retinal artery occlusion
   c. Central retinal vein occlusion
   d. Optic neuritis

3. This is the fundus picture of a 50-year-old patient with history of hypertension and diabetes. What is the diagnosis?

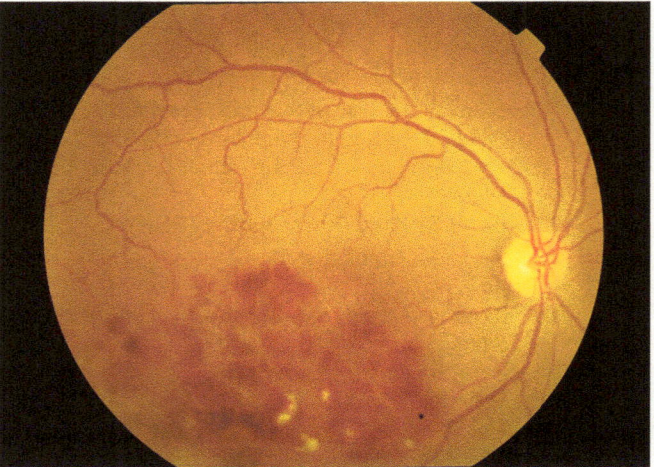

   a. Central retinal vein occlusion
   b. Diabetic retinopathy
   c. Hypertensive retinopathy
   d. Branch retinal vein occlusion

4. This is the fundus photo of an 80-year-old man who presents with gradually progressive decrease in vision in both eyes. On examination he is pseudophakic in both eyes. The fundus in both eyes looks as shown in the photo. What is the probable diagnosis?

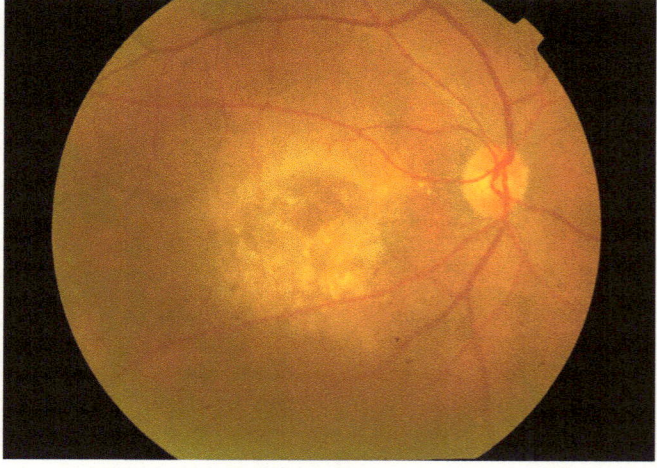

   a. Central serous retinopathy
   b. Cystoid macular edema
   c. Age-related macular degeneration
   d. Stargardt's disease

Answer Key: 1. b   2. b   3. d   4. c

5. This is the fundus photograph of an 80-year-old man who presents with sudden loss of vision in the right eye. What is the possible diagnosis?

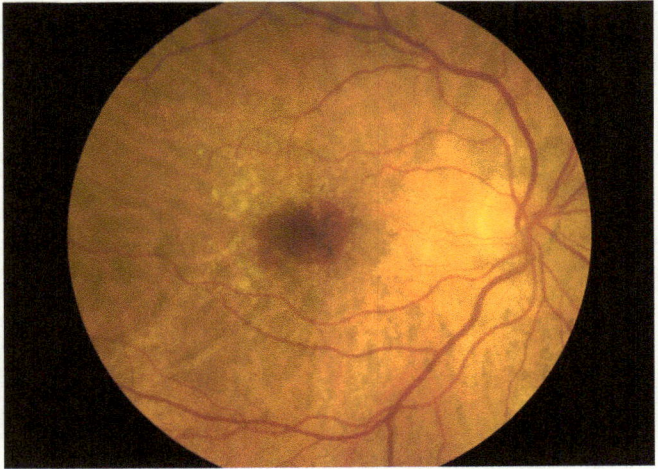

   a. Neovascular ARMD
   b. Dry ARMD
   c. Central serous retinopathy
   d. Stargardt's disease

6. This is the fundus photo of a 25-year-old man who presents with gradually progressive decrease in vision in both eyes, more in dim light and at night. His father and two other siblings have the same problem. What is the diagnosis?

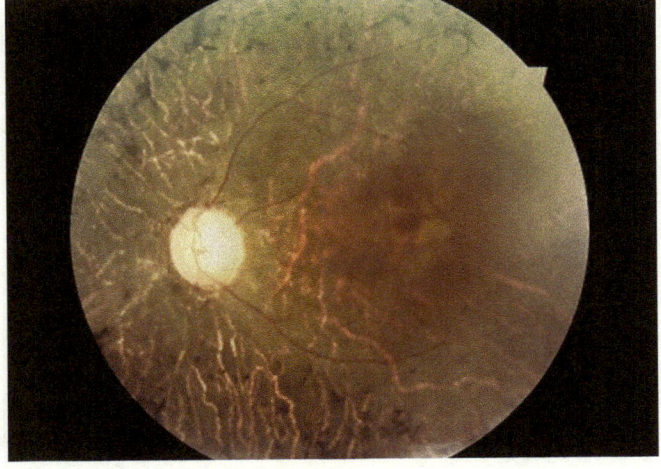

   a. Eales' disease
   b. Retinitis pigmentosa
   c. Stargardt's disease
   d. Best's disease

7. From the clinical photograph, identify the retinal dystrophy:

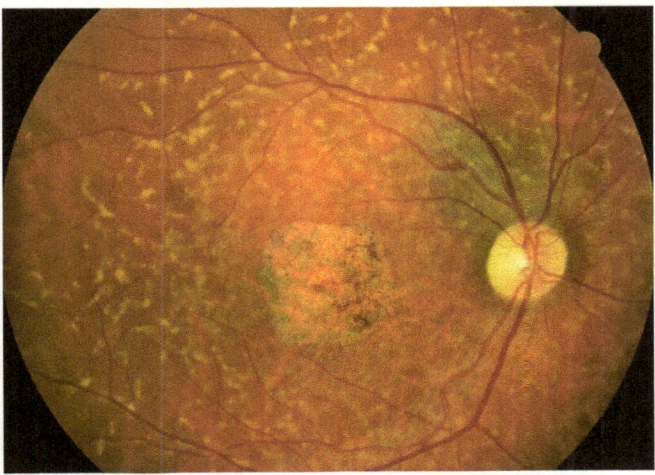

   a. Retinitis pigmentosa
   b. Stargardt's disease and fundus flavimaculatus
   c. Best's disease
   d. Congenital stationary night blindness

8. "Silent choroid" on FFA is a feature of: *(AIIMS 2017)*

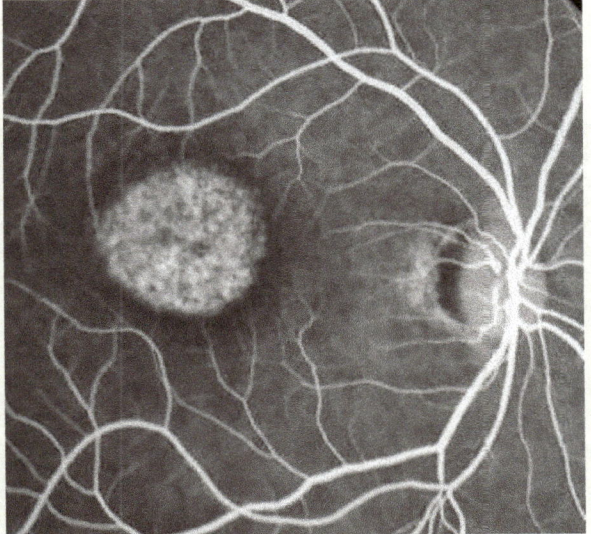

   a. Best's disease
   b. Stargardt's disease
   c. Age related macular degeneration
   d. Cystoid macular edema

Answer Key: 5. a 6. b 7. b 8. b

9. A 15-year-old girl presents with gradually progressive loss of vision in both eyes. The fundus photograph is given below. Her father is affected with the same condition. The diagnosis is confirmed by EOG. What is the diagnosis?

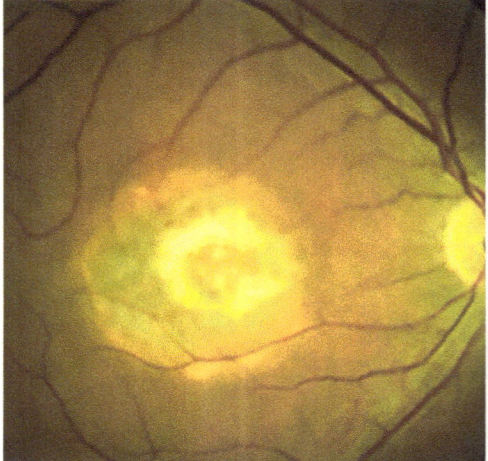

a. Retinitis pigmentosa
b. Fundus flavimaculatus
c. Congenital stationary night blindness
d. Best's disease

10. This is the fundus photo of a 50-year-old patient with history of diabetes mellitus for the past 8 years. The fundus in both eyes shows diabetic retinopathy. What is indicated by the black arrow in the photograph?

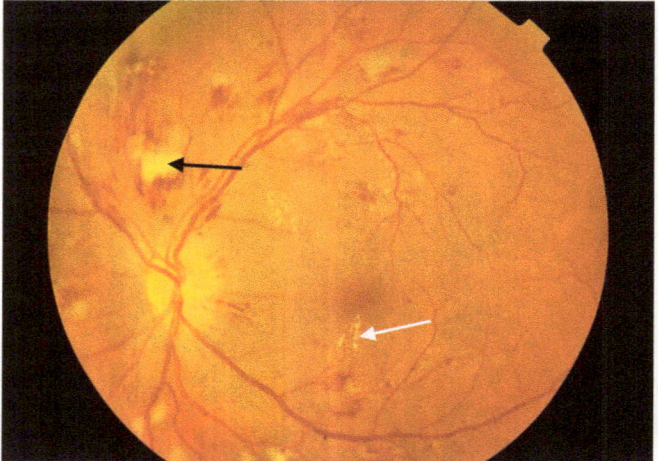

a. Hard exudates
b. Cotton wool spot
c. Neovascularization
d. Microaneurysm

11. From the fluorescein angiography picture, identify the diagnosis: *(Nov AIIMS 2017)*

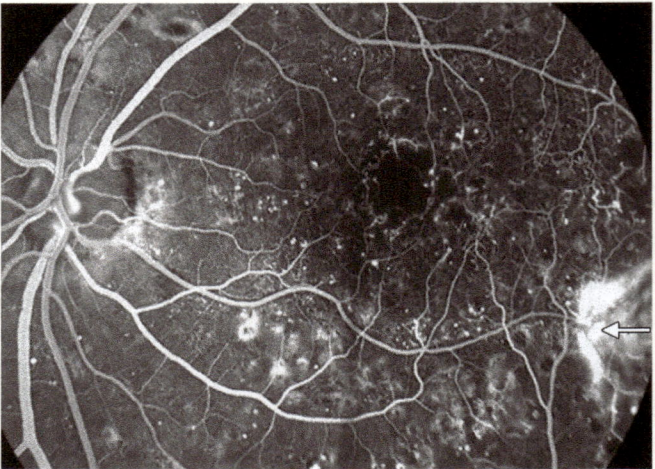

a. Non-proliferative diabetic retinopathy
b. Proliferative diabetic retinopathy
c. Familial dominant drusen
d. Birdshot choroidopathy

12. This is the fundus photo of a 6-year-old boy who presented with decrease in vision in the left eye. The right eye was normal. The left eye fundus showed areas of exudation as seen in the photograph. Telangiectatic vessels were also seen. What is the possible diagnosis?

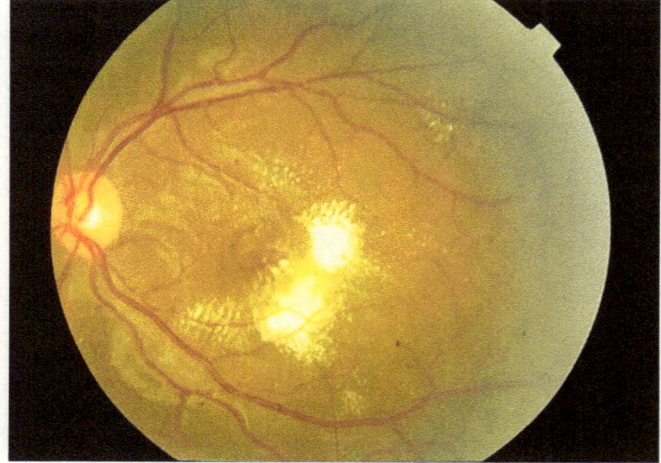

a. Eales' disease
b. Coat's disease
c. PHPV
d. Retinal artery macroaneurysm

Answer Key: 9. d 10. b 11. b 12. b

13. The device shown in the photograph is used for Indirect Ophthalmoscopy. What is the power of the lens that should be used with it to visualise the retina?
(Nov AIIMS 2016)

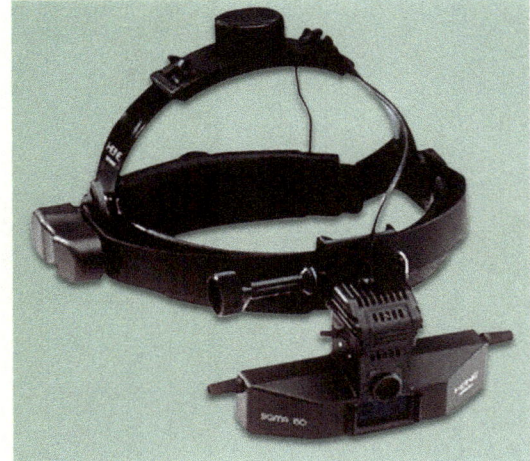

a. 90D
b. 58D
c. −55D
d. 20D

14. What magnification is achieved by viewing the retina by the instrument shown in the picture?

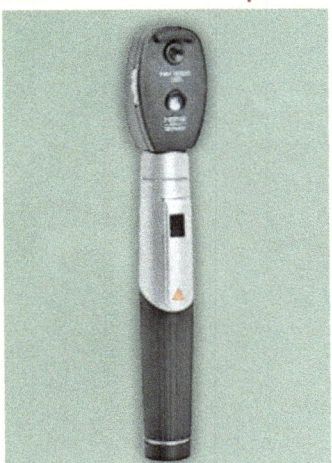

a. 5 times
b. 15 times
c. 3 times
d. No magnification

15. A 26-year-old male presented with sudden diminution of vision in left eye. The fluorescein angiography revealed a picture as shown below. A diagnosis of central serous retinopathy was made. The optical coherence tomography (OCT) image is shown below. Which of the retinal layers is indicated by the arrow in the photograph?
(Nov AIIMS 2016)

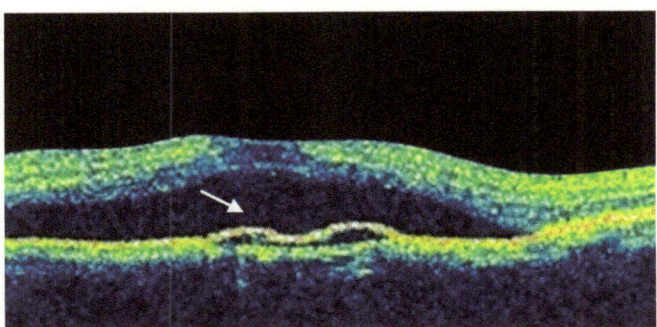

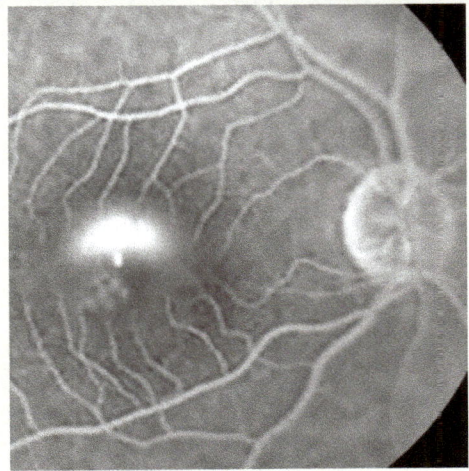

a. Retinal pigment epithelium
b. Outer plexiform layer
c. Inner nuclear layer
d. Nerve fiber layer

16. A diabetic patient complains of decrease in vision about 6 weeks posts-cataract surgery. The OCT macula of the patient is given below. What is the possible diagnosis?

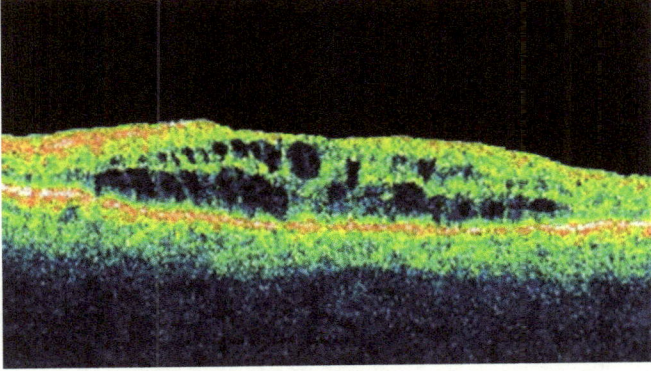

a. Central serous retinopathy
b. Cystoid macular edema
c. Macular hole
d. Epiretinal membrane

| Answer Key: | 13. d | 14. b | 15. a | 16. b |

Self Assessment and Review of Ophthalmology

17. A patient with a history of blunt trauma presents with decrease in vision in the right eye. The OCT macula of the patient is shown in the picture. What is the diagnosis?

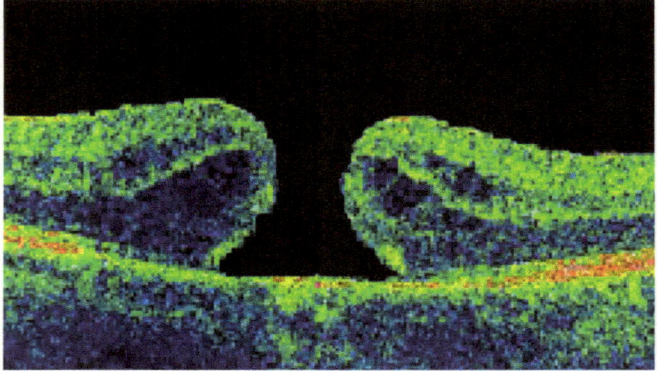

   a. Retinal detachment
   b. Macular hole
   c. Macular break
   d. Retinal dialysis

18. The OCT image of an 80-year-old patient presenting with gradually progressive decrease in vision in both eyes is given. What is the diagnosis?

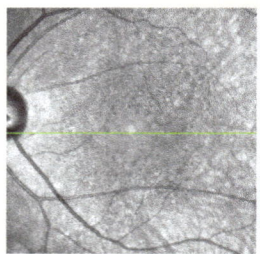 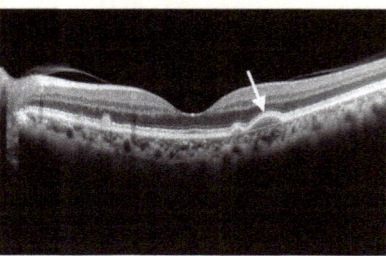

   a. Central serous retinopathy
   b. Dry ARMD
   c. Macular hole
   d. Cystoid macular edema

19. From the OCT image in the question, what is the diagnosis?

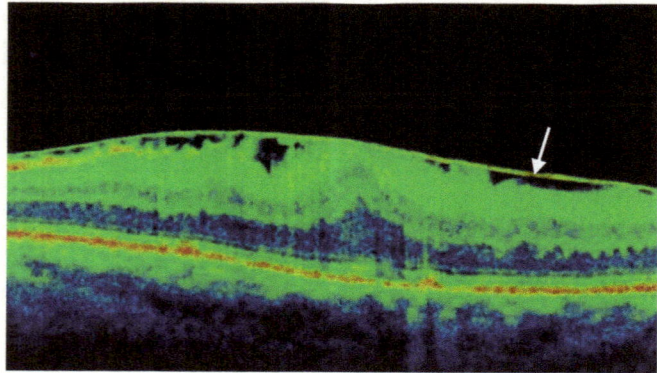

   a. Central serous retinopathy
   b. Cystoid macular edema
   c. Macular hole
   d. Epiretinal membrane

20. A high myopic patient presents with sudden loss of vision in the left eye. The loss of vision was preceded by flashes. From the photograph, what is the diagnosis?

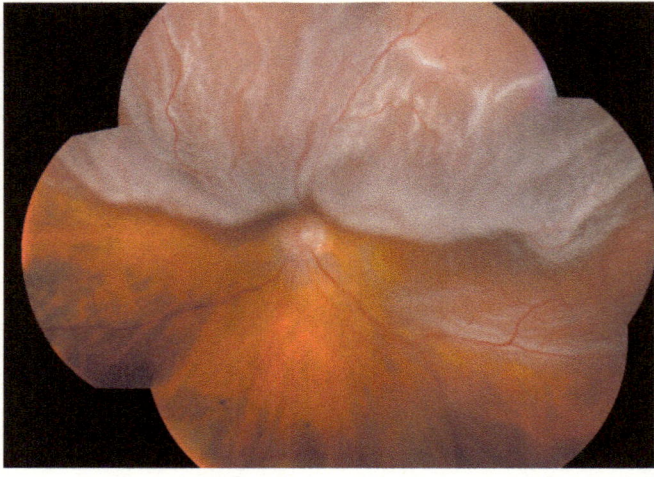

   a. Exudative retinal detachment
   b. Central serous retinopathy
   c. Rhegmatogenous retinal detachment
   d. Optic neuritis

21. What does the condition in the given clinical photograph predispose to?

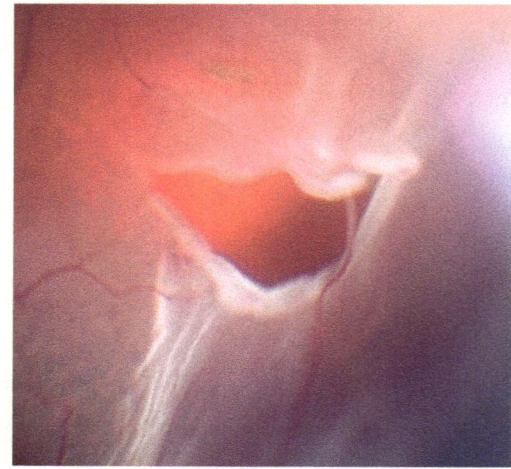

   a. Cystoid macular edema
   b. Tractional retinal detachment
   c. Rhegmatogenous retinal detachment
   d. Eales' disease

Answer Key: 17. b   18. b   19. d   20. c   21. c

22. What is the diagnosis from the above USG B-Scan of the patient:

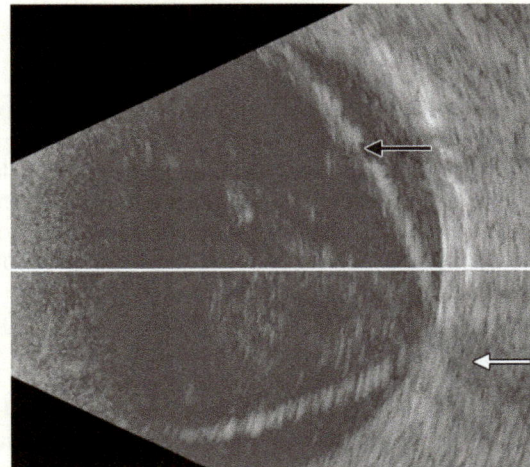

a. Normal
b. Posterior vitreous detachment
c. Retinal detachment
d. Choroiditis

23. A patient presents with severe loss of vision within 1 week of uneventful cataract surgery. On examination there is congestion, hypopyon and no view of the posterior segment. The USG B-Scan of the patient is given. What is the diagnosis?

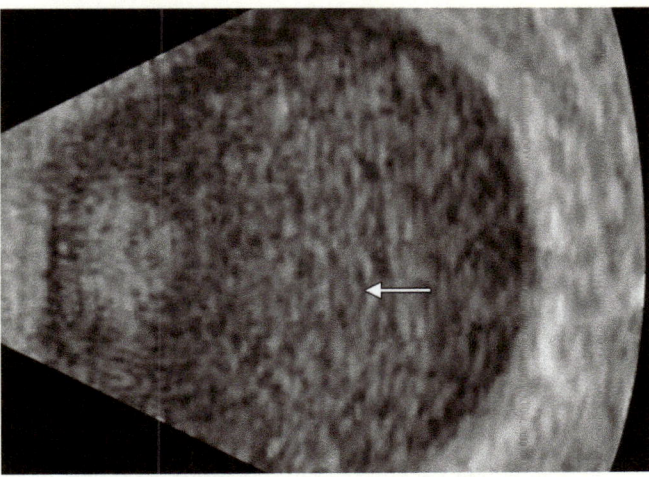

a. Dislocated IOL
b. Retinal detachment
c. Endophthalmitis
d. Macular edema

24. A patient who is on treatment for rheumatoid arthritis presents with complain of decrease in vision. The fundus picture and FFA picture of the patient are given. What is the probable diagnosis? *(AIIMS 2018)*

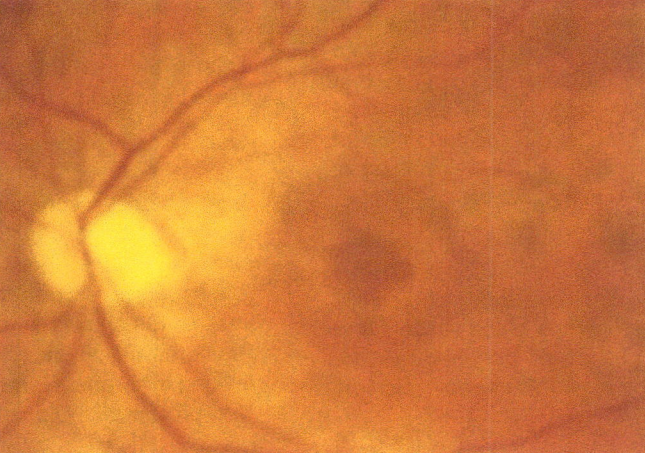

a. Cystoid macular edema
b. Central serous retinopathy
c. Bull's eye maculopathy
d. Age related macular degeneration

Answer Key: 22. c   23. c   24. c

ANSWERS AND EXPLANATIONS

1. **Answer: b. Central retinal vein obstruction**
   (Ref: Yanoff & Duker 4th edition p 526–28)
   This is the typical splashed tomato appearance of CRVO where the entire fundus is scattered with hemorrhages.

2. **Answer: b. Branch retinal artery occlusion**
   (Ref: Yanoff & Duker 4th edition p 518–23)
   The fundus photo shows whitening of the superior part of the retina whereas the lower half of the retina is normal. Hence the answer is branch retinal artery occlusion.
   In central retinal artery occlusion, the whole retina appears white due to ischemia with red foveal reflex or cherry red spot.

3. **Answer: d. Branch retinal vein occlusion**
   (Ref: Yanoff & Duker 4th edition p 531–32)
   In this fundus picture, hemorrhages are seen only along one arcade of vessels whereas the rest of the fundus is normal. Hence the answer is BRVO.
   In CRVO, the entire fundus is scattered with hemorrhages.

4. **Answer: c. Age related macular degeneration**
   (Ref: Yanoff & Duker 4th edition p 581–83)
   The yellowish dots seen at the macula in the fundus picture are drusens (Dry ARMD)

5. **Answer: a. Neovascular ARMD**
   (Ref: Peyman's Principles and Practice of Ophthalmology 2nd edition p 849)
   The photograph shows hemorrhage at the macula with surrounding yellowish dots or drusens. It suggests that the patient had Dry ARMD which gradually progressed to Wet/Neovascular ARMD resulting in the formation of Choroidal Neovascular Membrane (CNVM). Subretinal bleed from the CNVM is shown in the picture.

6. **Answer: b. Retinitis pigmentosa**
   (Ref: Yanoff & Duker 4th edition p 483–84)
   The fundus photo shows classical triad of retinitis pigmentosa with pale disc, attenuated blood vessels and bony spicules or pigments in the mid peripheral retina. The blackish dots seen are the pigments or bony spicules.

7. **Answer: b. Stargardt's disease and fundus flavimaculatus**
   (Ref: Peyman's Principles and Practice of Ophthalmology, 2nd edition, p 907–11)
   The photograph shows yellowish flecks scattered throughout the retina (Fundus flavimaculatus) with an atrophic area at the center of the macula typically called "**beaten bronze appearance**"[Q] (Stargardt's disease). Hence the answer.

8. **Answer: b. Stargardt's disease**
   (Ref: Kanski 8th edition p 654–55)
   Stargardt's disease and Fundus flavimaculatus are variants of the same retinal dystrophy characterized by diffuse RPE involvement due to accumulation of lipofuscin. Stargardt's disease mainly involves the center of macula and is hence called **juvenile macular dystrophy**. In early stages, there is mottling of the RPE with subsequent RPE atrophy.
   The FFA picture in the question shows a dark background with a hyperfluorescent (bright) area at the center of the macula. The dark background is due to masking of the choroidal fluorescence by diffuse RPE abnormality. Hence it is called 'silent choroid" or "dark choroid". Advanced RPE atrophy causes the hyperfluorescence at the center.

9. **Answer: d. Best's disease**
   (Ref: Peyman's Principles and Practice of Ophthalmology. 2nd edition, p 914–18)
   The photograph shows a yellowish lesion at the center of the macula. This is due to deposition of lipofuscin at the RPE level. The associated family history and the diagnosis by EOG points to the diagnosis of Best's disease.

10. **Answer: b. Cotton wool spot**
    (Ref: Yanoff & Duker 4th edition p 542–44)
    The photograph shows diabetic retinopathy with intraretinal hemorrhages, hard exudates and cotton wool spots. The small, well circumcumscribed white dots indicated by the white arrow are hard exudates. The larger ill-defined white areas indicated by the black arrow are cotton wool spots.

11. **Answer: b. Proliferative diabetic retinopathy**
    (Ref: Kanski 8th edition pg 529–31)
    The picture given in the question shows multiple hyperfluorescent (bright) spots which represent the leaking microaneurysms. Along the inferotemporal arcade there is a hyperfluorescent area showing leak from new blood vessels (as shown by the arrow). Hence the diagnosis is Proliferative Diabetic Retinopathy (PDR). However, if only leaking microaneurysms are present, the diagnosis will be Non-proliferative Diabetic Retinopathy (NPDR).

12. **Answer: b. Coat's disease**
    (Ref: Yanoff & Duker 4th edition p 560–61)
    Coat's disease is classically described in boys between 5-10 years of age. It is a unilateral condition presenting with telangiectatic vessels and exudation, usually in the inferotemporal quadrant of the retina.

13. **Answer: d. 20D** *(Ref: Yanoff & Duker 4th edition p 69)*
    The indirect ophthalmoscope is used to visualize the retina along with a 20D lens. Instruments used to visualize retina are:

- Direct Ophthalmoscope
  - **15 times magnification**^Q
  - Limited field of view : about 6 degrees
  - **Image is virtual and erect**^Q
  - Illumination is limited
  - **No stereoscopic view**
- Binocular Indirect Ophthalmoscope with condensing lens
  - The condensing lens commonly used is a **biconvex lens** of 20D. Other lenses used may be 13D or 30D
  - The magnification produced is Power of eye (60D) Power of converging lens. Hence magnification with 20D lens is 3 times. However it may range from **2–5 times** depending on the power of the converging lens.
  - Image is **real and inverted**^Q. Image is formed **between the observer and the converging lens**^Q
  - **Stereoscopic view**
  - Illumination is very strong, hence **useful in hazy media**
  - Field of view is up to the retinal periphery. Maximum field with minimum magnification will be achieved with 30D lens
- Slit lamp Biomicroscopy with fundus lens
  - The lenses commonly used are **biconvex lenses of 90D, 78D or 60D**. The magnification produced is Power of eye/ Power of the lens. Hence 90D and 78D lenses actually cause minification. **60D lens gives 1:1 magnification**^Q. Image is inverted.
  - **Hruby lens** is a **plano concave** lens of **minus 55D** which is attached to the slit lamp. **Image is erect**.
  - **Goldman's 3 mirror lens** may also be used. This lens has to be placed on the cornea and is a contact procedure
  - **Stereoscopic view.**

14. Answer: b. 15 times
(Ref: Yanoff & Duker 4th edition p 69)

The instrument shown in the picture is a direct ophthalmoscope which produces a magnification of around 15 times while viewing the retina.

15. Answer: a. Retinal pigment epithelium
(Ref: Yanoff & Duker 4th edition p 606–07)

- **Central serous retinopathy (CSR) or Central serous chorioretinopathy (CSCR)** is an idiopathic detachment of **neurosensory retina** in the area of the macula due to accumulation of serous fluid. It may also be associated with detachment of the **retinal pigment epithelium**.
- The fundus fluorescein angiography (FFA) image in the question shows the classical **Smoke-stack sign**^Q. It is also known as **Mushroom/Umbrella** pattern.

- The more commonly seen FFA pattern is **Ink-blot sign**^Q (Enlarging dot sign)

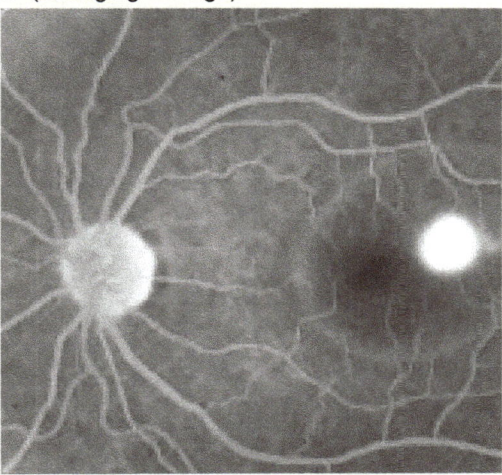

- OCT is an imaging technique which uses **infra-red light**^Q to create a three-dimensional image of different structures of the eye. Below is an image of OCT macula in a normal eye. It shows the different retinal layers with a depression at the centre of the macula which is the fovea

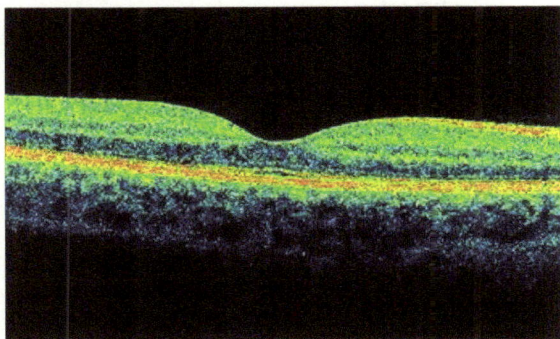

- The picture given in the question above is also an OCT image of the macula but you can now make out that it shows detachment of the neurosensory retina from the underling layers. Beneath the detached neurosensory retina, another small detachment is seen, as depicted by the arrow. This is the detachment of retinal pigment epithelium.

16. Answer: b. Cystoid macular edema
(Ref: Yanoff & Duker 4th edition p 453)

The OCT shows multiple cystic spaces within the retinal layers with increase in retinal thickness suggestive of cystoid macular oedema (CME). Diabetic patients undergoing cataract surgery are more prone to develop CME.

17. Answer: b. Macular hole
Ref.: Peyman's Principles and Practice of Ophthalmology 2nd edition, p 999-1000

The OCT image a defect at the centre of the macula extending up to the RPE. This is a full-thickness macular hole.

18. **Answer: b. Dry ARMD**

    (Ref: Peyman's Principles and Practice of Ophthalmology 2nd edition, p 845-48)

    The OCT shows irregularity at the RPE level suggestive of drusens. (indicated by arrow). Hence the answer is Dry ARMD

19. **Answer: d. Epiretinal membrane**

    The OCT picture shows a thick membrane above the retinal layers (indicated by arrow). Hence the diagnosis is epiretinal membrane.

20. **Answer: c. Rhegmatogenous retinal detachment**

    (Ref: Peyman's Principles and Practice of Ophthalmology 2nd edition, p 1021–25)

    The photograph shows bullous retinal detachment superiorly with corrugated appearance. This, along with the preceding history of flashes points to the diagnosis of rhegmatogenous retinal detachment.

21. **Answer: c. Rhegmatogenous retinal detachment**

    (Ref: Peyman's Principles and Practice of Ophthalmology 2nd edition, p 1021–25)

    The picture shows a horseshoe retinal tear which is an important risk factor for rhegmatogenous retinal detachment.

22. **Answer: c. Retinal detachment**

    The picture shows a membrane like structure detached from the retinochoroidal complex (indicated by black arrow) but attached at the optic nerve head (indicated by white arrow). This is the classical picture of retinal detachment.

    If the detached membrane is not attached to the optic nerve head, it is likely to be posterior vitreous detachment.

23. **Answer: c. Endophthalmitis**

    The USG B-Scan shows dense echoes in the vitreous cavity suggestive of vitreous exudates, hence the diagnosis is endophthalmitis.

24. **Answer: c. Bull's eye maculopathy**

    (Ref: Peyman's Principles and Practice of Ophthalmology 2nd edition, p 906)

    Drug-induced maculopathy is caused mainly by the prolonged used of Chloroquine and less commonly by Hydroxy-chloroquine in the treatment of rheumatoid arthritis.

    The typical fundus picture is called Bull's eye maculopathy. The ocular side effects of Chloroquine are:

    - Drug induced keratopathy
    - Toxic cataract
    - Toxic optic neuropathy
    - Bull's eye maculopathy

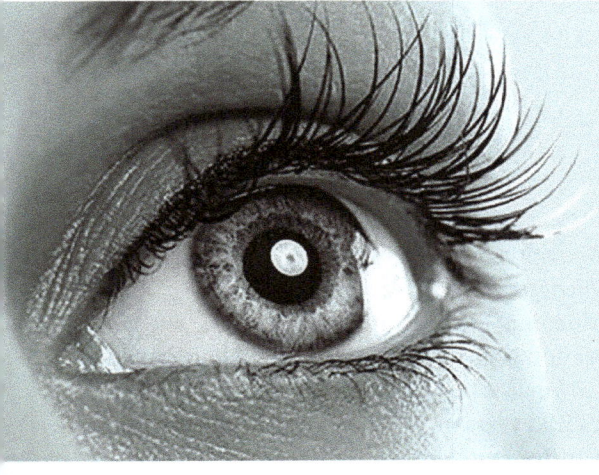

Uveal Tract

Uvea is the middle vascular coat of the eyeball comprising of the following parts
- Iris
- *Ciliary body*: It is divided into pars plicata and pars plana
- Choroid

UVEITIS

Uveitis refers to the inflammation of the uveal tract

Clinical Classification

- *Acute*: Sudden onset uveitis with limited duration
- *Recurrent*: Repeated episodes of uveitis separated by periods of inactivity lasting at least 3 months
- *Chronic*: Persistent inflammation which promptly recurs within 3 months when treatment is stopped.

Anatomical classification

Depending upon the anatomical part of the uveal tract which is involved, uveitis can be classified into
- *Anterior uveitis:* It involves the iris and pars plicata of the ciliary body, hence known as **iridocyclitis**[Q]
- *Intermediate uveitis:* It involves the pars plana of the ciliary body and the surrounding vitreous, hence known as **pars planitis**[Q]
- *Posterior uveitis*: It involves mainly the choroid with associated inflammation of the overlying retina and vitreous, hence called **chorioretinitis**

Pathological Classification

- Non-granulomatous
- Granulomatous

Causes of granulomatous uveitis

- **Tuberculosis**[Q]
- **Leprosy**[Q]
- **Syphilis**[Q]
- Herpetic uveitis

Contd...

Contd...
- Brucellosis
- Histoplasmosis, Cryptococcosis
- **Sarcoidosis**[Q]
- **Vogt Koyanagi Harada's disease**[Q]
- **Sympathetic Ophthalmitis**[Q]
- **Lens induced uveitis**[Q]
- **Foreign body uveitis**[Q]

Clinical Features

Anterior Uveitis

Clinical features of acute anterior uveitis are
- Pain, photophobia, redness associated with decrease in vision
- Circumciliary congestion
- *Keratic precipitates (KPs)*[Q]: These are proteinaceous deposits on the back of the cornea. They are usually present in a triangular area in the lower part of the cornea, known as **Arlt's triangle**[Q]. They are divided into
    - *Mutton fat KPs*: Large KPs seen in **granulomatous uveitis**[Q]. They are composed of **epithelioid cells and macrophages**[Q]
    - *Medium and small sized KPs*: Seen in non-granulomatous uveitis. They are composed of lymphocytes
    - Pigmented KPs-Seen in old uveitis
    - *Red KPs*: Seen in haemorrhagic uveitis
- Anterior chamber
    - *Aqueous cells*: They are inflammatory cells in the aqueous humour
    - *Aqueous flare*: This is due to the disruption of the blood-aqueous barrier and increase in the protein content of the aqueous humour. The flare becomes clinically detectable due to a phenomenon known as **Tyndall effect**[Q]
- Pupillary Signs
    - Constriction of the pupil due to ciliary spasm
    - *Posterior synechiae*: Segmental adhesions between the iris and the anterior capsule of the lens occurs due to prolonged inflammation. Dilatation of

this pupil gives a distorted appearance known as **festooned pupil**^Q
- *Ring synechiae*: When synechiae are formed around 360 degrees of the pupillary margin, it is called ring synechiae or **seclusio pupillae**^Q. When the pupillary area is covered by an inflammatory membrane it is known as **occlusio pupillae**^Q
- *Iris nodules*: Seen in **granulomatous inflammation**
  - *Koeppe's nodules*^Q: Seen at the pupillary border
  - *Bussaca's nodules*^Q: Seen at the base of the iris

Intermediate Uveitis
- Patient mainly complains of floaters
- *Anterior segment*: May be quiet or associated with mild inflammation
- *Posterior segment*: Whitish vitreous exudates are seen surrounding the pars plana, more prominent inferiorly. These exudates are known are **snow-ball opacities.** They coalesce to form an inflammatory plaque around the pars plana which is referred to as **snow-banking**^Q

Posterior Uveitis
- Decrease in vision is the common complaint. Pain, photophobia and redness are generally absent
- Anterior chamber is generally quiet
- *Posterior chamber*: It shows the following features
  - Vitritis
  - *Choroiditis*: It may be unifocal or multifocal
  - Periphlebitis
  - Neuroretinitis

Complications of uveitis
- *Complicated cataract:* Most common complication of **recurrent anterior uveitis**^Q
- Secondary glaucoma
  - *Pupillary block glaucoma:* Formation of seclusio or occlusio pupillae does not allow the aqueous to move to the anterior chamber. As the result the iris bulges forward forming **iris bombe** leading to secondary angle closure
  - *Open angle glaucoma:* This occurs due to blockage of the trabecular meshwork by the inflammatory cells
- *Cystoid macular oedema:* It is mainly seen in intermediate uveitis^Q
- *Exudative retinal detachment:* It is seen in posterior uveitis^Q
- *Band shaped keratopathy:* It is seen in chronic cases
- *Iris atrophy, rubeosis:* It is seen in chronic cases
- *Phthisis bulbi:* It is seen in chronic cases

Treatment
- Anterior uveitis
  - *Topical steroids*: Drug of choice^Q
  - Periocular steroid in the form of sub-tenon injection is given in severe or unresponsive cases
  - *Mydriatric -cycloplegic like atropine*: This relieves the **ciliary spasm**^Q and **prevents the formation of posterior synechiae**^Q
- Intermediate uveitis
  - Periocular steroid
  - Systemic steroids
- Posterior uveitis
  - Systemic steroids
- Panuveitis
  - Systemic steroids
  - *Cytotoxic agents and Immunomodulators*: These are given in cases like **Sarcoidosis, Sympathetic Ophthalmitis, VKH**^Q

Causes of Uveitis

Different causes of uveitis affect the eye in different ways. The basic presentation is that of uveitis but with certain special characteristics for each. We have to memorize these salient features for MCQ examinations

JUVENILE RHEUMATOID ARTHRITIS
- It has three varieties
  - *Pauciarticular*: **Pauciarticular Seronegative**^Q variety has the **most common** association with uveitis
  - Polyarticular
  - *Systemic*: **Systemic variety**^Q or **Still's disease** has **least common** association with uveitis
- Presents as **bilateral non-granulomatous anterior uveitis**
- This anterior uveitis is not associated with circumcorneal congestion, hence also known as **white eye uveitis**^Q
- Associated with **complicated cataract**, extensive posterior synechiae and band shaped keratopathy
- **IOL insertion is generally avoided**^Q after cataract surgery in these cases due to possibility of severe inflammatory reaction.

HLA B-27 ASSOCIATED UVEITIS
- It is associated with diseases like **Ankylosing Spondylitis**^Q, Reiter's Syndrome and Psoriatic Arthritis
- **Acute severe recurrent non-granulomatous anterior uveitis**^Q is seen

Uveal Tract

FUCH'S HETEROCHROMIC IRIDOCYCLITIS
- It is a distinctive entity seen in young females
- Associated with **unilateral non-granulomatous anterior uveitis**
- **Diffusely distributed stellate white keratic precipitates**^{Q}
- **Absence of posterior synechiae**^{Q}
- **Spontaneous hyphaema** due to rupture of small filiform vessels seen in the angle. This is called **Amsler's sign**^{Q}
- Iris heterochromia is seen

POSSNER SCHLOSSMAN SYNDROME
- It is a distinctive entity seen in young males
- **Mild non-granulomatous anterior uveitis is associated with severe rise of IOP (about 50-60 mm Hg)**^{Q}
- It is also called **glaucomatocyclitic crisis**^{Q}

BEHCET'S DISEASE
- It is associated with **HLA B-5**^{Q}
- **Bilateral non-granulomatous anterior and posterior uveitis**
- **Associated with transient hypopyon**^{Q}
- Features of posterior segment involvement like vitritis, periphlebitis, retinitis may be present

TOXOPLASMOSIS
- Toxoplasma is an obligate intracellular parasite where cat is the definitive host and human being is the intermediate host
- Infection occurs usually in the foetal life
- **Unilateral non-granulomatous anterior and posterior uveitis is seen.**
- In the posterior segment, there is severe vitritis associated with **a focal necrotising retinochoroiditis**^{Q}, usually at the macula. This is called **headlight in fog appearance**^{Q}
- Treatment is Clindamycin Cotrimoxazole/Pyrimethamine along with steroids

SARCOIDOSIS
- **Bilateral chronic granulomatous panuveitis is seen. Sometimes it may present as only intermediate uveitis**
- Vitritis with **snow ball opacities**
- *Periphlebitis*: Sheathing of vessels is seen due to periphlebitis. This is known as **candle wax dripping**^{Q}
- Posterior segment nodules known as **Lander's Sign**^{Q} may be seen
- Choroidal granuloma may be seen
- Optic nerve head granuloma may also be seen

VOGT-KOYANAGI-HARADA'S DISEASE
- It is an **oculo-neuro-cutaneous** condition. It is associated with HLA DR4
- The cutaneous features are
  - Alopecia
  - Vitiligo
  - Poliosis
- The neurological features are
  - Meningismus
  - Encephalopathy
  - Tinnitus
- The ocular features are
  - **Bilateral granulomatous panuveitis**^{Q}
  - Bilateral multiple areas of exudative retinal detachment
  - Perilimbal vitiligo, known as **Suguira's sign**
  - In chronic cases, the fundus has a dull yellow colour known as **sunset glow fundus**

SYMPATHETIC OPHTHALMITIS
- It is a distinctive condition where **severe penetrating trauma**^{Q} to the area of the **ciliary body**^{Q} in one eye leads to **bilateral granulomatous panuveitis**
- The eye which has suffered the trauma is called the **exciting eye** and the other eye is called as the **sympathising eye**
- The first symptom of sympathising ophthalmitis is blurring of near vision^Q due to loss of accommodation
- The first sign is retrolental flare^Q
- Anterior and intermediate uveitis are seen
- In the posterior segment, yellowish white subretinal granulomas called as **Dalen Fuch's nodules**^{Q} are seen
- To prevent sympathetic ophthalmia, severely traumatised eyes with no visual potential may be **enucleated**

HIV ASSOCIATED UVEITIS
- HIV associated uveitis is a **bilateral non-granulomatous panuveitis**^{Q}.
- Anterior and intermediate uveitis may be present but involvement is mainly posterior
- In the posterior segment, the most commonly seen feature is **HIV microangiopathy**^{Q} which presents as **cotton wool spots**^{Q}
- Treatment is anti-retroviral therapy associated with steroids

- HIV is associated with certain opportunistic infections which also give rise to various types of uveitis. These are
  - *Cytomegalovirus retinitis (CMV)*: This mainly causes **posterior uveitis**. It is characterised by severe retinal vasculitis, haemorrhages and opacification. This is called **sauce and cheese retinopathy**[Q] or **pizza-pie retinopathy.** The vasculitis extends along the blood vessels relentlessly like a fire to reach the optic nerve head, hence also called **brushfire retinopathy.** The treatment is intravenous Gancyclovir/ Cidofovir/ Foscarnet. Intravitreal Gancyclovir and Cidofovir are also given
  - **Pneumocystitis carinii associated chorioretinitis**
  - *Progressive outer retinal necrosis (PORN)*: This is a type of **necrotising retinochoroiditis** seen in HIV patients due to fulminant infection by **varicella zoster virus.** It initially involves only the outer retinal layers but rapidly progresses to full-thickness involvement and necrosis. Treatment is intravenous ganciclovir
  - **Cryptococcus associated chorioretinitis**
  - **Tuberculosis, leprosy, syphilis** associated **panuveitis** is also seen in HIV patients.

HERPES SIMPLEX ASSOCIATED UVEITIS

- **Granulomatous anterior uveitis**, usually associated with high IOP.
- It is associated with **extensive iris atrophy**[Q]
- Posterior uveitis is also seen
- *Acute retinal necrosis (ARN)*: It is a typical **necrotising retinitis** seen in young male patients due to HSV infection. It is a retinal vasculitis with multiple focii of chorioretinitis which rapidly progresses to necrosis. The posterior pole is usually spared. Treatment is intravenous acyclovir along with steroids

White dot syndromes

This is a broad term which encompasses different entities which are associated with posterior uveitis giving rise to multiple white dots in the chorioretina. These are actually microgranulomas composed of lymphocytes and macrophages. The important causes of white dot syndromes are

Contd...

- Acute posterior multifocal placoid pigment epitheliopathy
- Serpiginous choroidopathy
- Birdshot retinochoroidopathy
- Punctuate inner choroidopathy
- Progressive subretinal fibrosis and uveitis
- Presumed ocular histoplasmosis syndrome (POHS)
- Multiple evanescent white dot syndrome (MEWDS)

Causes of anterior uveitis

- Juvenile rheumatoid arthritis[Q]
- HLA B27 associated uveitis[Q]
- Fuch's heterochromic iridocyclitis[Q]
- Possner Schlossman syndrome[Q]
- Inflammatory bowel disease
- Herpes simplex
- Lens induced uveitis
- Behcet's disease

Causes of posterior uveitis

- Toxoplasmosis
- Herpes simplex associated acute retinal necrosis
- Behcet's disease
- HIV associated uveitis
- CMV retinitis
- White dot syndromes

Causes of intermediate uveitis

- Sarcoidosis
- Toxocariasis
- Candidiasis
- Multiple sclerosis

Causes of panuveitis

- Sarcoidosis[Q]
- Vogt- Koyanagi- Harada's disease[Q]
- Sympathetic ophthalmitis[Q]
- Tuberculosis[Q]
- Leprosy[Q]
- Syphilis[Q]
- Herpes zoster[Q]

Contd...

MASQUERADE SYNDROME

These are conditions which mimic uveitis. They are
- Intraocular malignancies like retinoblastoma, choroidal melanoma, choroidal metastasis
- Leukaemia
- Lymphoma
- Amyloidosis

Ophthalmia nodosum: Granulomatous uveitis due to caterpillar hair[Q]

> **Must Remember**
> - *Amsler's sign:* Fuch's Heterochromic Iridocyclitis
> - *Candle-wax dripping sign:* Sarcoidosis
> - *Bilateral hypopyon uveitis:* Behcet's disease
> - *Lander's sign:* Sarcoidosis
> - *Dalen Fuch's nodules:* Sympathetic ophthalmitis
> - *Sunset glow fundus:* Vogt Koyanagi Harada's disease

QUESTIONS

1. **True about ciliary body is:** *(PGI 2013)*
   a. Located about 10 mm from the corneoscleral junction
   b. Consists of pars plana and pars plicata
   c. Contraction of the ciliary body helps in accommodation
   d. Secretes aqueous humour
   e. Derives its blood supply from the short posterior ciliary arteries

2. **Granulomatous uveitis is seen in:** *(PGI)*
   a. Vogt- Koyanagi Harada's disease
   b. Fuch's heterochromic iridocyclitis
   c. Behcet's disease
   d. Sarcoidosis
   e. Psoriatic arthritis

3. **Koeppe's and Busacca's nodules are characteristic of:** *(Jipmer)*
   a. Granulomatous uveitis
   b. Non-granulomatous uveitis
   c. Recurrent uveitis
   d. Chronic uveitis

4. **Mutton fat keratic precipitates are seen in:** *(APPG 2006)*
   a. Non-granulomatous uveitis
   b. Granulomatous uveitis
   c. Posterior uveitis
   d. Intermediate uveitis

5. **Mutton fat keratic precipitates are not seen in:** *(Manipal 2009)*
   a. Tuberculosis
   b. Fuch's heterochromic iridocyclitis
   c. Sarcoidosis
   d. Fungal infections

6. **Anterior uveitis is characterized by all except:** *(AIIMS 2000)*
   a. Aqueous flare
   b. Shallow anterior chamber
   c. Circumcorneal congestion
   d. Miosis

7. **The type of synechiae in iris bombe is:** *(AIPG)*
   a. Ring
   b. Total
   c. Filiform
   d. Goniform

8. **What is the most common complication of recurrent anterior uveitis?** *(AIIMS 2000)*
   a. Staphyloma
   b. Cataract
   c. Glaucoma
   d. Vitreous haemorrhage

9. **Drug of choice for acute iridocyclitis:** *(DPG 2009)*
   a. Steroids
   b. Acetazolamide
   c. Atropine
   d. Antibodies

10. **Primary objective of use of atropine in anterior uveitis is:** *(AIIMS 2000)*
    a. Relaxation of ciliary muscle
    b. Increase blood flow
    c. Prevent posterior synechiae formation
    d. Increase supply of antibodies

11. **Which drug should not be used in raised IOP with uveitis:** *(PGI)*
    a. Timolol
    b. Pilocarpine
    c. Atropine
    d. Acetazolamide

12. **Snow banking is seen in:** *(PGI/ DNB 2014)*
    a. Pars planitis
    b. Endophthalmitis
    c. Coat's disease
    d. Eales' disease

13. **In a patient of anterior uveitis, decrease in vision due to posterior segment involvement may be because of:** *(AIIMS 2012)*
    a. Vitreous floaters
    b. Inflammatory disc oedema
    c. Exudative retinal detachment
    d. Cystoid macular oedema

14. **Iridocyclitis is a feature of:** *(AIIMS 2002)*
    a. Juvenile rheumatoid arthritis with systemic features
    b. Seropositive pauciarticular JRA
    c. Seronegative pauciarticular JRA
    d. Seropositive polyarticular JRA

15. **Most common cause of chronic iridocyclitis in children:** *(DNB 2015)*
    a. Juvenile idiopathic arthritis
    b. Sjogren's Syndrome
    c. Behcet's disease
    d. SLE

16. **A 25-year-old man has pain, redness and mild diminution of vision in one eye for the past 3 days. There is also history of low backache for the past one year. On examination there is circumcorneal congestion, few keratic precipitates on the corneal endothelium, 2+ cells in the anterior chamber. Intraocular pressure is within normal limits. The patient is likely to be suffering from:** *(AIIMS 2005)*
    a. Acute angle closure glaucoma
    b. HLA B-27 associated anterior uveitis
    c. JRA associated anterior uveitis
    d. Herpetic keratitis

17. **All of the following are true regarding anterior uveitis in ankylosing spondylitis except:** *(SGPGI)*
    a. More common in female
    b. Recurrent attacks are seen
    c. Fibrinous reaction in anterior chamber is seen
    d. Narrowing of joint spaces in sacroiliac joints is a feature

18. **HLA B5 is associated with:** *(APPG 2014)*
    a. Vogt-Koyanagi Harada's disease
    b. Possner Schlossman syndrome
    c. Behcet's disease
    d. Reiter's syndrome

Uveal Tract

19. In Fuch's heterochromic iridocyclitis, true is :
    (Manipal)
    a. 60% cases develop glaucoma
    b. Show a good response to steroids
    c. Lens implantation following cataract surgery is contraindicated
    d. Hyphaema during cataract surgery is seen

20. A young patient presents with gradual blurring of vision in the left eye. Slit lamp reveals fine stellate keratic precipitates, aqueous flare and posterior subcapsular cataract. No posterior synechiae are seen. The most likely diagnosis is:
    a. Intermediate uveitis
    b. Heerfordt's disease
    c. Heterochromic iridocyclitis of Fuch
    d. Subacute iridocyclitis

21. Skin depigmentation, bilateral uveitis and tinnitus is a feature of: *(AIIMS 2011)*
    a. Waardenberg syndrome
    b. Vogt Koyanagi Harada disease
    c. Alport's syndrome
    d. Werner's syndrome

22. A 32-year-old male presents with blurring of vision in the right eye. On examination there is mid iritis, severe vitritis and a focal necrotic lesion on the macula. The most likely diagnosis is: *(AIIMS)*
    a. Multiple evanescent white dot syndrome
    b. Ocular toxoplasmosis
    c. Multifocal choroiditis
    d. Ocular sarcoidosis

23. Most rapid and accurate method to diagnose CMV retinitis: *(AIIMS 2013)*
    a. Virus isolation in intraocular fluid
    b. Viral antigen detection in vitreous
    c. Viral nucleic acid detection in intraocular fluid
    d. Viral antibody in blood by ELISA

24. Ocular manifestations of HIV are all except: *(PGI)*
    a. Predisposition to bacterial, viral and fungal infections
    b. Kaposi sarcoma
    c. CMV retinitis
    d. Cotton wool spots
    e. Intraocular lymphoma

25. Most common ocular lesion in HIV : *(DNB 2015)*
    a. CMV retinitis
    b. Cotton wool spots
    c. Kaposi sarcoma
    d. Choroiditis

26. Treatment of CMV retinitis is: *(DNB 2015)*
    a. Oseltamivir
    b. Valgancyclovir
    c. Amantadine
    d. Fludrabine

27. Sauce and cheese retinopathy is seen in: *(DNB 2013)*
    a. Toxoplasmosis
    b. CMV retinitis
    c. Tuberculosis
    d. Sarcoidosis

28. Headlight in fog appearance is characteristic of: *(DNB 2013)*
    a. CMV retinitis
    b. Tuberculosis
    c. Toxoplasmosis
    d. Sarcoidosis

29. In which of these conditions is intraocular pressure very high with minimum inflammation? *(Maharashtra 2010/ NEET 2016)*
    a. Acute iridocyclitis
    b. Glaucomatocyclitic crisis
    c. Acute angle closure glaucoma
    d. Hypertensive uveitis

30. Sympathetic ophthalmitis is: *(AIIMS)*
    a. U/L suppurative uveitis
    b. B/L suppurative uveitis
    c. U/L non-suppurative uveitis
    d. B/L non-suppurative uveitis

31. Earliest symptom of sympathetic ophthalmitis is: *(AIIMS)*
    a. Photophobia
    b. Pain
    c. Loss of near vision
    d. Loss of distant vision

32. A 20-year-old man complains of difficulty in reading newspaper in the right eye 4 weeks after gunshot injury in the left eye. The likely diagnosis is: *(AIPG 2001)*
    a. Macular oedema
    b. Sympathetic ophthalmitis
    c. Optic nerve avulsion
    d. Delayed vitreous haemorrhage

33. First sign in sympathetic ophthalmitis: *(AIIMS 2001)*
    a. Aqueous flare
    b. Keratic precipitates
    c. Retrolental flare
    d. Constriction of the pupil

34. Dalen Fuch's nodules are seen in: *(AIIMS/PGI)*
    a. Sympathetic ophthalmitis
    b. Myopia
    c. Spring catarrh
    d. Retinal detachment

35. Which of the following is incorrect regarding phthisis bulbi? *(AIPG 2009)*
    a. The intraocular pressure is increased
    b. Calcification of the globe is common
    c. Sclera is thickened
    d. Size of the globe is reduced

36. Uveal effusion syndrome is associated with all except: *(AIPG 2009)*
    a. Myopia
    b. Ciliochoroidal detachment
    c. Structural defects in the sclera
    d. Nanophthalmos

ANSWERS AND EXPLANATIONS

1. b. **Consists of pars plicata and pars plana, c. Contraction of ciliary body helps in accommodation, d. Secretes aqueous humour**

   (Ref: Yanoff & Duker 4th edition, p 687-88)

   The ciliary body begins about 1.5 mm posterior to the limbus in the horizontal meridian and 2 mm posterior to the limbus in the vertical meridian. It ends about 7-8 mm posterior to the limbus (7 mm superiorly, nasally, inferiorly and 7.5-8 mm temporally)

   It is supplied by the long posterior ciliary arteries and the anterior ciliary arteries which form the major arterial circle at the root of the iris

2. a. **Vogt Koyanagi Harada's disease, d. Sarcoidosis** *(Ref: Kanski 7th edition, p 422, 65)*
3. a. **Granulomatous uveitis** *(Ref: Yanoff & Duker 4th edition, p 694-95)*
4. b. **Granulomatous uveitis** *(Ref: Yanoff & Duker 4th edition, p 695)*
5. b. **Fuch's heterochromic iridocyclitis** *(Ref: Kanski 7th edition, p 465)*
6. b. **Shallow anterior chamber** *(Ref: Yanoff & Duker 4th edition, p 694-95)*
7. a. **Ring** *(Ref: Yanoff & Duker 4th edition, p 695)*
8. b. **Cataract** *(Ref: Yanoff & Duker 4th edition, p 695)*
9. a. **Steroids** *(Ref: Yanoff & Duker 4th edition, p 697-98)*
10. a. **Relaxation of the ciliary muscle** *(Ref: Yanoff & Duker 4th edition, p 697-98)*

    Atropine is the adjuvant drug that must be given in all cases of uveitis. The main role of atropine is to relieve the ciliary spasm which makes the patient comfortable

11. b. **Pilocarpine** *(Ref: Kanski 7th edition, p 364)*

    Pilocarpine causes miosis and ciliary spasm. It also increases intraocular inflammation. Hence it is not preferred in inflammatory glaucoma

12. a. **Pars planitis** *(Ref: Yanoff & Duker 4th edition, p 695)*
13. d. **Cystoid macular oedema** *(Ref: Yanoff & Duker 4th edition, p 699)*

    Cystoid macular oedema is more common with intermediate uveitis but may also occur with anterior uveitis

14. c. **Seronegative pauciarticular JRA** *(Ref: Yanoff & Duker 4th edition, p 750)*
15. a. **Juvenile idiopathic arthritis** *(Ref: Yanoff & Duker 4th edition, p 750)*
16. b. **HLA-B27 associated anterior uveitis** *(Ref: Yanoff & Duker 4th edition, p 748)*
17. a. **More common in female** *(Ref: Yanoff & Duker 4th edition, p 748)*
18. c. **Behcet's disease** *(Ref: Yanoff & Duker 4th edition, p 758)*
19. d. **Hyphaema during cataract surgery is seen** *(Ref: Yanoff & Duker 4th edition, p 772)*
20. c. **Heterochromic iridocyclitis of Fuch** *(Ref: Yanoff & Duker 4th edition, p 772)*
21. b. **Vogt Koyanagi Harada's disease** *(Ref: Yanoff & Duker 4th edition, p 761-62)*
22. b. **Ocular toxoplasmosis** *(Ref: Yanoff & Duker 4th edition, p 739)*

    This is a classical description of ocular toxoplasmosis or "headlight in fog appearance"

23. c. **Viral nucleic acid detection in intraocular fluid** *(Ref: Yanoff & Duker 4th edition, p 706)*

    PCR for detection of viral nucleic acid in intraocular fluid is the best investigation for CMV retinitis

24. e. **Intraocular lymphoma** *(Ref: Kanski 7th edition, p 442)*

    HIV may be associated intraocular lymphoma rarely but if one option has to be chosen, then this is the one.

25. b. **Cotton wool spots** *(Ref: Kanski 7th edition, p 442)*
26. b. **Valgancyclovir** *(Ref: Yanoff & Duker 4th edition, p 707)*
27. b. **CMV retinitis** *(Ref: Yanoff & Duker 4th edition, p 704-05)*
28. c. **Toxoplasmosis** *(Ref: Yanoff & Duker 4th edition, p 739)*
29. b. **Glaucomatocyclitic crisis (explained in the chapter on glaucoma)**
30. d. **B/L non-suppurative uveitis** *(Ref: Yanoff & Duker 4th edition, p 767)*
31. c. **Loss of near vision**

Uveal Tract

32. b. **Sympathetic ophthalmitis** *(Ref: Yanoff & Duker 4th edition, p 767)*
33. c. **Retrolental flare** *(Ref: Yanoff & Duker 4th edition, p 767)*
34. a. **Sympathetic ophthalmitis** *(Ref: Yanoff & Duker 4th edition, p 767)*
35. a. **The intraocular pressure is increased**

    Pthisis bulbi occurs as the end stage of severe ocular disease. It is described as a shrunken and hypotonous globe with atrophic and disorganised ocular tissue.

    Causes are chronic uveitis, perforating injuries, panophthalmitis, multiple ocular surgeries etc.

    Features are
    - No visual potential
    - Globe is small and shrunken with disorganised ocular tissue so that ocular structures cannot be identified clearly
    - Ciliary body shutdown leading to hypotony
    - Thickening of the sclera
    - It may be associated with intraocular calcification

    A shrunken, hypotonous globe with nil visual potential where ocular structures can be identified is called as **atrophic bulbi**

36. a. **Myopia** *(Ref: Kanski 7th edition, p 709)*

    Uveal effusion is seen in Nanophthalmos or Dwarf eye. It is a condition where the axial length of the eyeball is less than 19 mm. The features are
    - Familial variety may be autosomal dominant or recessive
    - High hypermetropia
    - Lens thickness is disproportionate to the axial length of the eyeball
    - Shallow anterior chamber with occludable angles
    - Predisposition to angle closure glaucoma
    - Thickened sclera which obstructs the outflow through the vortex veins leading to uveal effusion
    - Ciliochoroidal detachment
    - Exudative retinal detachment

IMAGE BASED QUESTIONS

1. This is the anterior segment photograph of a 20-year-old man who presented with acute anterior uveitis. Looking at the picture, which one of the following seems the least likely diagnosis?

   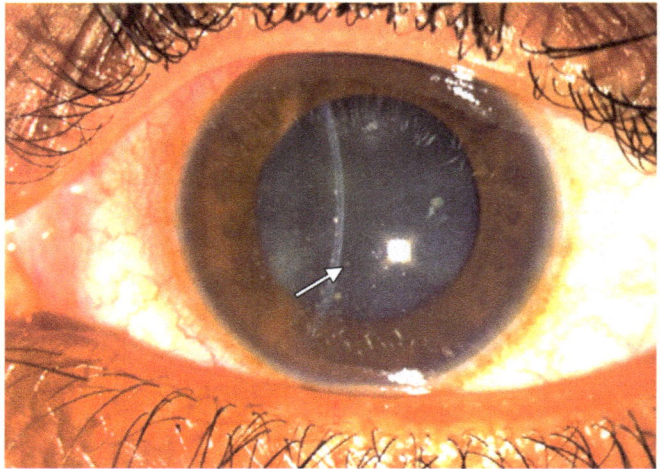

   a. Tuberculosis b. Ankylosing spondylitis
   c. Sarcoidosis   d. Leprosy

2. A 25-year-old man presents with complains of pain, redness and decrease in vision in the right for the past one week. On examination, the visual acuity in the right eye is 6/18. The anterior segment is normal. The posterior segment shows vitritis and the fundus photograph is given above. The left eye is normal. What can be the possible diagnosis?

   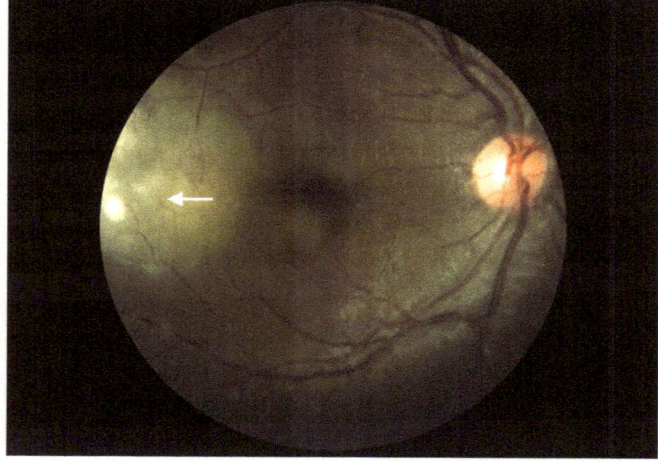

   a. Retinal detachment b. Coat's disease
   c. Posterior uveitis   d. Eales' disease

3. The fundus photograph of a patient is given. What is the diagnosis?

   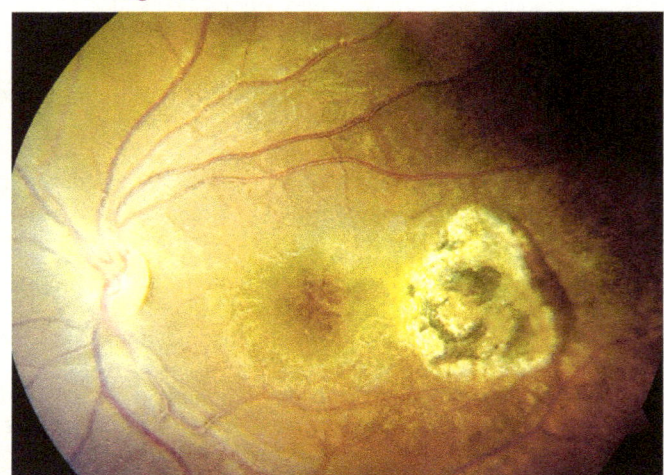

   a. Healed toxoplasma retinochoroiditis
   b. Active toxoplasma retinochoroiditis
   c. Candida endophthalmitis
   d. CMV retinitis

4. A patient with history of back pain presents with recurrent episodes of pain and redness in both eyes. The clinical picture is given. What is the investigation that should be ordered for the patient?

   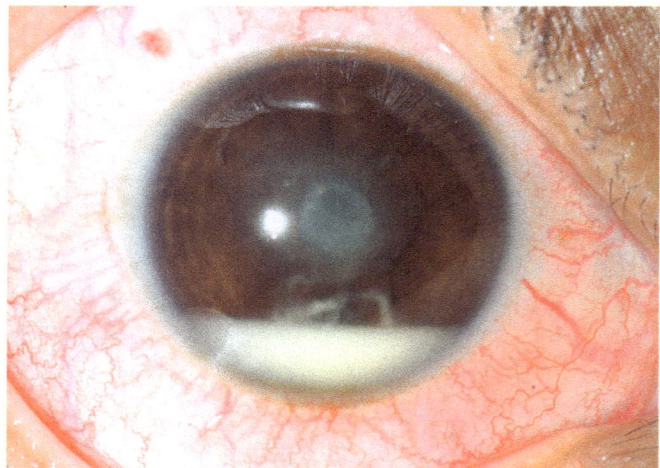

   a. HLA DR 5
   b. Mantoux test
   c. HLA B-27
   d. ANA

Answer Key: 1. b   2. c   3. a   4. c

Uveal Tract

5. A patient presents with bilateral chronic granulomatous panuveitis. The clinical picture is given. What is the possible diagnosis?

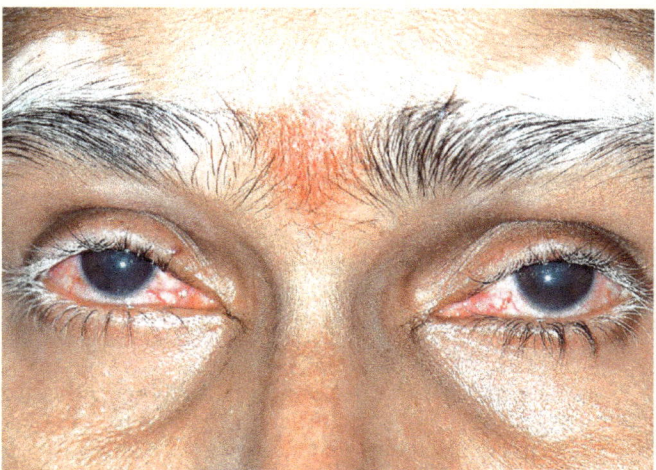

a. Sarcoidosis
b. Systemic lupus erythromatosus
c. Vogt Koyanagi Harada (VKH) syndrome
d. Behcet's disease

6. An HIV-positive patient with low CD-4 count presents with sudden painless loss of vision. From the fundus picture, what is the likely diagnosis?

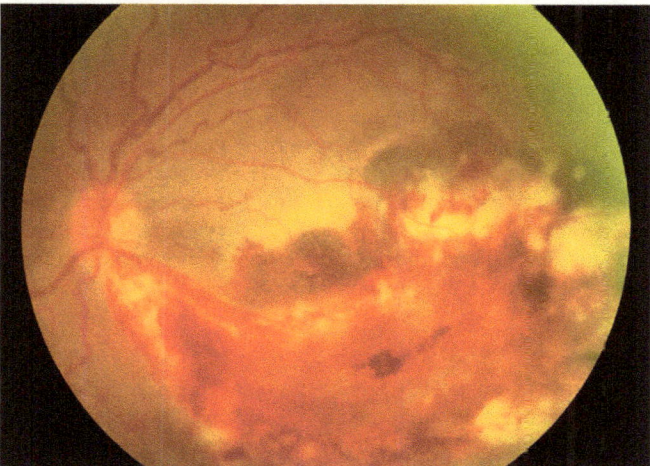

a. Candida endophthalmitis
b. CMV retinitis
c. Pneumocystis carinii choroiditis
d. HIV vasculopathy

Answer Key: 5. c   6. b

ANSWERS AND EXPLANATIONS

1. **Answer: b. Ankylosing spondylitis**
   (Ref: Yanoff & Duker 4th edition p 748-49)
   The black arrow in the picture points to brownish deposits on the corneal endothelium. These are called keratic precipitates. Here these KPs are large and greasy (mutton- fat KPs) suggestive of granulomatous uveitis. Ankylosing spondylitis causes non-granulomatous uveitis and hence is the answer.

2. **Answer: c. Posterior uveitis**
   (Ref: Yanoff & Duker 4th edition p 740-41)
   The patient presents with pain, redness and decrease in vision. Examination shows vitritis. The arrow in the photograph points to the patch of choroiditis. Hence the answer is posterior uveitis or choroiditis.

3. **Answer a. Healed toxoplasma retinochoroiditis**
   (Ref: Peyman's Principles and Practice of Ophthalmology, 2nd edition pg 1359)
   This is a classical picture of healed toxoplasma retinochoroiditis. It is a well-circumscribed punched out lesion on the posterior pole with irregular pigmentation.

4. **Answer c. HLA B-27**
   (Ref: Peyman's Principles and Practice of Ophthalmology, 2nd edition p 1359)
   The picture shows severe non-granulomatous (Note the absence of mutton fat keratic precipitates on the corneal endothelium) anterior uveitis with fibrinous reaction and hypopyon. Recurrent severe non-granulomatous uveitis with history of back pain suggests the possibility of Ankylosing spondylitis and hence HLA B-27 is the answer.

5. **Answer c. Vogt Koyanagi-Harada(VKH) syndrome**
   (Ref: Peyman's Principles and Practice of Ophthalmology, 2nd edition p 1359)
   The photograph shows evidence of vitiligo with poliosis. In a patient with bilateral chronic granulomatous panuveitis, this points to the diagnosis of VKH syndrome.

6. **Answer b. CMV retinitis**
   (Ref: Peyman's Principles and Practice of Ophthalmology, 2nd edition p 1371)
   This is a classical picture of **brushfire retinopathy** described in CMV retinitis. A large patch of hemorrhage is seen inferiorly with areas of retinitis (yellowish lesions).

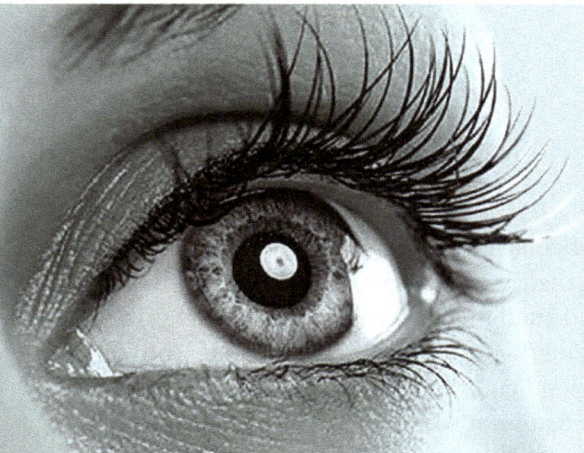

7 Optics and Refraction

Basics of refraction in the eye

- The **total refractive power** of the eye is **58–60 diopters**[Q]
- The refractive power of the **cornea** is **44–45 diopters**[Q]
- The refractive power of the **lens** is **15–16 diopters**[Q]
- The refractive indices of the different ocular media are
  - *Cornea:* 1.376[Q]
  - *Aqueous humor:* 1.336
  - *Lens:* 1.386[Q]
  - *Vitreous humor:* 1.336

The eye may be considered as a convex or converging lens of 58–60 D power and the retina is like a screen, which is located at its principal focus. So the parallel rays of light coming from infinity are brought to focus at a point on the retina. But the eye is capable of adjusting its refractive power according to the distance at which an object is to be viewed. For example, rays of light coming from a near object are divergent rays. So more refractive power is needed by the eye to converge these rays to the retina. This ability to adjust or increase the refractive power so as to focus at near objects is called accommodation.

Accommodation: The changes that occur during accommodation are:
- Contraction of the ciliary muscle
- Relaxation of the ciliary zonules
- Increase in the anterior curvature of the lens
- Increase in the refractive power of the eye.

Presbyopia

It is defined as a **physiological decrease in the amplitude of accommodation with age**[Q] which results in difficulty in near vision. The factors responsible are
- Decrease in the tone of the ciliary zonules[Q]
- Rigidity of the zonules with age[Q]
- Thickening of the lens with age which decreases its flexibility to change its shape[Q]

Hence, presbyopes are to be given **convex lenses for near work**[Q]

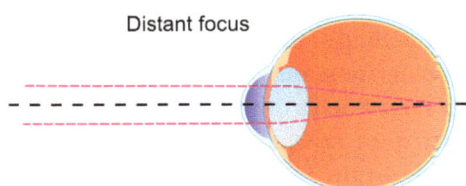
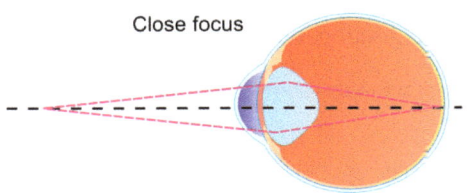

Fig. 1: Emmetropic eye

ERRORS OF REFRACTION

Myopia

In myopia, parallel rays of light coming from infinity, in the absence of accommodation, converge to a point in front of the retina. This means that the refractive power of the myopic eye is more than what it needs. Hence myopia is treated with **minus or concave lenses**[Q]. The different types of myopia are
- *Axial*: Due to increased axial length
- *Curvatural*: Due to increase in corneal curvature, as in keratoconus
- *Index*: Due to increase in refractive index of the eye, as in nuclear cataract.

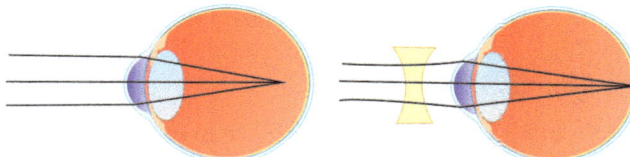

Fig. 2: Myopic eye

Childhood myopia can be broadly divided into
- *Simple myopia*: Refractive error is usually less than –6D with no degenerative changes in the eye
- *Pathological myopia*: Refractive error may increase up to 20–25D with degenerative changes in the eye.

Changes in the myopic eye[Q]

- Pseudoproptosis due to large eyeball
- Exotropia or divergent squint[Q]
- Thin cornea[Q]
- Increased risk of open angle glaucoma
- Subluxation and dislocation of lens[Q]
- Complicated cataract
- Vitreous degeneration
- Fundus changes
  - Myopic crescent temporal to the disc due to stretching of the eyeball
  - **Posterior staphyloma**[Q]
  - **Foster Fuch's maculopathy**[Q]
  - **Lacquer cracks**[Q] **and choroidal neovascular membrane (CNVM)**
  - Peripheral retinal degenerations like lattices, breaks and holes
  - Rhegmatogenous retinal detachment[Q]

Hypermetropia

In this condition, the parallel rays of light coming from infinity, in the absence of accommodation, converge to a point behind the retina. Thus, a hypermetropic eye has less refractive power than it needs and so it is treated with **plus lenses or convex lenses**[Q]. Hypermetropia is divided into:

- *Latent hypermetropia*: This is masked by the tone of the ciliary body
- *Facultative hypermetropia*: This is masked by the voluntary accommodative effort of the individual
- *Absolute hypermetropia*: This is the hypermetropia which is apparent

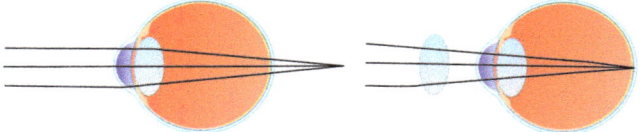

Fig. 3: Hypermetropic eye

Astigmatism

In this condition, there is a difference in refractive powers in the two principal meridians of the eye. As a result, the rays in the two meridians are focused at different points leading to a blurred image. Based on the axis of the two principal meridians, astigmatism is of two main types

- *Regular astigmatism*: Here the two meridians are perpendicular to each other. If the horizontal axis is steeper than vertical, it is called **"against the rule"** astigmatism. If the vertical is steeper than horizontal, it is called **"with the rule"** astigmatism. If the axes are perpendicular but obliquely inclined, it is called **oblique astigmatism.**
- *Irregular astigmatism*: Here the two meridians are not perpendicular to each other.

Astigmatism is treated with **cylindrical lenses**[Q] **(lenses with power only in one axis)**.

Anisometropia

This is a condition where there is a significant difference in the refractive power of the two eyes. As a result of this, **there is a significant difference in the image size of the two eyes. This is called aniseikonia**[Q]. To avoid this, high anisometropia should be treated with contact lenses (Contact lenses produce less change in image size as compared to spectacles).

TREATMENT OF REFRACTIVE ERRORS

- Spectacles.
- *Contact lenses*: Contact lenses are lenses worn on the surface of the eye for the correction of refractive error. The different types of contact lenses are:
  - *Soft lenses*: These are made up of **hydroxyethylmethacrylate (HEMA)**[Q] and used for the correction of myopia, hyperopia and low astigmatism
  - *Rigid gas permeable lenses (RGP)*: These are made up of **cellulose acetate butyrate (CAB)**[Q]. They are used for **high astigmatism.** Irregular astigmatism has to be corrected with RGP lenses.

Advantages of contact lenses

- Less change in image size, hence useful in high degree of anisometropia
- Useful for correcting irregular astigmatism which is not amenable to spectacles
- Greater field of vision
- High power spectacles have aberrations like spherical, chromatic, prismatic etc. These are minimum with contact lenses

Optics and Refraction

> **Complications with contact lenses**
>
> - **Giant papillary conjunctivitis**[Q]
> - *Corneal hypoxia with vascularization:* The corneal epithelium receives its oxygen from the air and glucose from the aqueous and limbal vessels. **Contact lenses reduce the availability of oxygen to the cornea**[Q]. As a result, the metabolism shifts from aerobic to anaerobic. **So the content of lactate and pyruvate in the cornea are increased**[Q].
> - Corneal abrasion
> - *Microbial infections:* Most common organism is **Pseudomonas**[Q]
> - Overwear syndrome also called as contact lens warpage

Other uses of Contact Lenses
- Bandage contact lenses are used in non-healing epithelial defects of the cornea, excessive thinning of the cornea, impending perforation
- Contact lenses are also used as a vehicle for drug delivery.

➢ *Refractive surgery*: Surgeries to correct refractive errors may be cornea-based or lens based. The cornea based surgeries are more common.

Cornea-based surgeries	Lens-based surgeries
- LASIK (laser assisted in situ keratomileusis) - Photorefractive keratectomy (PRK) - LASEK (laser assisted surface epithelial keratomileusis) - Femtosecond LASIK - SMILE (Small incision lenticule extraction) - FLEx (Femtosecond lenticule extraction) - Intracorneal ring segments	- Phakic IOL - Clear lens extraction

Cornea-based Surgeries

➢ *LASIK (laser assisted in situ keratomileusis)*: In LASIK, a flap of the cornea is raised and the underlying stromal bed is ablated with laser. This **photoablation** is done by **Excimer laser**[Q]. Hence, at the end of the procedure, **the shape of the cornea is altered, the thickness is decreased** and the refractive error is corrected.

The **eligibility criteria**[Q] for LASIK are:
- Age> 18 years
- Stability of refraction for at least 6 months
- **Minimum corneal thickness of 500 microns**[Q]
- **Residual stromal depth of 250 microns**[Q]
- Absence of any other corneal pathology like keratoconus
- Absence of other ocular pathologies like glaucoma, retinal degenerations, etc.

➢ *Photorefractive keratectomy (PRK)*: This procedure is used for patients with low to moderate myopia (–2 to –6), hyperopia and astigmatism whose corneal thickness is not adequate for LASIK. Here the corneal epithelium is manually removed instead of making a flap so that more stroma is available for ablation. **Main disadvantages are pain, delayed post-operative recovery, corneal haze and regression of refractive error**

➢ *LASEK (laser assisted surface epithelial keratomileusis)*: Used in patients with thin corneas which makes them ineligible for LASIK

➢ *Femtosecond LASIK*: This is the recent advancement in laser refractive surgery where Femtosecond laser is used for flap creation in LASIK or for lenticule extraction in SMILE and FLEx.

Lens-based Surgeries

➢ This type of refractive surgery is considered in patients with very high refractive errors when they are not eligible for corneal refractive surgery
➢ The commonly performed surgery is **phakic IOL** where a corrective lens is placed in the eye in front of the crystalline lens.
➢ The main eligibility criteria would be
   - Age> 18 years with stable refraction for at least 6 months
   - Not eligible for cornea based surgery
   - Open angles on gonioscopy
   - Minimum anterior chamber depth of 2.8 mm
   - No evidence of cataract.

ERRORS OF ACCOMMODATION

➢ *Presbyopia*: described earlier
➢ *Pseudomyopia*[Q]: This is also called **spasm of accommodation**. It is seen in children especially during their examination when they are doing excessive near work. Due to excess accommodation, there is a myopic shift. **So the near vision is good but the distance vision is poor**[Q]. Treatment is to relax the accommodation with cycloplegics.
➢ *Inertia of accommodation*: In this condition, there is difficulty in changing the focus from distance to near and vice versa. This is because the accommodative system is slow in making a change.

➢ *Paralysis of accommodation*: The possible causes are cycloplegics, third nerve palsy, etc.
➢ *Insufficiency of accommodation*: This is a condition where the amplitude of accommodation is less than the normal physiological limit according to the patient's age.

REFRACTION

The process of determining and correcting the refractive error of a patient is called refraction. At first an **objective assessment of the refractive error**[Q] is done by **retinoscopy**[Q]. Then, verification of retinoscopy is done by subjective acceptance.

Method of Retinoscopy

➢ Retinoscopy is a method of determining the refractive status of an individual by the method of neutralization.
➢ The patient is made to sit at a distance of 1 m from the examiner and instructed to look at a distant target so as to relax his accommodation. Ideally, cycloplegic drop should be instilled to relax the patient's accommodation completely.
➢ With the help of a retinoscope, light is shown in the patient's eye and the examiner observes the red reflex in the patient's pupillary area. The reflex moves along with the movement of the retinoscope mirror. The direction of movement of the reflex depends upon the refractive error of the patient.
  ♦ **Movement of reflex in the direction of the mirror: Hypermetropia or Myopia <1D**[Q]
  ♦ **Movement of reflex opposite to the direction of the mirror: Myopia > 1D**[Q]
➢ Next, the movement of the reflex is neutralized by using plus lenses (with movement) or minus lenses (against movement). The final readings are noted. The same process is carried out in both meridians/axes of the eye.
➢ Estimation of refractive error from retinoscopy is done by adjusting for the distance
  ♦ For **a distance of 1 m, the deduction made is 1**[Q]
  ♦ For **a distance of 2/3 m, the deduction made is 1.5**[Q]
  ♦ The closer the examiner moves to the patient, greater is the deduction
➢ If a cycloplegic has been used to relax the accommodation, then the retinoscopy value has to be adjusted according to the cycloplegic used
  ♦ For **atropine as cycloplegic, the deduction made is 1**
  ♦ For cyclopentolate, the deduction is 0.75
  ♦ For homatropine, the deduction is 0.5

➢ Thus if retinoscopy done at 1 m under atropine gives reading of +5, the corrected reading would be +5-1 (for 1 m distance) -1 (for atropine) = +3.

Prescription of Glasses from Retinoscopy Readings

Let us take a few examples.

Example 1

The retinoscopy findings of a child are given below. The refraction is done from a distance of 1 m after instilling atropine. Prescribe the glasses for the child.

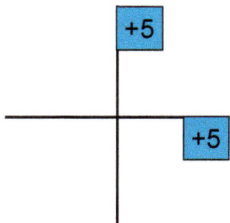

Answer: The question shows a retinoscopy cross indicating the neutralization values during retinoscopy in both the vertical and horizontal meridians is +5. So the patient has a spherical refractive error.
The corrected retinoscopy value would be
+5-1 (deduction for distance) -1(deduction for atropine) = +3
Hence, the patient is to be prescribed glasses of +3 sphere (DS).

Example 2

The retinoscopy findings of a child are given below. The refraction is done from a distance of 1 m after instilling atropine. Prescribe the glasses for the child.

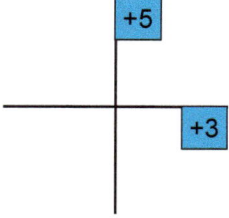

Answer: The question shows a retinoscopy cross indicating the neutralization values during retinoscopy in both the vertical and horizontal meridians. In the vertical meridian, the value is +5 and in the horizontal meridian it is +3.

The corrected retinoscopy values are
In the vertical meridian: **(+5) -1 (deduction for distance) -1 (deduction for atropine) = + 3**
In the horizontal meridian: **(+3) -1 (deduction for distance) -1(deduction for atropine) = +1**
So, the corrected retinoscopy cross is

Optics and Refraction

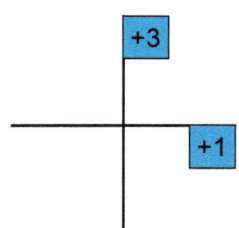

Now, this means that both meridians of the eye have a refractive error but they are not equal. So, there is a component of astigmatism and the prescription will be a spherocyclinder (combination of sphere and cylinder).

The simplest method to arrive at the answer is:
The smaller integer is prescribed as the sphere: +1 (in this case)
The cylinder = Difference in power between the two meridians
$= (+3) - (+1)$
$= +2$ (in this case)

Axis of cylinder: The axis which shows the smaller integer = 180 degrees (in this case because +1 is in the horizontal axis)
So the prescription reads as
+1 sphere (DS)/ +2 cylinder (DC) * 180 degrees

Example 3

The retinoscopy findings of a child are given below. The refraction is done from a distance of 1 m after instilling atropine. Prescribe the glasses for the child.

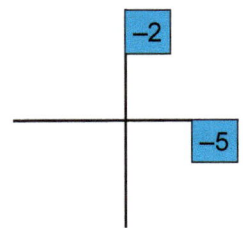

Answer: The question shows a retinoscopy cross indicating the neutralization values during retinoscopy in both the vertical and horizontal meridians. In the vertical meridian, the value is –2 and in the horizontal meridian it is –5

The corrected retinoscopy values are
In the vertical meridian: **(–2)** –1 (deduction for distance) –1 (deduction for atropine) = **–4**
In the horizontal meridian: **(–5)** –1 (deduction for distance) –1 (deduction for atropine) = **–7**
So, the corrected retinoscopy cross is

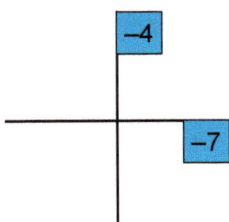

Now, this means that both meridians of the eye have a refractive error but they are not equal. So, there is a component of astigmatism and the prescription will be a spherocyclinder (combination of sphere and cylinder).

The simplest method to arrive at the answer is:
The smaller integer is prescribed as the sphere: –4 (in this case)
The cylinder = Difference in power between the two meridians
$= (-7) - (-4)$
$= -3$ (in this case)

Axis of cylinder: The axis which shows the smaller integer
= 90 degrees (in this case because –4 is in the vertical axis)
So the prescription reads as
–4 sphere (DS)/ –3 cylinder (DC)* 90 degrees

Cycloplegics

Cycloplegics are used to relax the accommodation of the patient so as to get an accurate assessment of the refractive error in retinoscopy.

- **Atropine (1% ointment)**[Q]: It is the **longest acting**[Q] dilator- cycloplegic with duration of action of about **10–14 days.** It is used for refraction in children less than 3 years of age and patients with squint
- **Tropicamide (0.5% eye drops)**: It is the **shortest acting**[Q] dilator - cycloplegic with a duration of action of **4–6 hours.** It is used for refraction in adults
- **Homatropine (2% eye drops)**: It has a duration of action of 3–4 days and is used in school going children
- **Cyclopentolate (1% eye drops)**: It has a duration of action of 12–24 hrs
- **Phenylephrine**: This is a **dilator with no cycloplegic action**[Q].

> **Must Remember**
> - *Foster Fuch's maculopathy*: Degenerative myopia
> - *Lattice degeneration/Paving-stone degeneration*: Myopia
> - *Silk retina*: Hypermetropia
> - *Pseudopapillitis/Pseudopapilloedema*: Hypermetropia
> - *Refractive error which is causes maximum amblyopia*: Hypermetropia
> - *First line management of amblyopia*: Occlusion therapy

QUESTIONS

Refraction in the Eye

1. **Maximum contribution to the refractive power of the eye is by:** *(Nov AIIMS 2016)*
   a. Anterior surface of cornea
   b. Anterior surface of lens
   c. Posterior surface of cornea
   d. Posterior surface of lens

2. **Normal power of the reduced eye:** *(Maharashtra)*
   a. +6D   b. +17D
   c. +43D   d. +60D

3. **Most important factor determining convergence of light rays on the retina is:** *(DNB 2014)*
   a. Length of the eyeball
   b. Refractive power of the lens
   c. Curvature of the cornea
   d. Physical state of the vitreous

4. **Which component of the eye has maximum refractive index:** *(AIIMS 2010)*
   a. Anterior surface of lens
   b. Posterior surface of lens
   c. Center of lens
   d. Cornea

5. **True statements about accommodation:** *(PGI 2013)*
   a. Mainly occurs due to increase in posterior curvature of the lens
   b. Helps to improve stereopsis
   c. It is abolished by sympathomimetic drugs
   d. Mainly due to increase in anterior curvature of the lens
   e. Elasticity of the capsule has a bearing on accommodation

Refractive Errors

6. **Most common type of refractive error in older children:** *(COMEDK 2015)*
   a. Hypermetropia   b. Myopia
   c. Presbyopia   d. Astigmatism

7. **The most common cause of myopia is:** *(DPG 2010)*
   a. Increase in axial length of the eyeball
   b. Increase in thickness of the lens
   c. Increase in viscosity of aqueous humor
   d. Increase in viscosity of vitreous humor

8. **Which of the following is a serious complication of degenerative myopia?** *(UPSC 2009)*
   a. Retinal detachment   b. Posterior staphyloma
   c. Myopic crescent   d. Vitreous liquefaction

9. **Which of the following is true about degenerative myopia?** *(AIIMS 2013)*
   a. More common in males as compared to females
   b. Myopic degeneration can lead to retinal detachment
   c. It is seen in <6 diopters of myopia
   d. Retinal tear is less common and is a late complication

10. **Foster Fuch's spots are seen in:** *(Kerala PG)*
    a. Myopia   b. Hypermetropia
    c. Sympathetic ophthalmia d. Astigmatism

11. **Subretinal hemorrhage at the macula in myopes is known as:** *(NEET 2016)*
    a. Posterior staphyloma   b. Retinoschisis
    c. Foster Fuch's spot   d. Lattice degeneration

12. **Pseudopapillitis is seen in:** *(DPG 2008)*
    a. Hypermetropia   b. Myopia
    c. Squint   d. Presbyopia

13. **Silk retina is seen in:** *(DNB 2015)*
    a. Myopia   b. Hypermetropia
    c. Astigmatism   d. Presbyopia

14. **Regular astigmatism means:** *(DNB 2015)*
    a. The two meridians are perpendicular
    b. The two meridians are parallel
    c. Asymptomatic astigmatism
    d. Astigmatism after cataract surgery

15. **True about presbyopia:** *(PGI)*
    a. Age related error of refraction
    b. Age related defect in accommodation
    c. Concave lens is used
    d. Convex lens is used
    e. Cylindrical lens is used

16. **Aniseikonia means:** *(AIIMS 2003)*
    a. Difference in axial length in the two eyes
    b. Difference in the curvature of the cornea in the two eyes
    c. Difference in the size of the pupil in the two eyes
    d. Difference in the size of the image formed by the two eyes

17. **Spasm of accommodation mimics:** *(NEET 2016)*
    a. Myopia   b. Hypermetropia
    c. Presbyopia   d. Amblyopia

Contact Lens and Refractive Surgery

18. **Treatment options for myopia are:** *(PGI 2014)*
    a. Radial keratotomy   b. LASIK
    c. Epikeratophakia   d. Keratoplasty
    e. Photorefractive keratectomy (PRK)

19. **Soft contact lens is made up of:** *(APPG 2015)*
    a. PMMA   b. HEMA
    c. Silicon   d. Glass

20. **Laser used in the treatment of myopia:** *(DNB 2015)*
    a. Nd-YAG   b. Excimer
    c. Argon   d. Krypton

21. **All of the following are treatment options for myopia except:** *(DNB 2015)*
    a. LASIK   b. Radial keratotomy
    c. Phakic IOL   d. Nd: YAG laser therapy

Optics and Refraction

22. A lady wants LASIK surgery for her daughter. Which of the following is not an eligibility criteria for LASIK? *(AIPG 2005)*
    a. Myopia of 4 D
    b. Age of 15 years
    c. Stable refraction for 1 year
    d. Corneal thickness of 600 microns

23. Oblate shape of the cornea is seen in: *(NEET 2016)*
    a. Post myopic LASIK
    b. With the rule astigmatism
    c. Against the rule astigmatism
    d. Oblique astigmatism

Refraction

24. Concentration of tropicamide: *(AIIMS 2013)*
    a. 0.01
    b. 0.02
    c. 0.03
    d. 0.04

25. Which of the following is not a cycloplegic? *(AIPG 2007)*
    a. Phenylephrine
    b. Atropine
    c. Tropicamide
    d. Homatropine

26. Mydriatic to be used in a 3-year-old child for refraction: *(Maharashtra PG)*
    a. 1% Atropine drops
    b. 1% Atropine eye ointment
    c. 0.5% Tropicamide eye drops
    d. 2% Homatropine eye drops

27. Cyclopentolate is used for refraction in the age group of: *(NEET 2016)*
    a. 0–3 years
    b. 5–10 years
    c. >20 years
    d. >50 years

28. Cycloplegic action of atropine lasts up to: *(NEET 2016)*
    a. 1 day
    b. 2 days
    c. 1 week
    d. 2 weeks

29. Objective assessment of refraction is termed as: *(COMEDK 2013)*
    a. Gonioscopy
    b. Retinoscopy
    c. Ophthalmoscopy
    d. Keratoscopy

30. In retinoscopy, for a distance of 1 m the correction factor is –1D. What is the correction factor for retinoscopy done at 66 cm? *(Kerala PG)*
    a. –2
    b. –1
    c. –0.5
    d. –1.5

31. On performing retinoscopy using a plane mirror in a patient who has a refractive error of –3D sphere with –2 cylinder at 90 degrees from a distance of 1 m, the reflex would move: *(AIIMS)*
    a. With the movement in the horizontal axis and against the movement in the vertical axis
    b. With the movement in both the axes
    c. Against the movement in both the axes
    d. With the movement in the vertical axis and against the movement in the horizontal axis

32. On performing retinoscopy using plane mirror in a patient with myopia of 0.5D from a distance of 1 m, the reflex will move: *(AIIMS 2001)*
    a. Move with the mirror
    b. Move opposite to the mirror
    c. No movement
    d. May move to either side

33. Cross cylinder is: *(PGI)*
    a. One plus cylinder and one minus cylinder of equal strength
    b. One plus and one minus cylinder of unequal strength
    c. Two plus cylinders
    d. Both minus cylinders
    e. One spherical and one cylindrical lens

Miscellaneous

34. A 35-year-old man has 6/5 vision in each eye unaided. His cycloplegic refraction is 0.00. He complains of blurring of newsprint at 30 cm which clears up in about 2 minutes. The probable diagnosis is: *(AIPG 2005)*
    a. Hypermetropia
    b. Presbyopia
    c. Accommodative inertia
    d. Cycloplegia

35. A 35-year-old man has normal distance vision but complains of difficulty in near vision. His retinoscopy shows +2D sphere. The probable diagnosis is: *(AIIMS/ AIPG 2002)*
    a. Hypermetropia
    b. Presbyopia
    c. Myopia
    d. Accommodative inertia

36. A 10-year-old boy is brought to the doctor with complains of squeezing his eyes to see the blackboard in school. What is the probable diagnosis? *(Manipal)*
    a. Hypermetropia
    b. Myopia
    c. Astigmatism
    d. Accommodative inertia

37. A 9-year-old boy is brought with complaints of difficulty in vision for distance. On examination, the visual acuity on Snellen's chart is 6/36 but it improves to 6/6 with pin-hole. What is the diagnosis?
    a. Malingering
    b. Refractive error
    c. Developmental cataract
    d. Amblyopia

38. Treatment of choice for aphakia: *(AIPG/ UPPG 2007)*
    a. Spectacles
    b. Contact lenses
    c. IOL
    d. Laser therapy

39. 1 mm change in the axial length would change the refractive power of the eye by: *(DNB 2015)*
    a. 1D
    b. 2D
    c. 3D
    d. 5D

40. Lensometer detects: *(DNB 2015)*
    a. Correct power of glasses
    b. IOL power
    c. Corneal topography
    d. Biochemical constitution of lens

ANSWERS AND EXPLANATIONS

1. a. Anterior surface of cornea (Ref: Optics of the human eye, p 15–20)
2. d. +60D (Ref: Optics of the human eye, p 15–20)
3. c. Curvature of the cornea (Ref: Optics of the human eye, p 15–20)
   The total refractive power of the eye is about 60D of which 44–45D comes from the cornea. Thus the cornea is the most important refracting medium responsible for convergence of light rays to the retina
4. c. Center of the lens (Ref: Optics of the human eye, p 15–20)
5. d. Mainly due to increase in anterior curvature of the lens, e. Elasticity of the capsule has a bearing on accommodation
6. b. Myopia (Ref: Khurana 4th edition, p 32)
7. a. Increase in axial length of the eyeball (Ref: Khurana 4th edition, p 32)
8. a. Retinal detachment (Ref: Kanski 6th edition, p 706)
9. b. Myopic degeneration can lead to retinal detachment (Ref: Kanski 6th edition, p 706)
   Myopia>6 D is associated with peripheral retinal holes, tears and degenerations like lattice. This may predispose the patient to develop rhegmatogenous retinal detachment
10. a. Myopia
11. c. Foster Fuch's spot
12. a. Hypermetropia
    In hypermetropia, the optic disc appears small and hyperemic. The disc margins also appear slightly blurred, giving a false impression of papillitis. Hence the name pseudopapillitis
13. b. Hypermetropia
14. a. The two meridians are perpendicular (Ref: Khurana 4th edition, p 119)
15. b. Age-related defect of accommodation, d. Convex lens is used
16. d. Difference in the size of the image formed by the two eyes
17. a. Myopia
18. a. Radial keratotomy, b. LASIK, e. Photorefractive keratectomy (PRK) (Ref: Yanoff &Duker 4th edition p 84–90)
    Radial keratotomy is an old and abandoned procedure for myopia correction. In this, radial cuts are made in the cornea of about 90% depth and extending from the paracentral region to the limbus. These cuts lead to corneal flattening and correction of myopia. The complications are
    - Corneal perforation
    - Epithelial ingrowth
    - Irregular corneal scarring leading to irregular astigmatism
    - Unpredictable results
    - Regression of myopia after about 10 years

    Hence this procedure is not done nowadays. Thus options for myopia correction now are LASIK, PRK, LASEK, Femtosecond LASIK and Phakic IOL.

    Epikeratophakia is a surgery for hypermetropia where a lenticule from a donor cornea is placed on the recipient cornea. It is rarely done.
19. b. HEMA (Ref: Yanoff &Duker 4th edition p 52)
20. b. Excimer (Ref: Yanoff &Duker 4th edition p 81)
21. d. Nd: YAG laser therapy (Ref: Yanoff &Duker 4th edition p 84–90)
22. b. Age of 15 years (Ref: Yanoff &Duker 4th edition p 92–93)
23. a. Post myopic LASIK
    The shape of the cornea is prolate which means that the center is steeper than the periphery. In myopic LASIK, the central part of the cornea is flattened and the periphery effectively becomes steeper. The shape of the cornea thus becomes oblate.
24. a. 0.01
    The concentration of Tropicamide is usually 0.5–1% (0.005–0.01)

Optics and Refraction

25. a. **Phenylephrine**
26. b. **1% Atropine eye ointment**
27. b. **5–10 years**
28. d. **2 weeks**
29. b. **Retinoscopy** *(Ref: Yanoff & Duker 4th edition p 47–50)*
30. d. **−1.5** *(Ref: Yanoff & Duker 4th edition p 47–50)*
31. c. **Against the movement in both the axes** *(Ref: Yanoff & Duker 4th edition p 47–50)*
    As the refractive error is myopia >1D in both axes, the movement of the reflex will be against the mirror in both the axes
32. a. **Move with the mirror** *(Ref: Yanoff & Duker 4th edition p 47–50)*
    As the refractive error is myopia <1 D, the reflex will move with the mirror
33. a. **One plus cylinder and one minus cylinder of equal strength, e. One spherical and one cylindrical lens**
    Cross cylinder is an instrument used to refine the power and axis of cylinder during subjective refraction. It consists of one plus and one minus cylinder of same power but in opposite axis
    The combination of a cylinder and a sphere of opposite and double power produces the same effect
34. c. **Accommodative inertia**
    The question suggests that the patient has good distance and near vision but has difficulty in adjusting from one distance to another. This is accommodative inertia
35. a. **Hypermetropia**
36. b. **Myopia**
    The question suggests that the boy has poor distance vision and so he tries to squeeze his eyes to see better. Hence the answer is myopia
37. b. **Refractive error** *(Ref: Yanoff & Duker 4th edition p 41)*
    A pinhole is a blocker with a small aperture of diameter 1 mm at the center. When placed in front of the eye, it allows only the central rays to pass whereas all the paraxial rays are blocked.
    In refractive errors, visual acuity improves with pinhole.
    In cataract and macular disorders, visual acuity decreases with pinhole.
38. c. **IOL**
    Aphakia means absence of crystalline lens. **The refractive status in aphakia is high hypermetropia^Q (+10 to +12 diopters).**
    In the early days of cataract surgery, the lens was removed in toto and the patient was left aphakic. Postoperatively, the patient was advised high convex lenses. But these glasses have some important drawbacks. They are
    * **High magnification**: The high power convex lenses cause a magnification of the image size by **25–30%^{Q}**. These glasses cannot be prescribed in unilateral aphakia because they cause aniseikonia.
    * Limited field of vision
    * Spherical and chromatic aberration
    * **Prismatic aberration^Q**: This causes **roving-ring scotoma or Jack in the box^Q** effect as a result of which objects keep appearing and disappearing in the field of view.
    * **Pin cushion effect^Q**: Straight lines appear curved and images are distorted
    Aphakia may be corrected by contact lenses but the **treatment of choice is IOL^Q**
39. c. **3D**
40. a. **Correct power of glasses**

IMAGE BASED QUESTIONS

1. Identify the refractive error: *(Nov AIIMS 2017)*

   a. Hypermetropia   b. Myopia
   c. Astigmatism   d. Presbyopia

2. The fundus picture of a patient is given. All of the following may be seen in this patient except

   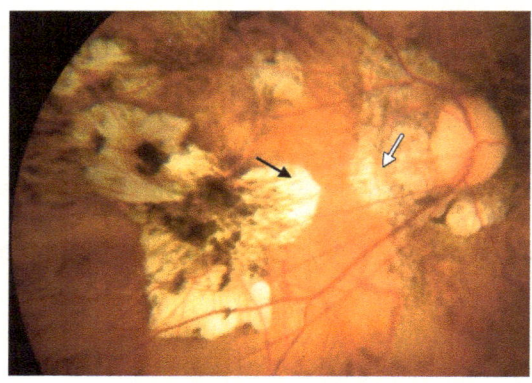

   a. Retinal tears
   b. Rhegmatogenous retinal detachment
   c. Silk retina
   d. Foster Fuch's spot

3. Identify the type of glasses given in the photograph

   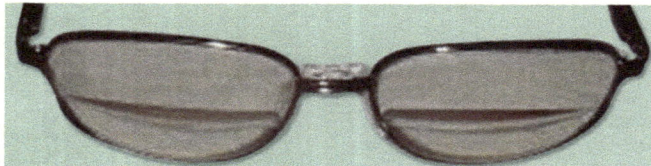

   a. Single vision glasses
   b. D-bifocal
   c. C-bifocal
   d. Executive bifocal

4. Identify the type of glasses given in the photograph

   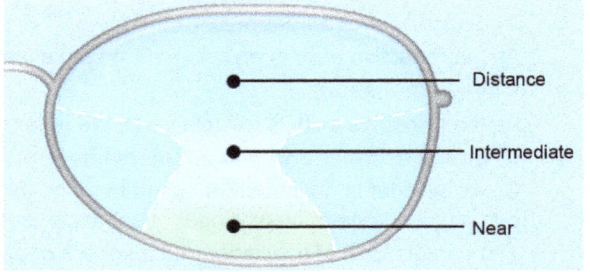

   a. Single vision glasses
   b. Executive bifocal
   c. Progressive addition lenses
   d. C-bifocal

5. What is the procedure shown in the picture?

   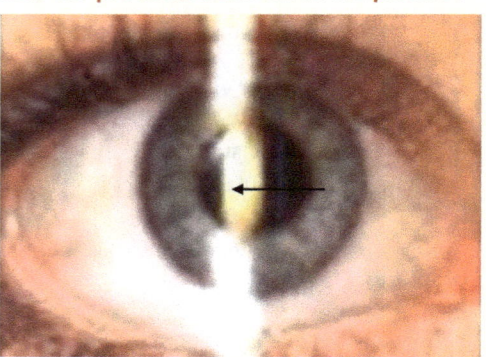

   a. Retinoscopy   b. Subjective refraction
   c. Ophthalmoscopy   d. Slit lamp examination

6. All of the following are true about the device shown in the picture except

   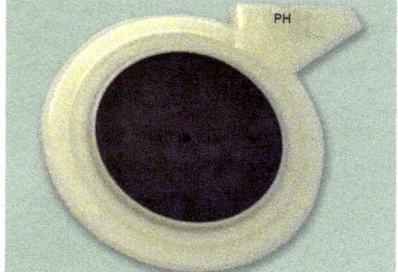

   a. The diameter of the central aperture is around 1 mm
   b. Improvement of visual acuity with the device indicates only myopia
   c. Worsening of visual acuity with the device indicates macular pathology
   d. It allows only the central rays to pass through

Answer Key: 1. b   2. c   3. d   4. c   5. a   6. b

Optics and Refraction

7. What is the use of the device shown in the picture

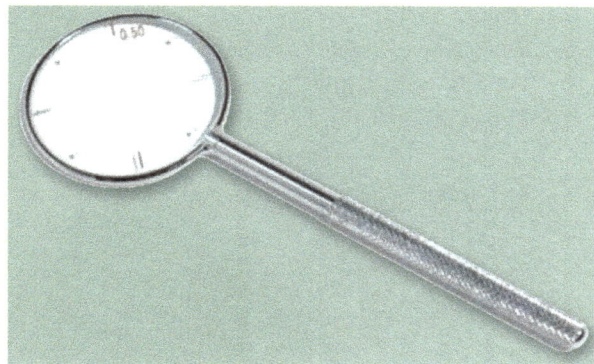

   a. Pinhole test
   b. To check the accuracy of cylindrical power and axis
   c. To examine the anterior segment of the eye
   d. Duochrome test

8. Identify the test shown in the photograph

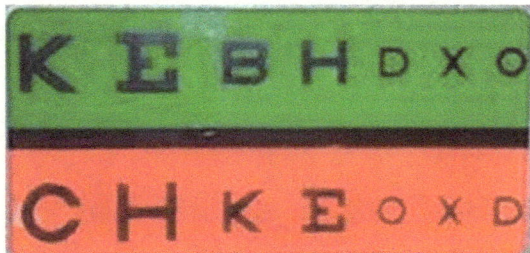

   a. Pinhole test
   b. Objective refraction
   c. Retinoscopy
   d. Duochrome test

9. What is the type of contact lens shown in the picture?

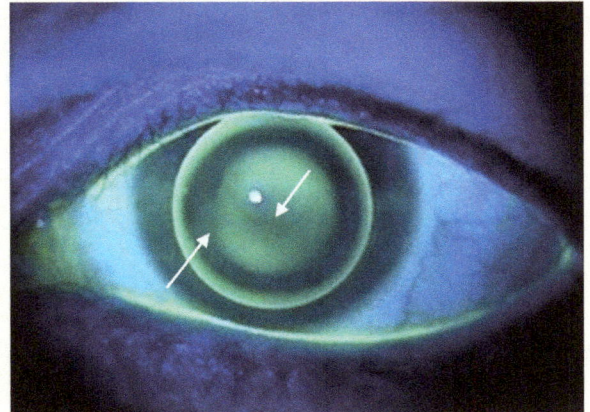

   a. Soft contact lens   b. RGP contact lens
   c. Prosthetic contact lens   d. Orthokeratology lens

10. Which is the type of contact lens shown in the picture?

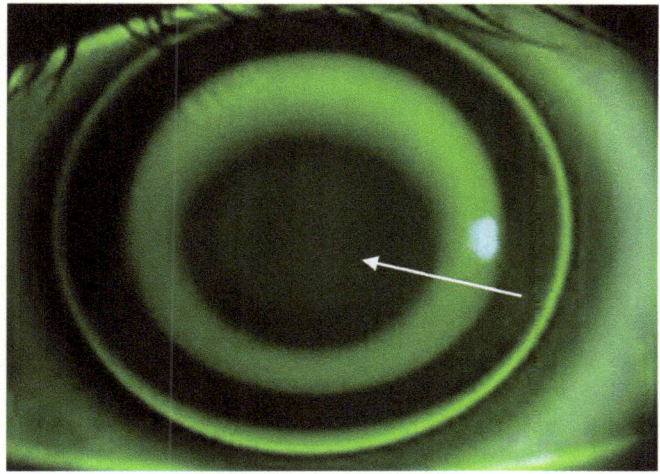

   a. Soft contact lens
   b. RGP contact lens
   c. Prosthetic contact lens
   d. Orthokeratology lens

11. A patient who has history of prolonged use of soft contact lenses complains of severe itching, irritation and intolerance to the lenses for the past 1 month. The clinical picture is given. What is the possible diagnosis?

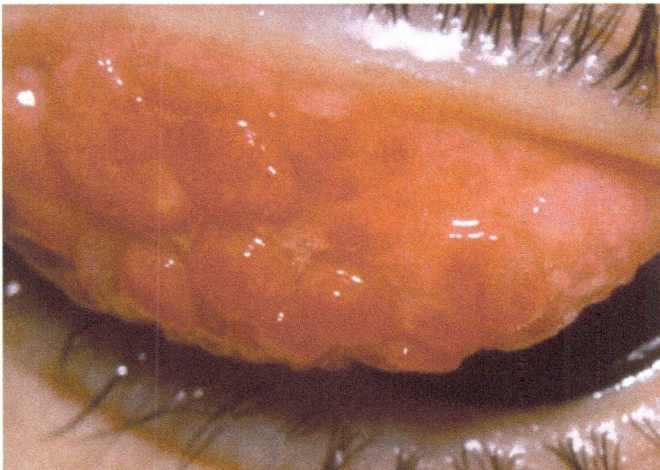

   a. Vernal keratoconjunctivitis
   b. Phlyctenular conjunctivitis
   c. Giant papillary conjunctivitis
   d. Angular conjunctivitis

Answer Key: 7. b   8. d   9. b   10. d   11. c

Self Assessment and Review of Ophthalmology

12. What is the surgical procedure shown in the picture?

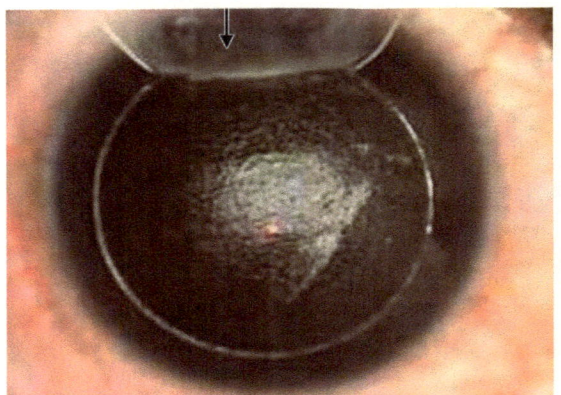

   a. PRK
   b. LASIK
   c. Penetrating keratoplasty
   d. Phakic IOL

13. Identify the device in the photograph

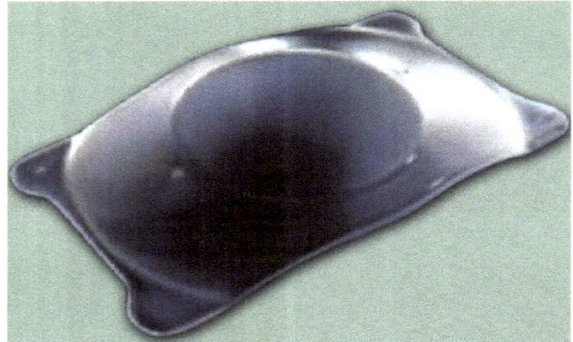

   a. Multifocal IOL   b. Phakic IOL
   c. RGP contact lens   d. Orthokeratology lens

14. What is the procedure shown in the photograph

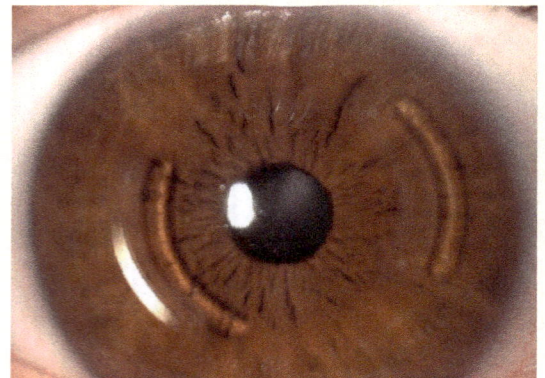

   a. LASIK
   b. PRK
   c. Intra-corneal ring segments
   d. Penetrating keratoplasty

15. What is the use of the instrument shown in the picture
   a. Refraction
   b. Evaluation of anterior segment
   c. Fundus evaluation
   d. Evaluation of IOP

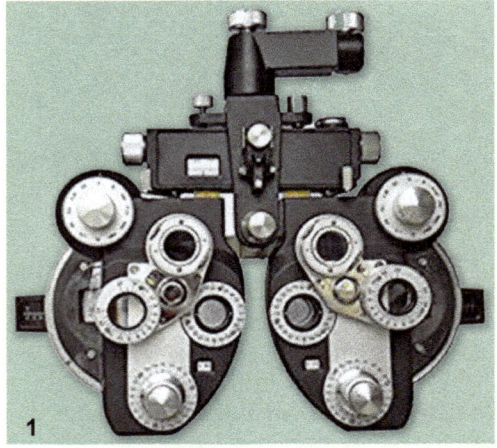

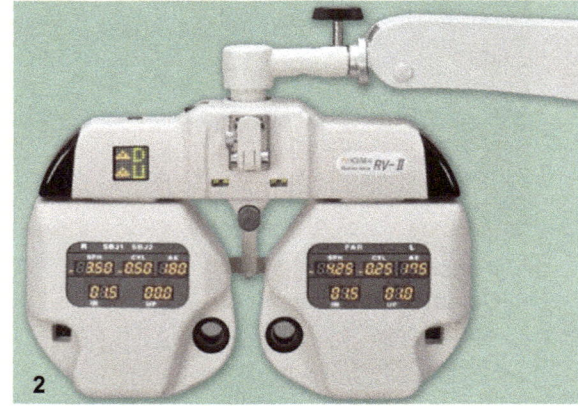

Answer Key: 12. b   13. b   14. c   15. a

Optics and Refraction

ANSWERS AND EXPLANATIONS

1. **Answer: b. Myopia**
   The picture shows rays of light focusing in front of the retina; hence the answer is myopia

2. **Answer c. Silk Retina**
   The photograph shows myopic fundus with myopic crescent (white arrow), posterior staphyloma and chorioretinal atrophic patches (black arrow)
   Hence, the answer is silk retina which is seen in hypermetropia.

3. **Answer d. Executive bifocals**
   Bifocal glasses are used in patients for whom refractive correction has to be prescribed for both distance and near vision. They have two separate optical segments with separate powers for distance and near. They are available in different varieties. **Executive bifocals provide maximum field of vision for near and are used in children**.

4. **Answer c. Progressive addition lenses**
   Progressive addition lenses (PAL) contain separate power for distance and near along with an intermediate corridor. They are better than bifocal lenses because they provide refractive correction for intermediate distance also. They are particularly useful for **computer work**.

5. **Answer a. Retinoscopy**
   The picture shows a reflex in the pupillary area (indicated by arrow). This is called retinoscopy reflex. Movement and neutralization of the reflex helps to assess the refractive error.

6. **Answer b. Improvement of visual acuity through the device indicates only myopia**
   The device shown in the picture is a **pinhole**

Pinhole test
• The size of the aperture at the centre is around 1 mm
• It blocks all the peripheral rays and allows only the axial rays to enter into the eye
• **Improvement** in visual acuity with pinhole indicates **refractive error**[Q]
• **Worsening** in visual acuity with pinhole indicates **macular pathology**[Q]
• **No change** in visual acuity with pinhole indicates ocular pathology
• **Improvement in visual acuity over spectacles** with pinhole indicates that refractive correction needs to be refined.

7. **Answer b. To check the accuracy of cylindrical power and axis**
   The device shown in the picture is **Jackson's cross cylinder**[Q]

Jackson's cross cylinder
• It is a **spherocyclinder**
• It is a combination of one plus and **one minus cylinder of same power** (generally 0.5D) at **right angles** to each other
• It is used for **subjective refinement of the magnitude and axis of the cylinder**[Q]

8. **Answer d. Duochrome test**

Duochrome test
• This test is useful for refinement of spherical refractive error.
• If the letters on the **red** background appear more **clear**, the patient has **myopia**.
• If the letters on the **green** background appear more **clear**, the patient has **hypermetropia**
• If both the letters are equally clear, the patient has emmetropia
• The basic rule is that myopes should be slightly uncorrected and hypermetropes should be fully corrected.

9. **Answer b. RGP contact lens**
   Rigid gas permeable (RGP) contact lenses are used for correction of high spherical and cylindrical errors and irregular corneal astigmatism.
   The fitting of RGP lens is assessed by fluorescein staining and examination under cobalt blue filter as shown in the picture.
   The ideal fit is indicated by a light feather central touch (indicated by arrow) with surrounding pooling of dye (green area), mid-peripheral touch (indicated by arrow) and peripheral edge lift (green area)

10. **Answer d. Orthokeratology lens**
    Orthokeratology (Ortho-K) lens
    - Ortho-K lenses are rigid gas permeable lenses which worn **overnight** flatten the corneal surface so as to correct **myopia**. Hence, by wearing lenses at night, the patient becomes free of refractive correction during the day.
    - They are **reverse geometry lenses**. So the fitting, when assessed on fluorescein staining shows large area of central touch (black area indicated by arrow) unlike routine RGP lens (Refer to question no 9)
    - They are also called **myopia control lenses**. It has been observed in several studies that use of Ortho-K lens decreases the progression of myopia in children and adolescents.

11. **Answer c. Giant papillary conjunctivitis**
    Giant papillary conjunctivitis is one of the most common complications due to prolonged use of soft contact lens leading to redness, irritation and lens intolerance.

Self Assessment and Review of Ophthalmology

12. **Answer b. LASIK**
    The picture shows a corneal flap with a hinge or attachment.
    In LASIK, a corneal flap (indicated by arrow) with hinge is raised either with the help of a microkeratome blade or Femtosecond laser. After raising the flap, treatment of the stromal bed is done with Excimer laser to correct the refractive error. The stromal bed is then thoroughly irrigated and then the flap is repositioned.

13. **Answer b. Phakic IOL**
    The photograph shows a lens called Implantable Collamer Lens (ICL) which is a type of Phakic IOL. The lens is placed in between the iris and crystalline lens. It is a lens based refractive surgery useful in patients with high refractive error and thin cornea who are unsuitable for corneal refractive surgery

14. **Answer c. Intra-corneal ring segments**
    Intra-corneal ring segments are a new modality of treatment to correct **irregular astigmatism** caused by corneal ecstatic disorders like keratoconus, pellucid marginal degeneration, post LASIK ectasia, etc. These rings modify the corneal curvature and help to correct irregular astigmatism.

15. **Answer: Refraction**
    The picture shows an instrument called **Phoropter**. This is the one of the latest devices for assessment of refractive error. It may be manual (Picture 1) or automated (Picture 2)

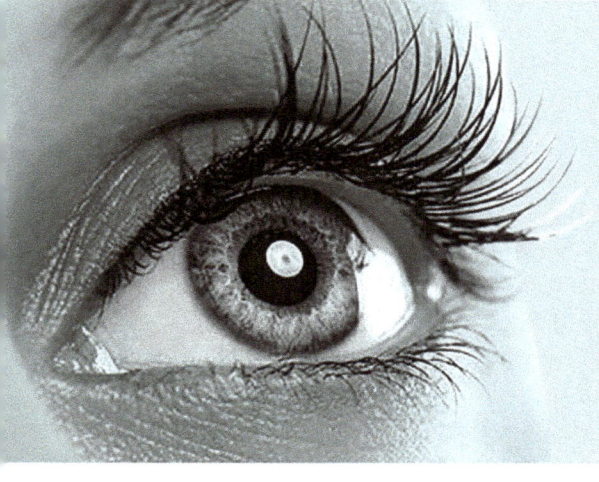

Strabismus

EXTRAOCULAR MUSCLES

The important extraocular muscles are:
- *Four recti*: Superior rectus (SR), medial rectus (MR), inferior rectus (IR) and lateral rectus (LR)
- *Two obliques*: Superior oblique (SO) and inferior oblique (IO)

	Recti	Superior oblique	Inferior oblique
Origin	Annulus of Zinn[Q] (common tendinous ring at orbital apex, encircling optic foramina and medial part of superior orbital fissure)	Body of sphenoid[Q] at the apex of the orbit	Orbital plate of maxilla at the floor of the orbit[Q]
Insertion	Inserted into sclera at different distances away from the limbus. **The distances from limbus are** **MR: 5.5 mm** **IR: 6.5 mm** **LR: 6.9 mm** **SR: 7.7 mm**	First travels antero-medially, and then turns backwards at the trochlea. It then travels posterolaterally to insert in the sclera in the **upper temporal quadrant of the globe**[Q]	Travels backwards and laterally to insert into the **lower temporal quadrant of the globe**[Q]

Few important facts
- Rectus muscle closest to limbus: MR[Q]
- Rectus muscle farthest from limbus: SR[Q]
- Longest extraocular muscle: SO
- Shortest extraocular muscle: IO
- **The Spiral of Tillaux is the line joining the points of insertion of the rectus muscles**[Q]

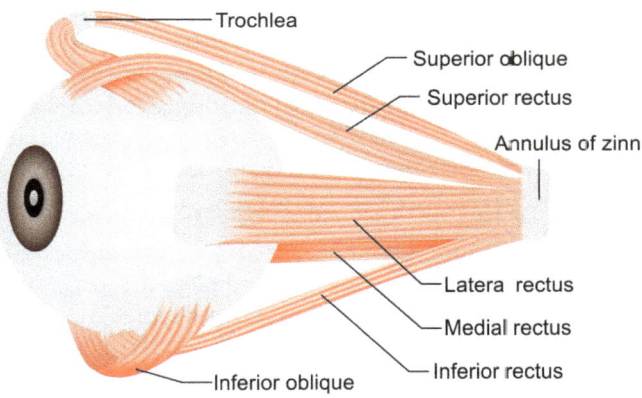

Fig. 1: Extraocular muscles

Nerve Supply
- LR is supplied by sixth cranial nerve
- SO is supplied by fourth cranial nerve
- MR, IR, SR, IO are supplied by third cranial nerve
- Remembered as **SO4 LR6**[Q]

Actions of the Extraocular Muscles

Muscle	Action			Nerve supply
	Primary	Secondary	Tertiary	
MR	Adduction			III
IR	Depression	Extorsion	Adduction	III
LR	Abduction			VI
SR	Elevation	Intorsion	Adduction	III
SO	Intorsion	Depression	Abduction	IV
IO	**Extorsion**	Elevation	Abduction	III

Points to Remember
- **SIN - Superiors are Intorters**[Q] (SR and SO)
- **RAD - Recti are Adductors**[Q] (SR and IR)
- The superior oblique functions **only as depressor in adducted position** and **only as intorter in abducted position**[Q]
- The inferior oblique functions **only as elevator in adducted position** and **only as extorter in abducted position**[Q]

Self Assessment and Review of Ophthalmology

OCULAR MOVEMENTS

- *Ductions*: These are monocular movements like adduction, abduction, elevation and depression
- *Versions*: These are binocular conjugate movements (in the same direction)
  - Dextroversion (right sided gaze)
  - Levoversion (left sided gaze)
  - Dextroelevation (up and right gaze)
  - Levoelevation (up and left gaze)
  - Dextrodepression (down and right gaze)
  - Levodepression (down and left gaze)
- *Vergence*: These are binocular disjugate movements (both eyes move in opposite directions) like convergence. Convergence is the ability of the two eyes to move inwards. It has two components: voluntary and reflex. Reflex convergence again has four components.
  - *Tonic convergence*: Due to basal tone of muscle
  - *Proximal convergence*: Induced by psychological awareness of a near object
  - *Fusional convergence*
  - *Accommodative convergence*: It is induced by the effort of accommodation. For each diopter of accommodation, a fairly constant increment in accommodative convergence occurs **(AC/A Ratio)**. AC/A ratio denotes the amount of convergence measured in **prism diopter** per unit change in accommodation. **Normal value is 4:1 (1 D of accommodation is associated with 4 prism diopters of convergence)**[Q]. High AC/A ratio leads to excessive convergence and esotropia. Low AC/A ratio leads to exotropia.

Points to Remember

- *Agonist-antagonist*: Muscles of same eye which have opposite functions, e.g. MR and LR of the same eye
- *Synergist*[Q]: Muscles of the same eye which move the eye in the same direction, e.g. SR and IO of the same eye are synergists in elevation
- *Yoke muscles*[Q]: A pair of muscles of opposite eyes which produce a conjugate ocular movement, e.g. LR of right eye and MR of left eye are yoke muscles for dextroversion

Laws of ocular motility

- *Herring's law of equal innervation*[Q]: During any conjugate movement, equal & simultaneous innervation flows to a pair of yoke muscles.
- *Sherrington's law of reciprocal innervation*[Q]: Increase in innervation and contraction of a muscle is associated with reciprocal decrease in innervation and relaxation of its antagonist

YOKE MUSCLES FOR CARDINAL POSITIONS OF GAZE

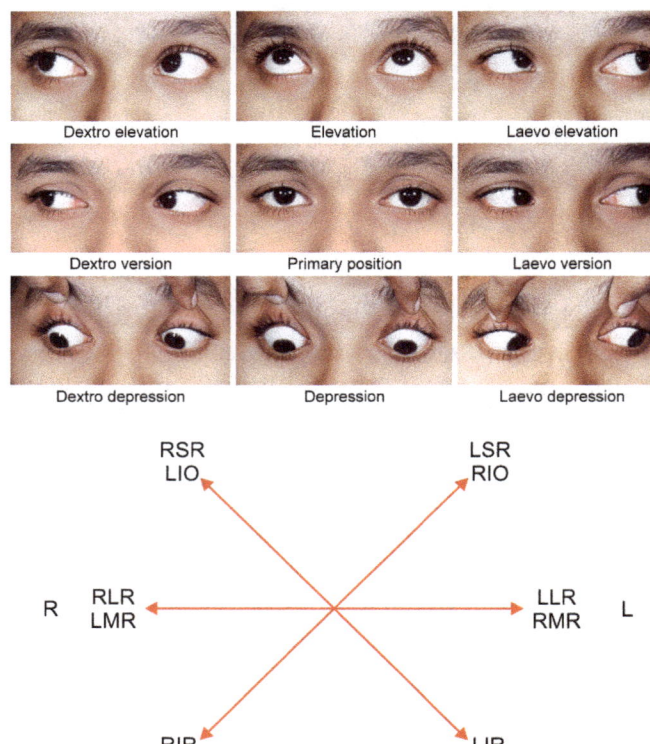

Fig. 2: Yoke Muscles

	Nature of movement	Yoke muscles
Dextroversion	Abduction for right eye Adduction for left eye	Right lateral rectus Left medial rectus
Dextroelevation	Elevation in abduction for right eye Elevation in adduction for left eye	Right superior rectus Left inferior oblique
Dextrodepression	Depression in abduction for right eye Depression in adduction for left eye	Right inferior rectus Left superior oblique
Levoversion	Abduction for left eye Adduction for right eye	Left lateral rectus Right medial rectus
Levoelevation	Elevation in abduction for left eye Elevation in adduction for right eye	Left superior rectus Right inferior oblique
Levodepression	Depression in abduction for right eye Depression in adduction for left eye	Left inferior rectus Right superior oblique

Binocular single vision (BSV)

BSV is achieved by use of the two eyes together. By this, slightly dissimilar images arising in each eye are appreciated as a single image.

Grades of binocular vision
- *Grade I:* Simultaneous Macular Perception (SMP)^Q
- *Grade II:* Fusion^Q
- *Grade III:* **Stereopsis**^{Q}: Ability to obtain an impression of depth

DOUBLE VISION/DIPLOPIA

The pre-requisite for binocular single vision is perfect ocular alignment. Strabismus or any ocular deviation hence may result in diplopia. But the individual undertakes certain adaptations in order to overcome this diplopia. The compensatory mechanisms vary according to the type of diplopia and the age of the individual.

Adaptations in Strabismus

- *Suppression*: It occurs in children with squint where the image formed on the retina by the squinting eye is suppressed by the visual cortex. This leads to the development of **amblyopia**.
- *Abnormal retinal correspondence (ARC)*: This is an adaptation where non-corresponding retinal areas are paired together to achieve an anomalous binocular vision in the presence of small degrees of squint
- *Compensatory head posture*: This is a feature of paralytic strabismus where the head is turned in the direction of field of action of the weak/paralysed muscle. The type of head posture depends upon the type of diplopia and the muscle involved
    - For horizontal muscle palsy like LR palsy, the patient develops a **face turn**^{Q}
    - For vertical muscle palsy like SR or IR, the patient develops **chin elevation or chin depression**^{Q}
    - For oblique muscle palsy like SO, the patient develops a **head tilt**^{Q}

CLASSIFICATION OF SQUINT

- *Pseudostrabismus*: This is not actually a deviation but gives an impression of ocular deviation. It is seen in prominent **epicanthic fold, hyperteleorism** etc.
- *Latent squint (Phoria)*: In this condition, the tendency of the eyes to deviate is kept in check by the fusional ability of the individual. If the fusion is broken by prolonged occlusion of one eye, deviation becomes manifest. This is also called **phoria**, e.g. **Esophoria** (latent convergent squint) and **Exophoria** (latent divergent squint)
- *Manifest squint (Tropia)*: In this condition, the deviation of the eye is evident on observation, e.g. **Esotropia** (manifest convergent squint) or **Exotropia** (manifest divergent squint). It is of two types
    - *Concomitant squint*: The degree of deviation is the **same in all gazes**^{Q}
    - *Incomitant squint*: The common type is **paralytic squint** where there is paralysis of one or more extraocular muscle. **The deviation is maximum in the direction of action of the paralysed muscle**^{Q}.

	Concomitant squint	Incomitant squint
Deviation	Same in all gazes	Maximum in the direction of gaze of the affected muscle^Q
Extraocular movements	Normal	Limitation in the direction of action of the affected muscle
Amblyopia	May be **present in children**^{Q}	Absent
Head posture	Usually absent	Usually present
Primary(P) and Secondary deviation(S)	Both are same	Secondary deviation> Primary Deviation^Q

Important points

- **Primary deviation is the deviation of the affected eye**^{Q}.
- **Secondary deviation is the deviation of the good eye under cover**^{Q}
- Secondary deviation> Primary deviation in paralytic squint is explained by Herring's law

ESOTROPIA OR CONVERGENT SQUINT

- Essential infantile esotropia
- Accommodative esotropia - It is of three types:
    - Refractive
    - Nonrefractive
    - Mixed
- Non accommodative esotropia
    - Sensory deprivation
    - Divergence insufficiency
    - Convergence excess or spasm
    - Consecutive.

Infantile Esotropia

- It presents within the **first six months of birth**^Q
- Common in children with hydrocephalus and cerebral palsy
- **Large and constant angle of squint**^Q
- **Minimum refractive error**^Q
- Alternate fixation in primary position and **cross fixation**^Q in side gaze
- **Nystagmus**^Q
- *Management is surgical.*

Accommodative Esotropia

It is esotropia associated with abnormality in the process of accommodation. **It usually manifests at the age of 2-3 yrs**^Q.

- *Refractive*: It is associated with high **hypermetropia**^Q. Due to excessive accommodative effort by the patient, there is excessive convergence leading to esotropia. **The angle of deviation is almost equal for both distance and near**^Q
- *Non Refractive*: In this condition, there is minimum refractive error but an **abnormally high AC/A ratio**^Q. This means that there is excessive convergence for a normal accommodative effort. **There is minimum deviation for distance but significant esotropia for near**^Q
- *Mixed*: This is a combination of high hypermetropia and high AC/A ratio
- Management
    - Spectacles for refractive type
    - Surgery for non-refractive type.

SPECIAL SQUINTS

Duanne's retraction syndrome

- It is a syndrome where there is failure of innervation of the lateral rectus by the sixth nerve and abnormal innervation of the lateral rectus by the third nerve. It has three types
    - TYPE I: Esotropia with limitation of abduction and relatively normal adduction^Q
    - TYPE II: Exotropia with limitation of adduction and relatively normal abduction^Q
    - TYPE III: Limitation of both abduction and adduction with minimal deviation^Q
- On attempted adduction there is retraction of the globe and narrowing of the palpebral fissure
- Treatment is not needed in most cases because deviation is not much and there is no amblyopia

Brown's superior oblique tendon sheath syndrome: Limitation of elevation in adduction and normal elevation in abduction.

Mobius syndrome: Congenital aplasia of VI, VII, IX, XII cranial nerve nuclei.

Double elevator palsy: Paresis of SR and IO of the same eye.

PRINCIPLES OF SQUINT SURGERY

The basic principle of squint surgery is weakening of the stronger muscle and strengthening of the weaker muscle. The weakening and strengthening procedures are

- **Weakening Procedures**
    - *Recession*: The insertion of the muscle is moved posteriorly towards its origin.
    - *Marginal myotomy*
    - *Myectomy*: Muscle is severed from its insertion but not reattached
- **Strengthening Procedures**
    - *Resection*: Pull of muscle is enhanced by making it shorter
    - Tucking
    - *Advancement*: Muscle is disinserted and advanced closer to the limbus.

AMBLYOPIA

Amblyopia is a unilateral or bilateral reduction of best corrected visual acuity in the absence of any organic cause.

Clinical Features

- Unilateral or bilateral reduced vision
- *Crowding phenomenon*^Q *may be seen*: The patient is able to identify a Snellen's chart character with the amblyopic eye when the character is presented in isolation. If the character is shown along with other letters, the patient may not be able to recognize it.
- *Neutral Density Filter Test (NDF)*: When the patient is asked to read through a NDF, the amblyopic eye shows no change, while in the normal eye, there is a drop in visual acuity
- Amblyopia treatment should be tried till the child is 12 years old. **Best results are seen between 5–8 years of age**^Q.

Types of Amblyopia

Strabismic amblyopia	Refractive amblyopia	Stimulus deprivation amblyopia
Caused by uncorrected squint where the protective mechanism of **suppression** leads to amblyopia	Caused by uncorrected refractive error	Caused by media opacity in the form of cataract or corneal opacity where amblyopia develops due to **visual form deprivation**.
Best prognosis[Q]	Good prognosis	**Worst prognosis**[Q]

Refractive Amblyopia

- *Anisometropic amblyopia*: It develops due to difference in refractive error between the two eyes. This leads to amblyopia in the eye with the larger refractive error if corrective glasses are not worn. **Hypermetropes are more prone to develop anisometropic amblyopia**[Q].
- Bilateral emetropic amblyopia can occur if the refractive error is high in both eyes and is not corrected
- Meridional amblyopia is the term used when amblyopia affects only one meridian due to high astigmatic error.

Treatment of Amblyopia

- *Occlusion*[Q]: Occlusion of the good eye forces the child to see with the amblyopic eye and helps in improving vision.
- *Penalization*[Q]: If a child is not co-operative to occlusion, penalization by instillation of atropine in the good eye is the next option
- Pleoptic therapy
- CAM stimulator.

Must Remember

- *Primary action of superior oblique:* Intorsion
- *Primary action of inferior oblique:* Extorsion
- *Test for latent squint/phoria:* Cover-uncover test
- *Hess chart:* Used in paralytic squint
- *Secondary deviation > Primary deviation:* Paralytic squint

QUESTIONS

Extraocular Muscles

1. Functions of superior oblique muscle are: *(PGI 2000)*
   a. Intorsion
   b. Extortion
   c. Abduction
   d. Adduction
   e. Depression

2. Function of superior oblique muscle is: *(AIPG)*
   a. Elevation with inward rotation
   b. Elevation with outward rotation
   c. Depression with inward rotation
   d. Depression with outward rotation

3. Which of the following muscles is an intorter? *(AIIMS 2000)*
   a. Inferior rectus
   b. Inferior oblique
   c. Superior rectus
   d. Lateral rectus

4. The superior oblique is supplied by: *(AIPG 2005)*
   a. IIIrd cranial nerve
   b. IVth cranial nerve
   c. VIth cranial nerve
   d. Vth cranial nerve

5. Primary function of superior oblique is: *(APPG 2013)*
   a. Elevation
   b. Depression
   c. Intorsion
   d. Extortion

6. IIIrd cranial nerve supplies: *(PGI)*
   a. Lateral rectus
   b. Levator palpebrae superioris
   c. Superior oblique
   d. Superior rectus
   e. Medial rectus

7. Action of right superior oblique is: *(PGI)*
   a. Dextroelevation
   b. Dextrodepression
   c. Levodepression
   d. Levoelevation

8. Functions of superior rectus are: *(DNB 2012)*
   a. Elevation, extorsion, adduction
   b. Elevation, intorsion, adduction
   c. Depression, intorsion, adduction
   d. Depression, extorsion, adduction

9. Functions of superior oblique are: *(NEET 2016)*
   a. Extorsion, depression, adduction
   b. Intorsion, depression, abduction
   c. Elevation, extorsion, abduction
   d. Elevation, intorsion, adduction

10. Which of the following muscles does not have adduction function? *(WBPG 2012)*
    a. Medial rectus
    b. Superior rectus
    c. Inferior oblique
    d. Inferior rectus

11. The yoke muscle of right superior oblique is: *(DNB 2014/ NEET 2016)*
    a. Right inferior oblique
    b. Left inferior oblique
    c. Right inferior rectus
    d. Left inferior rectus

12. Left superior oblique and left inferior rectus are: *(Kerala PG 2014)*
    a. Yoke muscles
    b. Agonists
    c. Antagonists
    d. Synergists

13. Which of the following is not true about inferior oblique muscle: *(DNB 2016)*
    a. It is the shortest muscle
    b. Its primary action is extorsion
    c. It originates from the annulus of Zinn
    d. It is supplied by the third cranial nerve

14. Which muscle inserts closest to the limbus? *(CET JUNE 2017)*
    a. Medial rectus
    b. Superior rectus
    c. Lateral rectus
    d. Inferior rectus

15. The reciprocal inhibition of antagonist muscle is explained by: *(AIIMS 2008)*
    a. Sherrington's law
    b. Laplace's law
    c. Hick's law
    d. Herring's law

16. Equal and simultaneous innervation of yoke muscles is explained by: *(DPG 2009)*
    a. Sherrington's law
    b. Fick's law
    c. Herring's law
    d. Von Graefe's law

Evaluation of Squint

17. Which of the following is not a grade of binocular single vision? *(Maharashtra PG 2010)*
    a. Simultaneous macular perception
    b. Retinal correspondence
    c. Fusion
    d. Stereopsis

18. Stereopsis means: *(DNB 2015)*
    a. Perception of different colours
    b. Perception of depth
    c. Perception of visual field
    d. Perception of the size of an object

19. Hirschberg test is used to detect: *(APPG 2013)*
    a. Diplopia
    b. Squint
    c. Refractive error
    d. Glaucoma

20. Cover test is used to detect: *(DNB 2013)*
    a. Manifest squint
    b. Paralytic squint
    c. Latent squint
    d. Pseudosquint

Esotropia

21. Pseudo convergent squint is seen in: *(PGI)*
    a. Thyrotoxicosis
    b. Broad epicanthus
    c. Abducens palsy
    d. Narrow interpupillary distance

22. Features of infantile esotropia are: *(PGI)*
    a. Present since birth
    b. Large angle esotropia
    c. Inferior oblique overaction
    d. Surgery is the treatment
    e. High refractive error

Strabismus

23. Which of the following are true about infantile esotropia? *(PGI 2015)*
    a. Onset after 1 year of age
    b. Amblyopia may develop
    c. Angle of deviation is large and fixed
    d. Surgery should be done only after 2 years
    e. Minimum refractive error

24. Treatment of refractive accommodative esotropia is: *(AIIMS 2000)*
    a. Surgery
    b. Occlusion therapy
    c. Convergence exercises
    d. Correction of refractive error

25. True regarding accommodative esotropia: *(PGI)*
    a. Glasses are used when miotics are ineffective
    b. Miotics are used when glasses are ineffective
    c. Miotics are used when AC/A ratio is high
    d. Surgery is the only treatment

26. Most common type of squint seen in myopes is: *(DNB 2015)*
    a. Intermittent exotropia
    b. Intermittent esotropia
    c. Esotropia hypotropia complex
    d. Exotropia hypotropia complex

27. A 3-year-old child has esotropia in the right eye. On retinoscopy there is +4.5D hyperopia in right eye and +4D hyperopia in the left eye. The AC/A ratio is normal. What is the probable diagnosis? *(JIPMER)*
    a. Infantile esotropia
    b. Refractive accommodative esotropia
    c. Non-refractive accommodative esotropia
    d. Duane's retraction syndrome

Miscellaneous

28. A 10-year-old complains of headache. His best corrected visual acuity in the right eye is 6/36 and in the left eye is 6/6. Retinoscopy shows +5D in right eye and +1D in left eye. All other ocular examination is normal. What is the possible diagnosis? *(DNB 2012)*
    a. Optic neuritis
    b. Cortical blindness
    c. Amblyopia
    d. Malingering

29. Secondary deviation> Primary deviation is a feature of: *(WBPG 2007)*
    a. Accommodative squint
    b. Paralytic squint
    c. Infantile esotropia
    d. Alternate exotropia

30. Secondary deviation > Primary deviation in paralytic squint is explained by which law? *(WBPG 2008)*
    a. Sherrington's law
    b. Herring's law
    c. Park's law
    d. Fick's law

31. Which of the following is not a feature of paralytic squint? *(DNB 2012)*
    a. Diplopia
    b. Compensatory head posture
    c. Amblyopia
    d. Secondary deviation is more than primary deviation

32. In squint surgery, muscle resection leads to: *(DNB 2015)*
    a. Weakening of muscle
    b. Strengthening of muscle
    c. Paralysis of muscle
    d. No effect

33. Amblyopia is best corrected by: *(AIPG)*
    a. <5 years
    b. <8 years
    c. <15 years
    d. <20 years

34. Treatment of choice for amblyopia is: *(AIIMS 2000)*
    a. Occlusion therapy
    b. Orthoptic exercises
    c. Spectacles
    d. Surgery

35. Which of the following is true regarding Duane's retraction syndrome Type? *(VBPG 2009)*
    a. Defective abduction with normal adduction
    b. Defective adduction with normal abduction
    c. Both adduction and abduction are defective
    d. Elevation is defective

36. Duanne's retraction syndrome is characterised by: *(CET JUNE 2017)*
    a. Decreased function of 6th nerve with limitation of abduction
    b. Increased intraocular pressure
    c. Weakness of superior oblique
    d. Increased corneal pigmentation

37. Limitation of both adduction and abduction is seen in: *(AIIMS)*
    a. Duane's Type I
    b. Duane's Type II
    c. Duane's Type III
    d. Double elevator palsy

38. A-V pattern squint: Which of the following is/are true? *(PGI 2015)*
    a. The terms 'A' or V pattern squint are labeled when the amount of deviation in squinting eye varies by more than 10° and 15°, respectively, between upward and downward gaze.
    b. The terms 'A or V pattern squint are labeled when the amount of deviation in squinting eye varies by more than 20° and 25° respectively, between upward and downward gaze.
    c. Usually, over action of the inferior oblique or weakness of superior oblique leads to A pattern & over action of the superior oblique or weakness inferior oblique to V pattern
    d. Usually, over action of the inferior oblique or weakness of superior oblique leads to V pattern & over action of the superior oblique or weakness of inferior oblique to A pattern
    e. Oblique muscle dysfunction is the commonest cause of AV pattern

ANSWERS AND EXPLANATIONS

1. a. Intorsion, c. Abduction, e. Depression *(Ref: Yanoff & Duker 4th edition, p 1183)*
2. c. Depression with inward rotation *(Ref: Yanoff & Duker 4th edition, p 1183)*
3. c. Superior rectus *(Ref: Yanoff & Duker 4th edition, p 1183)*
   Just remember SIN meaning Superiors are Intorters.
   So **superior rectus** and **superior oblique** are **intorters**
4. b. IVth cranial nerve *(Ref: Yanoff & Duker 4th edition, p 1183-84)*
5. c. Intorsion *(Ref: Yanoff & Duker 4th edition, p 1183)*
6. b. Levator palpebrae superioris, d. Superior rectus, e. Medial rectus *(Ref: Yanoff & Duker 4th edition, p 1183)*
   The muscles supplied by the IIIrd cranial nerve are
   - Levator palpebrae superioris
   - All recti except lateral rectus
   - Inferior oblique
   - Sphincter pupillae and ciliary muscles
7. c. Levodepression *(Ref: Yanoff & Duker 4th edition, p 1186)*
   The muscles involved in levodepression are left inferior rectus and right superior oblique
8. b. Elevation, intorsion, adduction *(Ref: Yanoff & Duker 4th edition, p 1183)*
9. b. Intorsion, depression, abduction *(Ref: Yanoff & Duker 4th edition, p 1183)*
10. c. Inferior oblique *(Ref: Yanoff & Duker 4th edition, p 1183)*
    Just remember RAD meaning recti are adductors except lateral rectus
11. d. Left inferior rectus *(Ref: Yanoff & Duker 4th edition, p 1186)*
12. d. Synergists *(Ref: Yanoff & Duker 4th edition, p 1186)*
13. c. It originates from the annulus of Zinn *(Ref: Yanoff & Duker 4th edition, p 1183)*
14. a. Medial rectus *(Ref: Yanoff & Duker 4th edition, p 1186)*
15. a. Sherrington's law *(Ref: Yanoff & Duker 4th edition, p 1186)*
16. c. Herring's law *(Ref: Yanoff & Duker 4th edition, p 1186)*
17. b. Retinal correspondence *(Ref: Yanoff & Duker 4th edition, p 1201–03)*
18. b. Perception of depth *(Ref: Yanoff & Duker 4th edition, p 1201)*
19. b. Squint *(Ref: Kanski 6th edition, p 755)*

    Clinical tests for squint
    - *Hirschberg test:* This test is used to measure the angle of manifest squint or tropia [Q]. Light is shown on the eye. If there is no squint, the reflex should appear centrally on the pupil in both eyes. If there is esotropia or medial deviation of the eye, the reflex will fall temporally. If there is exotropia or lateral deviation of the eye, the reflex will fall nasally. If the reflex falls at the pupillary margin, the angle of deviation is around 15 degrees. If it falls at the limbus, the angle of deviation is around 45 degrees
    - *Krimsky test or Prism Bar test:* This test is also used to measure the angle of manifest squint[Q] by using prisms
    - Cover-Uncover test: This test is used to detect latent squint or heterophoria[Q]. Here one eye is covered in order to break the fusion. When the cover is removed, the eye under cover will show deviation if there is a phoria
    - *Alternate cover test:* In this test the two eyes are alternately covered to detect phoria in either eye
    - *Maddox rod test:* This test is used to detect torsional deviation[Q]
    - *Hess charting:* This test is used to confirm the paretic eye in cases of paralytic squint[Q]

20. c. Latent squint *(Ref: Kanski 6th edition, p 757)*
21. b. Broad epicanthus *(Ref: Kanski 6th edition, p 757-58)*
22. b. Large angle esotropia, c. Inferior oblique overaction, d. Surgery is the treatment *(Ref: Yanoff & Duker 4th edition, p 1207-08)*
23. b. Amblyopia may develop, c. Angle of deviation is large and fixed, e. Minimum refractive error
    (Ref: Yanoff & Duker 4th edition, p 1207-08)
    Surgery should be done as early as possible in infantile esotropia to restore ocular alignment and prevent the development of strabismic amblyopia

Strabismus

24. d. **Correction of refractive error** *(Ref: Yanoff & Duker 4th edition, p 1210)*
25. c. **Miotics are used when AC/A ratio is high** *(Ref: Yanoff & Duker 4th edition, p 1210)*

    Miotics like pilocarpine may be used as a modality of management in non-refractive accommodative esotropia. But it is not a very popular method

26. a. **Intermittent exotropia** *(Ref: Yanoff & Duker 4th edition, p 1215)*
27. b. **Refractive accommodative esotropia** *(Ref: Kanski 6th edition, p 770)*

    The question describes a patient with the following features
    - Age 3 years
    - Esotropia
    - Hypermetropic refractive error
    - Normal AC/A ratio

    Hence the answer is refractive accommodative esotropia

    In infantile esotropia, there is minimum refractive error and associated features like cross fixation, nystagmus will be present

    In non- refractive accommodative esotropia, there will be minimum refractive error with high AC/A ratio

28. c. **Amblyopia** *(Ref: Kanski 6th edition, p 746)*

    In this question, the patient has anisometropia because the refractive error in the right eye is +5D and in the left eye is +1D. The vision in right eye is 6/36 but the ocular examination is normal. This means that there is no organic cause for decreased vision in the right eye. Hence the answer is amblyopia. This is a type of refractive amblyopia (anisometropic)

29. b. **Paralytic squint** *(Ref: Yanoff & Duker 4th edition, p 1225)*

    Paralytic squint is a type of incomitant squint. In incomitant squint secondary deviation is more than primary deviation

30. b. **Herring's law**
31. c. **Amblyopia** *(Ref: Yanoff & Duker 4th edition, p 1225)*
32. b. **Strengthening of muscle** *(Ref: Yanoff & Duker 4th edition, p 1247)*
33. b. **<8 years** *(Ref: Yanoff & Duker 4th edition, p 1242)*
34. a. **Occlusion therapy** *(Ref: Yanoff & Duker 4th edition, p 1242)*
35. a. **Defective abduction with normal adduction** *(Ref: Yanoff & Duker 4th edition, p 1211)*
36. a. **Decreased function of 6th nerve with limitation of abduction** *(Ref: Yanoff & Duker 4th edition, p 1211)*
37. c. **Duane's Type III** *(Ref: Yanoff & Duker 4th edition, p 1211)*
38. a. **The terms 'A' or V pattern squint are labeled when the amount of deviation in squinting eye varies by more than 10° and 15°, respectively, between upward and downward gaze.**
    d. **Usually, over action of the inferior oblique or weakness of superior oblique leads to V pattern & over action of the superior oblique or weakness of inferior oblique to A pattern**
    e. **Oblique muscle dysfunction is the commonest cause of AV pattern**

    The above described features are seen in pattern strabismus *(Ref: Yanoff & Duker 4th edition, p 1221)*

IMAGE BASED QUESTIONS

1. From the picture, estimate the grade of squint:

   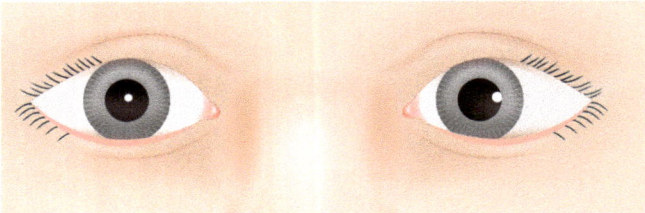

   a. 15 degrees Esotropia
   b. 15 degrees Exotropia
   c. 30 degrees Esotropia
   d. 30 degrees Exotropia

2. What is the device in the picture used for?

   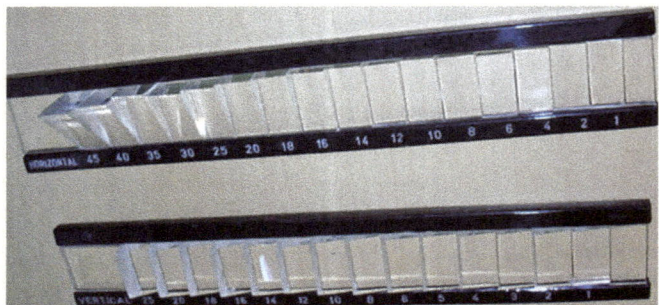

   a. Hirschberg test
   b. Prism bar cover test
   c. Worth's four dot test
   d. Stereopsis test

3. What does the picture in the test indicate?

   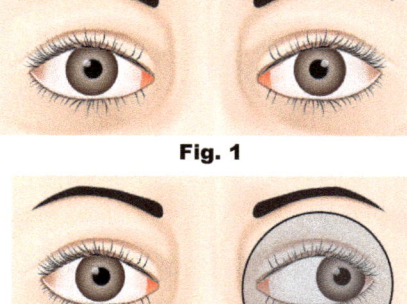

   Fig. 1

   Fig. 2

   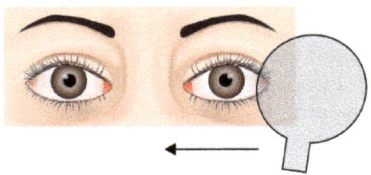

   Fig. 3

   a. Cover-uncover test indicating exophoria
   b. Cover-uncover test indicating esophoria
   c. Alternate cover test indicating esotropia
   d. Alternate cover test indicating exotropia

4. What does the picture in the question indicate?

   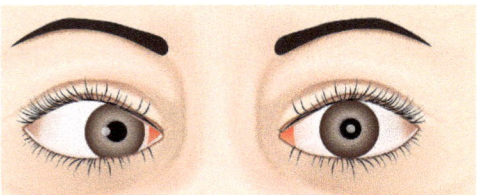

   Fig. 1

   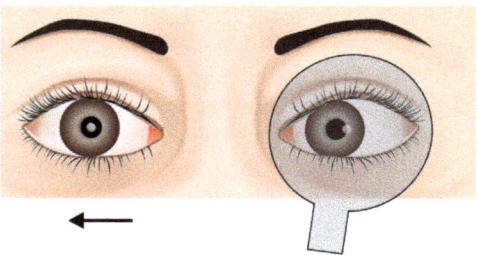

   Fig. 2

   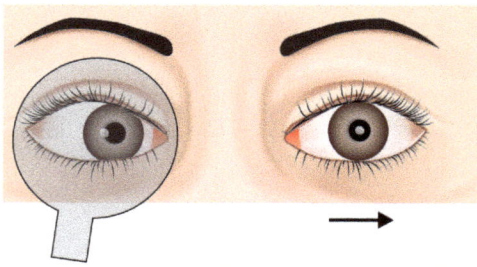

   Fig. 3

   a. Cover-Uncover test
   b. Alternate cover test showing right esotropia
   c. Alternate cover test showing right exotropia
   d. Alternate cover test showing alternate esotropia

| Answer Key: | 1. a | 2. b | 3. a | 4. d |

5. A patient reports the given result on Worth's Four Dot test. What does this mean?

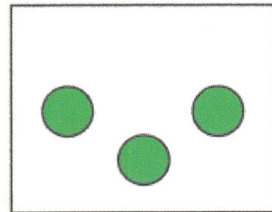

   a. Right eye suppression
   b. Left eye suppression
   c. Normal
   d. Diplopia.

6. Identify the device shown in the picture:

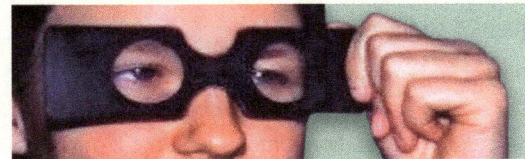

   a. Worth's four dot
   b. Bagolini's striated glasses
   c. Red-green goggles
   d. Titmus fly test

7. The test in the picture is used for the evaluation of:

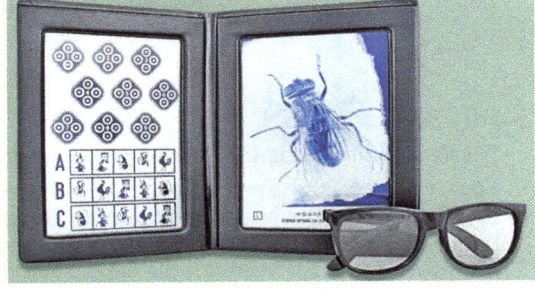

   a. Suppression
   b. Abnormal retinal correspondence
   c. Stereopsis
   d. Phoria

8. A child is undergoing patching/occlusion therapy for amblyopia. The picture is given. Which of the following statements is true?

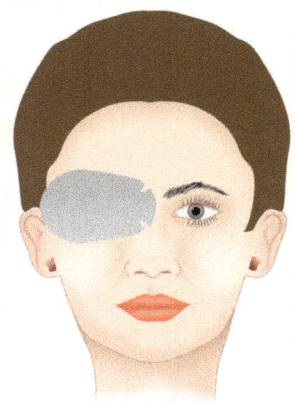

   a. Right eye is amblyopic
   b. Left eye is amblyopic
   c. Both eyes are amblyopic
   d. It is not known which eye is amblyopic

9. The clinical photographs of a child with and without glasses are given. What is the possible diagnosis?

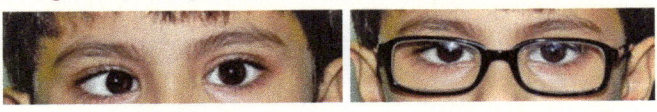

   a. Infantile esotropia
   b. Accommodative esotropia
   c. Intermittent exotropia
   d. Duanne's retraction syndrome

Answer Key: 5. a   6. b   7. c   8. b   9 b

Self Assessment and Review of Ophthalmology

ANSWERS AND EXPLANATIONS

1. **Answer: a. 15 degrees Esotropia**

   (Ref: Yanoff & Duker 4th edition p 1193)

   The picture represents the **Hirschberg test**^Q. It is used to detect **manifest squint** ^Q and get a rough **estimate of the degree of squint**.

   When a torch is shown in front of the eye, the reflex of the torch falls at the centre of the pupil in both eyes, if there is no squint (Fig. 1).

   If there is a convergent squint or **esotropia**, the reflex in that eye will be moved **temporally** (as the eye is shifted inwards).

   If there is a divergent squint or **exotropia**, the reflex in that eye will be moved **nasally** (as the eye is shifted outwards).

   The basic rules of Hirschberg test are
   - If the reflex falls at the edge of the pupil in the squinting eye, the deviation is 15 degrees (Fig. 2)
   - If the reflex falls at the limbus of the squinting eye, the deviation is 45 degrees (Fig. 4)
   - If the reflex falls in between the edge of pupil and the limbus, the deviation is around 30 degrees (Fig. 3)

   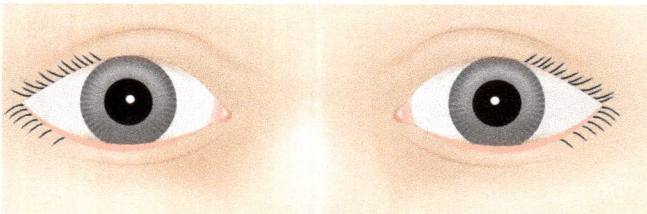

   Fig. 1

   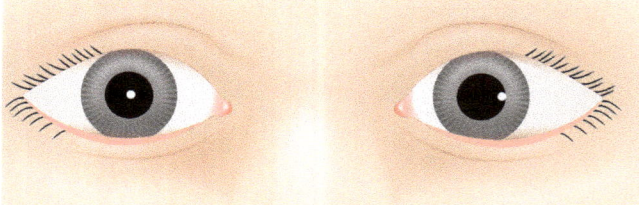

   Fig. 2

   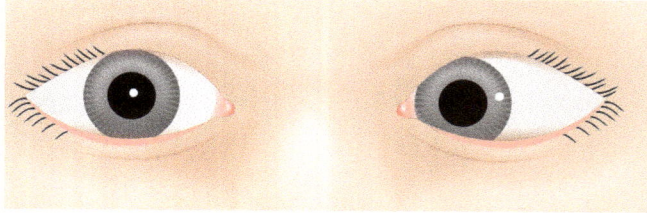

   Fig. 3

   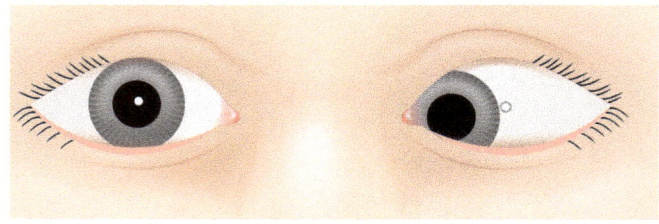

   Fig. 4

   From the picture in the question, it is evident that the left eye is deviated inwards and the reflex falls at the margin of the pupil. So the left eye has esotropia or convergent squint of about 15 degrees.

2. **Answer: b. Prism bar cover test**

   (Ref: Yanoff & Duker 4th edition p 1193-95)

   The picture shows horizontal and vertical prism bars.

   Prism bar cover test (PCT) is used for **quantitative evaluation of manifest squint.**

   Prisms of increasing power are placed in front of the eye till the deviation is neutralized.

   About **1 degree of squint = 2 prism diopters**

3. **Answer: a. Cover-uncover test indicating exophoria**

   (Ref: Peyman's Principles and Practice of Ophthalmology. 2nd edition, p 1310–13)

   Cover-uncover test
   - It is very useful to detect **latent squint** or **phoria**
   - The occluder is placed in front of one eye and then removed. (Cover-uncover). As the occluder is removed, the behavior of the eye which was occluded is observed.
   - If there is a phoria, the occluded eye deviates under cover and regains fixation when the occluder is removed.

   Figure 1 shows that there is no manifest squint as both eyes are straight.

   Figure 2 shows that on occluding the left eye, it deviates outward under cover.

   Figure 3 shows that when the occluder is lifted from the left eye, it moves inwards to regain fixation.

   So the test depicts latent divergent squint or exophoria of the left eye detected on cover-uncover test.

4. **Answer: d. Alternate cover test showing alternate esotropia**

   (Ref: Peyman's Principles and Practice of Ophthalmology. 2nd edition, p 1310–13)

Strabismus

Alternate cover test
- In this test, the occluder is switched back and forth from one eye to the other.
- It helps to measure the **total or maximum deviation**^{Q}
- It also helps to detect **alternating deviation**^{Q}

In the question, the occluder is shifted from one eye to another, so it depicts alternate cover test.

Figure 1 shows that the right eye is deviated inwards indicating right esotropia with left eye fixating.

Figure 2 shows that when the left eye is occluded, the right eye moves outwards to take fixation but the left eye deviates inwards under cover.

Figure 3 shows that when the occluder is shifted to the right eye, the left eye which was deviated inwards, now moves outwards to take fixation. The right again deviates inwards under cover.

So the alternate cover test shows that both the eyes deviate inwards under cover and move outwards to take fixation when occluder is shifted to the other eye. This is alternate esotropia.

5. **Answer: a. Right eye suppression**

   (Ref: Peyman's Principles and Practice of Ophthalmology. 2nd edition, p 1308)

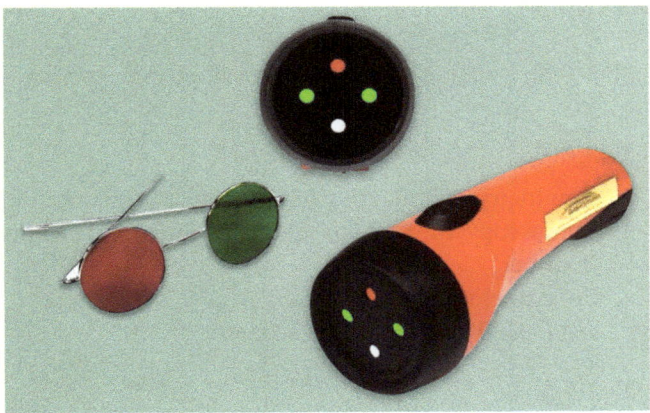

Worth's Four Dot Test

Worth's Four Dot Test
- It is a test for **binocular vision** and **sensory adaptation to strabismus**
- The patient is made to wear **red-green goggles** (red in front of right eye and green in front of left eye) to provide dissociation. He is then instructed to look at the Worth's four dot target which contains 1 red, 1 white and 2 green dots.
- The results are interpreted as follows

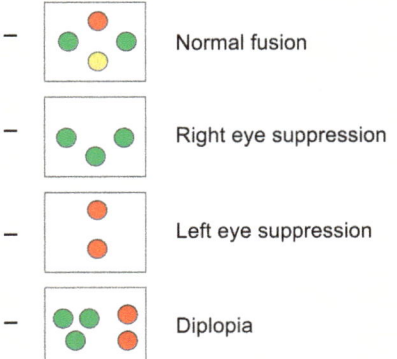

6. **Answer: b. Bagolini's striated glasses**

   (Ref: Peyman's Principles and Practice of Ophthalmology. 2nd edition, p 1308)

   Bagolini's striated glasses are used to evaluate **binocular vision** and **sensory adaptation to strabismus**. They help to diagnose **abnormal retinal correspondence** and **suppression**.

7. **Answer: c. Stereopsis**

   The picture shows **Titmus fly test** which is used for evaluation of stereopsis.

The tests used for stereopsis are:
• Titmus fly test with polaroid glasses
• Lang's test
• Random dot stereoacuity test
• TNO test
• Frisby test

8. **Answer: b. Left eye is amblyopic**

   The picture shows a child with patch in the right eye. In occlusion therapy, **the normal eye is occluded** to stimulate visual activity in the other eye, which is amblyopic. So, in this case, right eye is normal and left eye is amblyopic.

9. **Answer: b. Accommodative esotropia**

   (Ref: Peyman's Principles and Practice of Ophthalmology. 2nd edition, p 1330–41)

   The photograph shows esotropia in the right eye which disappears after wearing glasses. So it is likely to be accommodative esotropia.

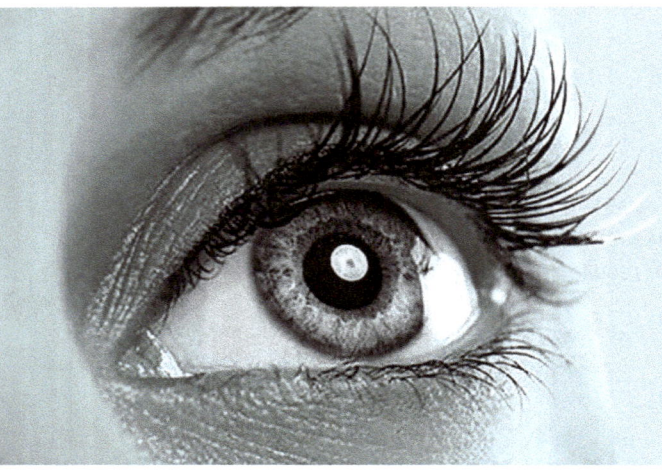

Glaucoma

Glaucoma is a type of **optic neuropathy** occurring in response to **raised intraocular pressure** and characterized by typical changes in the optic disc and the visual field. Glaucomatous optic neuropathy is also called **Cavernous Optic Atrophy**[Q].

AQUEOUS HUMOUR DYNAMICS

Aqueous humour is basically an ultrafiltrate of the plasma. The site of production is the **ciliary processes of the pars plicata**[Q]. Each ciliary process is lined by two layers of epithelium namely pigmented and non-pigmented. At the centre of the ciliary process is a rich capillary network within the surrounding stroma. Aqueous humour production involves the following steps:

- Formation of a plasma filtrate from the capillary network within the stroma by the process **of ultrafiltration**[Q]
- Transfer of this plasma filtrate from the ciliary stroma into the aqueous compartment across the epithelium. This involves two processes namely **diffusion**[Q] and **active secretion**[Q]
- Rate of aqueous production is **2–3 µL/min**
- Substances whose concentration in aqueous is less than plasma: **Protein, glucose, urea**[Q]
- Substances whose concentration in aqueous is more than plasma: **Ascorbate, lactate, pyruvate**[Q]

Aqueous humour flows from the posterior chamber to the anterior chamber through the pupil. From the anterior chamber it has two outflow pathways

- *Conventional or Trabecular pathway*[Q]: It operates through the angle of anterior chamber and accounts for **90%** of aqueous outflow. The structures in the pathway are **Trabecular meshwork → Schlemm's canal → Collector vessels→ Episcleral veins**[Q]. The site of maximum resistance in this pathway is the **juxtacanalicular part of the trabecular meshwork**[Q]
- *Unconventional or Uveoscleral pathway*[Q]: Accounts for remaining **10%** aqueous outflow:
    - Ciliary body → Suprachoroidal space → Episcleral veins
    - Ciliary body → Suprachoroidal space → Vortex veins

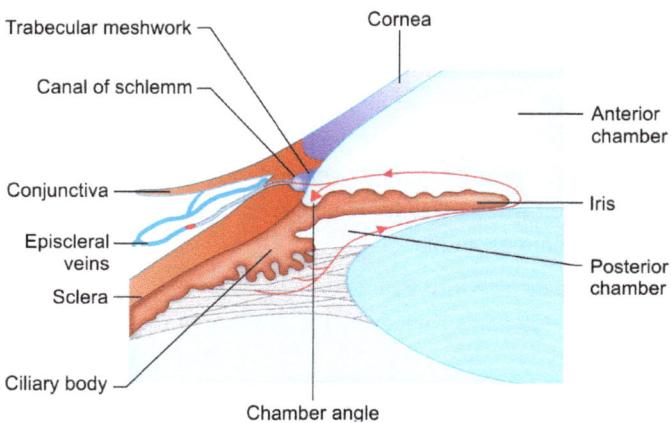

Fig. 1: Aqueous outflow through angle of anterior chamber

EVALUATION OF GLAUCOMA

- Tonometry or Evaluation of intraocular pressure (IOP)
- Gonioscopy or Evaluation of the angle of anterior chamber
- Optic disc evaluation
- Visual field evaluation or Perimetry

Tonometry

- *Normal*: 11 to 21 mm Hg or 15.5 + 2.5 mm Hg[Q]
- Diurnal variation is less than 5 mm Hg.

Types of Tonometers

- Indentation tonometer
    - *Schiotz tonometer*: It is widely used because it is portable and the technique is simple to learn. But the main disadvantage is that the reading is affected by **scleral rigidity**[Q]
- *Applanation tonometer*: It is based on **Imbert-Fick**[Q] law. The law states P = F/A where P = Pressure inside a sphere, F = Force and A = Area. In most applanation tonometers, the area (A) is fixed and the force (F) is variable.

Glaucoma

> **Types of applanation tonometer**
> - *Goldmann Applanation tonometer^Q*: It is the **gold standard tonometer^Q**. It gives accurate and reproducible readings. The main disadvantage is that the reading is dependent on **the corneal thickness**. Also its accuracy is decreased in **irregular corneas**
> - *Perkin's handheld tonometer*: It is a portable tonometer and **used mainly in children**
> - Tonopen: It is used in **irregular corneas**
> - *Mackay-Marg tonometer:* It is used in **irregular corneas^Q**
> - *Maklakov tonometer:* This is an applanation tonometer with **variable applanation area(A) and fixed force (F)^Q**

- *Non-contact tonometer*: This uses a puff of air to flatten the cornea and hence it is free from the risk of transmitting infection
- Newer tonometers
  - *Pascal's Dynamic Contour Tonometer*: It is the most accurate tonometer
  - *Rebound Tonometer*: It is a **home care tonometer or self use tonometer^Q**
  - *Transpalpebral Tonometer*: It is used in uncooperative patients

GONIOSCOPY

Gonioscopy means visualization of the angle of the anterior chamber. Light travelling from the anterior chamber angle is total internally reflected at the cornea-air interface because it is incident at an angle more than the critical angle for the two media. (**Critical angle for air-cornea interface is 46 degrees^Q**). Hence a lens called a gonioscope is required to overcome this total internal reflection.

> - *Direct gonioscopy lenses*: Koeppe, Barkan, Thorpe, Swan Jacob
> - *Indirect gonioscopy lenses*: Goldmann, Zeiss, Posner

Angle evaluation is clinically done with gonioscope but there are machines available for the same. They are:
- Anterior Segment OCT^Q
- Ultrasound Biomicroscopy (UBM)^Q

> **Structures visualized on gonioscopy (from anterior to posterior)**
> - **Schwalbe's line** which represents **the anterior limit of the Descemet's membrane^Q**
> - Trabecular meshwork
> - Scleral spur
> - Ciliary body and root of iris

Depending on the structures which are visible on gonioscopy, the angle is graded as open, occludable or closed

Shaffer's Grading of Angle Width

Grade	Angle	Structures visible	Configuration	Chances of closure
IV	35–45°	Schwalbe's line to ciliary body	Wide open	Nil
III	20–35°	Schwalbe's line to scleral spur	Open	Nil
II	20°	Schwalbe's line to trabecular meshwork	Moderately narrow	Possible^Q
I	10°	Schwalbe's line only	Narrow	High
0	0°	None	Closed	Closed

Optic Disc Evaluation

Glaucomatous disc damage is due to:
- Mechanical effect of raised IOP
- Compromised blood supply

Optic disc evaluation is clinically done by **Direct Ophthalmoscope/90D lens/60D lens.** The machines available for the same are:
- Optical Coherence Tomography (OCT)^Q
- Confocal Scanning Laser Polarimetry^Q

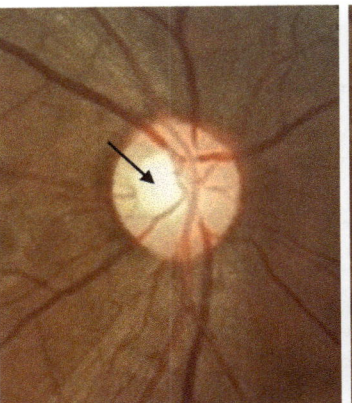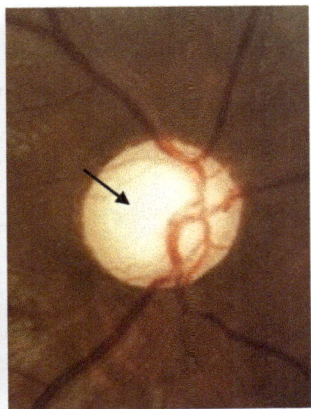

Fig. 2: Normal disc and Glaucomatous disc

> **Glaucomatous disc changes**
> - **Increase in Cup: Disc ratio due to enlargement of the optic cup^Q** (The physiological cup is a depression at the centre of the disc. The black arrows in the photographs point to the optic cup.

Contd...

Contd...

> As visible in the photographs here, the Cup:Disc ratio in the normal disc is around 0.3:1 whereas in the glaucomatous disc, it is very much increased)
> - Asymmetry of >0.2 in the C:D ratio between the two eyes
> - Thinning of neuroretinal rim which usually follows the **ISNT** rule (Inferior-Superior- Nasal- Temporal). Hence the upper and lower rims are thinned first making the cup **vertically oval**[Q].
> - *Laminar dot sign*[Q]: The pores of the lamina cribrosa become visible through the optic cup as the cup becomes deep.
> - Bayonetting of blood vessels
> - **Nasal shifting of vessels**[Q]
> - Nerve fibre bundle defects

Perimetry or Visual Field Evaluation

The normal visual field is:
- 50° superiorly
- 60° nasally
- 70° inferiorly
- 100°–110° temporally

Blind spot: Between 10°–20° temporally

> **Visual field changes in glaucoma**
> - Paracentral scotomas[Q]
> - Seidel scotoma
> - Nasal step of Roenne
> - **Arcuate or Bjerrum scotoma**
> - Ring scotoma
> - Total scotoma

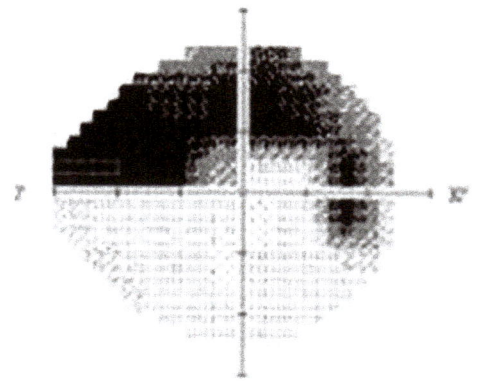

Fig. 3: Arcuate scotoma (characteristic scotoma of glaucoma)

> **Classification of Glaucoma**
> - Primary glaucoma
>   - Primary open angle glaucoma (POAG)
>   - Primary angle closure glaucoma (PACG)
> - Secondary glaucoma
> - Developmental glaucoma
>   - Primary congenital glaucoma or Buphthalmos
>   - Developmental glaucoma with associated anomalies

PRIMARY OPEN ANGLE GLAUCOMA

Primary open angle glaucoma (POAG) is a bilateral disease characterized by:
- Adult onset
- IOP> 21 mm Hg or diurnal variation> 8 mm Hg
- Open angles on gonioscopy
- Optic disc changes suggestive of glaucoma
- Visual field changes specific to glaucoma

> **Risk factors**
> - Age more than 65 years of age
> - Diabetes mellitus
> - Thyroid disorders
> - Family history
> - Myopia

Genetics: POAG is associated with six different locii on the human genome designated as **GLC1A-F**. The genes identified are **Myocillin**[Q] gene and **Optineurin**[Q] gene.

Mechanism of glaucoma: Trabecular meshwork sclerosis with reduction in intertrabecular spaces increases resistance to aqueous outflow. This results in increase in IOP.

Presentation: Patient is usually asymptomatic in the early stages. The patient may present with non-specific complaints of eye pain, headache and fatigue on near work. **Difficulty in vision at night may be a feature**[Q]. Blurring of vision, loss of visual field are complains in the advanced stage.

Diagnosis: IOP evaluation, Gonioscopy, Optic disc, Visual fields.

Treatment

- Medical therapy
- **Laser trabeculoplasty**[Q]

Glaucoma

- Filtering surgery (Trabeculectomy) when maximum tolerable medical therapy is not sufficient to control IOP

> **Variants of POAG**
>
> - *Ocular Hypertension (OHT):* This is a subset of POAG where IOP>21mm Hg with no evident damage to the optic nerve or visual field.
> - *Normal tension glaucoma (NTG)^Q:* It is considered to be a subset of POAG wherein the IOP does not rise beyond 21 mm Hg but optic disc and visual field changes specific to glaucoma are present. One additional risk factor is cardiovascular or hematologic abnormalities. **Optic nerve head hemorrhage is seen commonly in NTG^Q.**

PRIMARY ANGLE CLOSURE GLAUCOMA

Primary angle closure glaucoma (PACG) is a condition where optic nerve damage and visual field loss have resulted due to primary angle closure. Primary angle closure means elevation of IOP due to obstruction of aqueous outflow when the trabecular meshwork is occluded by the peripheral iris.

> **Risk factors**
>
> - Age more than 65 years
> - Sex – females
> - High hypermetropia^Q
> - Nanophthalmos^Q
> - Microcornea^Q
> - Thick lens
> - Plateau iris^Q

Pathogenesis

- *Pupillary block*: Dilatation of the pupil drags the iris tissue peripherally leading to crowding of the angle. Dilatation also makes the iris flaccid so that it touches the surface of the lens. This prevents aqueous from travelling from posterior to anterior chamber. Accumulation of aqueous behind the iris pushes the iris forward and closes the angle.
- *Synechiae formation*: Shallow anterior chamber with narrow angles leads to formation of anterior synechiae (adhesions between iris and cornea). This also leads to angle closure.

Stages of PACG

Angle Closure Suspect

- No symptoms are present.
- During a routine examination, shallow anterior chamber and narrow angles are identified on gonioscopy. This stage indicates a possibility of developing angle closure at a later date.
- Treatment is **prophylactic laser iridotomy^Q**.

Angle Closure Stage

- Intermittent attacks of angle closure are seen. These attacks are **usually precipitated by dim light^Q, stress, and mydriatic drugs which cause pupillary dilatation.**
- During the attack, there is sudden pain, redness and blurring of vision in the affected eye. Colored haloes may be present due to corneal epithelial edema. The attack resolves spontaneously when the pupil constricts.
- Treatment is **prophylactic laser iridotomy^Q**.

Acute Angle Closure Glaucoma^Q

In this condition, there is complete closure of the angle leading to severe rise in IOP. This is an ophthalmic emergency.

> **Features of acute angle closure glaucoma**
>
> - Severe pain in the eye, associated with headache
> - Nausea and vomiting
> - Severe decrease in vision associated with redness of the affected eye
> - Lid edema, chemosis, circumcorneal congestion
> - Cornea is **edematous and hazy^Q**
> - Anterior chamber is very shallow and may be associated with cells and flare.
> - Pupil is **vertically oval, mid dilated, fixed/non reacting^Q**
> - IOP markedly increased to 60-70 mm Hg

Treatment

- Immediate lowering of IOP with intravenous **Mannitol^Q** or oral **Acetazolamide^Q**
- Constriction of the pupil with 1% **Pilocarpine^Q** drops to break the attack
- Aqueous suppressant eye drops
- *Laser iridotomy^Q*: This is done when the acute attack has resolved and the corneal oedema has cleared. It is also done prophylactically in the other eye as the disease is bilateral.

Chronic Angle Closure Glaucoma

- Formation of peripheral anterior synechiae leads to constantly high IOP with associated damage to optic nerve and visual field loss.
- *Vogt's triad is characteristic*: **Pigment dispersion on corneal endothelium + Sectoral iris atrophy + Glaucomaflecken (Ant. capsular lens cataract)**[Q].
- Treatment is medical management followed by glaucoma filtration surgery.

Absolute Angle Closure Glaucoma

This is the stage of a painful blind eye due to permanently high IOP. Treatment is **cyclodestruction**[Q] by laser or cryotherapy

Provocative tests[Q]: Prior to the advent of gonioscopy, these tests were used to identify patients with occludable angles. If an increase in IOP> 8 mm Hg was seen, the test was considered positive and the angle as occludable. These tests are not done nowadays.

- Mydriatic provocative test
- **Dark Room test**[Q]
- Prone provocative test

PRIMARY CONGENITAL GLAUCOMA

Primary congenital glaucoma is a type of pediatric glaucoma where developmental anomaly of the angle of anterior chamber leads to obstruction of aqueous outflow and consequent rise in IOP. The distinctive feature of this condition is enlargement of the eyeball in response to the high IOP. This is called **Buphthalmos**[Q].

Symptoms

- Lacrimation[Q]
- Photophobia[Q]
- Blepharospasm[Q]
- This **triad** of symptoms is due to the corneal epithelial edema that results from increased IOP.

Signs

- Buphthalmos
- Increased corneal diameter: (>12 mm)
- Corneal edema is present associated with **Haab's striae**[Q] (Tears in the Descemet's membrane)
- Deep AC
- Enlargement of the eyeball leads to thin and bluish appearance of the sclera
- Antero-posteriorly flat lens, Subluxated lens
- Optic disc shows glaucomatous cupping
- Tonometry shows high IOP

Management

Surgery is the treatment[Q]. The options are
- Trabeculotomy
- Trabeculectomy

Trabeculotomy combined with Trabeculectomy[Q] is the best modality.

> **Developmental glaucoma with associated anomalies**
>
> - Associated with **irido-corneal dysgenesis**[Q]
>   - Axenfeld's anomaly
>   - Reigers anomaly
>   - Reigers syndrome
>   - Peter's anomaly
> - Associated with **Aniridia**[Q]
> - Associated with **Ectopia lentis**[Q]: Marfan, Weil-Marchesani and Homocystinuria
> - Associated with congenital ectropion uveae
> - Associated with **Nanophthalmos**[Q]
> - Associated with systemic conditions like
>   - **Naevus of Ota**[Q]
>   - Lowe's syndrome
>   - Phacomatosis like **Sturge-Weber syndrome**[Q]
>   - **Von-Recklinghausen's Disease**[Q]

SECONDARY GLAUCOMA

> **Lens induced glaucoma**
>
> - *Phacomorphic glaucoma*[Q]: It is a type of secondary angle closure glaucoma due to **intumescent cataract**[Q]. The swollen cataractous lens pushes the iris forward to occlude the angle.
> - *Phacolytic glaucoma*[Q]: It is a type of secondary open angle glaucoma due to **hypermature Morgagnian cataract**[Q]. It is also called **lens protein glaucoma**[Q]. The liquefied cortical protein matter leaks through the intact capsule and blocks the pores of the trabecular meshwork.
> - *Phacotoxic glaucoma*: This is seen in traumatic rupture of the capsule. The lens material in the anterior chamber blocks the pores of the trabecular meshwork.
> - *Phacoanaphylactic glaucoma*: This is seen in traumatic rupture of the capsule. The inflammatory reaction to the lens matter blocks the trabecular meshwork.
>
> Treatment of lens induced glaucoma is lowering of IOP with drugs followed by **cataract surgery**[Q].

Glaucoma

Irido-corneo-endothelial syndrome^Q

This is a condition characterized by **abnormal proliferation of corneal endothelium across the angle of anterior chamber**^Q. This membrane causes obstruction to aqueous outflow. It has three variants
- **Progressive iris atrophy**^Q
- *Chandler's syndrome:* Associated with abnormal corneal endothelium
- *Cogan Reese syndrome:* Associated with iris naevus

Treatment is **medical management and filtering surgery.**

Pigmentary glaucoma

- In this condition, there is loss of iris pigments which subsequently get deposited in different ocular tissues like cornea, lens capsule and trabecular meshwork. This is called **pigment dispersion**.
- Glaucoma results due to blockage of trabecular meshwork by these pigments
- It is common in **young males**^Q between 25-35 years of age with associated **myopia**^Q.
- **Iris heterochromia and transillumination defects**^Q are seen. **Krukenberg spindle**^Q (vertical spindle of pigments on corneal endothelium) is a characteristic feature.
- Treatment is **medical management, laser trabeculoplasty**^Q**, filtration surgery.**

Pseudoexfoliation Glaucoma

➤ Pseudoexfoliation is a condition where an **amorphous, eosinophilic material** produced from the **lens epithelium** is deposited in different ocular tissues like corneal endothelium, lens, zonules, pupillary margin and trabecular meshwork. Glaucoma results from blockage of the trabecular meshwork by this substance.

➤ Treatment is **medical management, laser trabeculoplasty**^Q **and filtration surgery.**

Neovascular Glaucoma

Glaucoma resulting from retinal ischaemic disorders like **Proliferative Diabetic Retinopathy, CRVO, Eales disease, ROP.** Treatment is **panretinal photocoagulation, glaucoma valve surgery.** (Explained in detail in the chapter on Retina)

Inflammatory/Uveitic Glaucoma

Glaucoma may be seen in acute or chronic uveitis especially uveitic syndromes like **Fuch's heterochromic iridocyclitis** and **Possner Schlossman syndrome**^Q. In these conditions, the inflammation is relatively mild but the rise of IOP is high. This is called **glaucomatocyclitic crisis**^Q. Treatment is **steroids and IOP lowering drugs.** (Explained in detail in the chapter on uveitis)

Steroid-induced Glaucoma

Steroids, mainly by **topical route of administration**^Q lead to glaucoma. Steroids increase the **synthesis of glycosaminoglycans**^Q which leads to thickening of the trabecular meshwork. Treatment is to discontinue steroids and medical control of IOP.

Traumatic glaucoma

Glaucoma may result from penetrating or blunt trauma. The different mechanisms are:
- **Hyphaema**^Q
- Inflammatory glaucoma
- Hemolytic glaucoma
- Hemosiderotic glaucoma
- Ghost cell glaucoma
- **Angle recession glaucoma**^Q
- Glaucoma associated with subluxation/dislocation of lens

Malignant glaucoma

- This is a type of **secondary angle closure glaucoma** which is seen after intraocular surgeries like trabeculectomy, cataract etc.
- The cause is **posterior misdirection of aqueous leading to expansion of vitreous volume**^Q. The expanded vitreous pushes the iris diaphragm forward causing angle occlusion.
- Treatment is **atropine**^Q**, laser hyloidotomy and vitrectomy**^Q

Self Assessment and Review of Ophthalmology

ANTIGLAUCOMA DRUGS

Beta blockers		
Timolol maleate[Q] (non selective Beta blocker) **0.5% drops**	**Aqueous suppressant**: Decreases production of aqueous by acting on beta receptors in the ciliary body[Q]	Hypotension Bradycardia Bronchospasm **Dry eye**[Q] **Superficial punctuate keratitis**[Q]
Levobunolol (0.5% drops)	Same	Same
Betaxolol (Selective Beta$_1$ blocker) (0.5% drops)	Same	Same but bronchospasm is avoided
Adrenergic agonists		
Brimonidine (0.2%, 0.1% drops)[Q]	**Aqueous suppressant**[Q]: Decreases aqueous production by acting on alpha2 receptors of the ciliary body Enhances outflow through the trabecular meshwork	**Allergic conjunctivitis**[Q] **CNS depression**[Q] **Cystoid macular edema**[Q] **Lid retraction**[Q]
Apraclonidine (0.5% drops)[Q]	Same	**Same but lid retraction is more**[Q] Tachyphylaxis[Q]
Cholinergics		
Pilocarpine (2% drops)[Q]	Increases trabecular meshwork outflow **In angle closure glaucoma, it breaks the pupillary block by miosis**[Q]	**Brow ache**[Q] Myopia (**accommodative spasm**)[Q] Retinal detachment[Q] Miosis **Iris cysts**[Q]
Cholinesterase inhibitors Echothiophate iodide Demecarium bromide	Increases availability of acetylcholine	Cataract **Iris cysts**[Q] **Posterior synechiae**
Carbonic anhydrase inhibitors		
Acetazolamide (250 mg tablet)[Q]	**Aqueous suppressant**: Decreases aqueous production by inhibition of carbonic anhydrase[Q]	**Parasthesias**[Q] GI upset Renal stones **Sulfa sensitivity**[Q] **Metabolic acidosis**[Q] Aplastic anemia
Dorzolamide (2% drops)[Q]	Same	**Endothelial decompensation**[Q] Bitter taste
Prostaglandin analogues		
Latanoprost (0.005% drops)[Q] Bimatoprost (0.03% drops)[Q] Travoprost (0.004% drops)[Q]	Increases uveoscleral outflow[Q]	**Iris pigmentation**[Q] Cystoid macular edema Anterior uveitis **Hypertrichosis**[Q]
Hyperosmotics		
Glycerol 50% oral	Decreases the vitreous volume by drawing water from the vitreous[Q]	Nausea, vomiting, Cardiac arrhythmia Cardiac overload
Mannitol 20% intravenous	Same	Electrolyte imbalance Congestive heart failure
Urea intravenous (rarely used)	Same	Same

Glaucoma

Laser Procedures

Laser Iridotomy	Selective Laser Trabeculoplasty (SLT)
Indications: Angle closure glaucoma^Q Prophylactic Iridotomy in the fellow eye of ACG^Q Laser used: Nd: YAG^Q	Indications: Primary Open angle glaucoma^Q Pseudoexfoliation glaucoma^Q Pigmentary glaucoma^Q Laser used: Double frequency Nd: YAG^Q

Glaucoma Surgeries

- Trabeculotomy (for congenital glaucoma)
- *Filtration surgery*: Trabeculectomy
- Filtration surgery with antimetabolites like MitomycinC
- *Non-penetrating filtration surgery*: Visco-canalostomy, Deep sclerectomy
- Glaucoma Valve surgery
- Express shunt surgery^Q
- Cyclodestructive surgery for absolute glaucoma

Glaucoma Valves

These are used in cases of refractory glaucoma or when filtering surgery has high chances of failure. These implants are placed subconjunctivally and have a drainage tube in the anterior chamber. This tube drains a controlled amount of aqueous to the subtenon space.

Indications

- Failed Trabeculectomy
- Neovascular glaucoma
- Uveitic glaucoma
- Post Keratoplasty glaucoma
- Post retinal surgery glaucoma
- Primary congenital glaucoma (intractable), e.g. Ahmed Glaucoma Valve (AGV)

> **Must Remember**
> - First-line management of Congenital Glaucoma: Surgery
> - First-line management of Primary Angle Closure Glaucoma (PACG): Laser Iridotomy
> - First-line management of Primary Open Angle Glaucoma (POAG): Medical management
> - Anti-glaucoma drug causing Heterochromia iridis: Latanoprost
> - Anti-glaucoma drug contraindicated in children: Brimonidine

Self Assessment and Review of Ophthalmology

QUESTIONS

Aqueous Humour

1. Cells affected in glaucomatous optic neuropathy are: *(AIIMS 2014/ 2013)*
   a. Amacrine cells
   b. Bipolar cells
   c. Ganglion cells
   d. Rods and cones

2. In the conversion of CO_2 and H_2O to form carbonic acid during formation of aqueous humour, the enzyme catalyzing the reaction is: *(AIIMS)*
   a. Carboxylase
   b. Carbamylase
   c. Carbonic anhydrase
   d. Carbonic dehydrogenase

3. Regarding aqueous humour, which of the following statements is/are true: *(PGI)*
   a. It is secreted at a rate of 2-3 microlitre/min
   b. Secreted by ciliary processes
   c. Has less protein than plasma
   d. Provides nutrition
   e. Normal IOP is 5-15 mm Hg

Glaucoma Investigations: Tonometry/Gonioscopy/Perimetry

4. Which of the following is used as self-tonometer? *(AIIMS 2014)*
   a. Diaton palpebral tonometer
   b. Rebound tonometer
   c. Perkin's tonometer
   d. Dynamic contour tonometer

5. Tonometer used in irregular cornea: *(AIIMS)*
   a. Mackay-Marg tonometer
   b. Rebound tonometer
   c. Draeger's tonometer
   d. Maklakov tonometer

6. Tonometer with variation in applanation surface is: *(AIIMS)*
   a. Maklakov tonometer
   b. Mackay-Marg tonometer
   c. Rebound tonometer
   d. Draeger tonometer

7. Goldmann tonometer is a type of: *(NEET 2016)*
   a. Applanation tonometer
   b. Rebound tonometer
   c. Indentation tonometer
   d. Non-contact tonometer

8. Critical angle of air-cornea interface: *(AIIMS)*
   a. 46 degrees
   b. 64 degrees
   c. 24 degrees
   d. 36 degrees

9. Which of the following procedures is not done in dilated pupil? *(AIIMS 2014)*
   a. Gonioscopy
   b. Fundoscopy
   c. Laser inferometry
   d. Electroretinogram

10. Schwalbe's line is: *(DNB 2015)*
    a. The posterior limit of the Descemet's membrane
    b. The posterior limit of the Bowman's membrane
    c. The anterior limit of the Descemet's membrane
    d. The anterior limit of the Bowman's membrane

11. Schwalbe's line represents: *(NEET 2016)*
    a. Junction of choroid and retina
    b. Termination of Descemet's membrane of cornea
    c. Junction of bulbar and palpebral conjunctiva
    d. Upper limit of the macula

12. Visual field abnormalities in the Bjerrum's area are seen in: *(Kerala PG 2015)*
    a. Cataract
    b. Glaucoma
    c. Keratitis
    d. Proptosis

13. Tonography is used to determine: *(AIPG 2002)*
    a. The rate of formation of aqueous
    b. The facility of aqueous outflow
    c. The IOP at different times
    d. None of the above

Congenital Glaucoma

14. True about Buphthalmos is/are: *(PGI)*
    a. Large cornea
    b. Shallow anterior chamber
    c. Haab's striae
    d. High IOP
    e. Medical management is the key

15. Which of the following is not true regarding primary congenital glaucoma: *(DNB 2015)*
    a. Photophobia is the most common symptom
    b. Haab's striae may be seen
    c. Thin and blue sclera may be seen
    d. Anterior chamber is shallow

16. A baby about 30 days old presents with excessive lacrimation and photophobia. He has large and hazy cornea in both eyes. His lacrimal system is normal. What is the probable diagnosis? *(AIIMS)*
    a. Congenital glaucoma
    b. Megalocornea
    c. Keratoconus
    d. Hunter's syndrome

17. The treatment of congenital glaucoma is: *(AIIMS 2003)*
    a. Essentially topical medication
    b. Trabeculoplasty
    c. Trabeculotomy with trabeculectomy
    d. Cyclocryotherapy

18. Earliest sign of congenital glaucoma is: *(DNB 2015)*
    a. Corneal oedema with watering
    b. Haab's striae
    c. Blue sclera
    d. Myopia

19. Descemet's membrane breach is seen in: *(DNB 2015)*
    a. Angle closure glaucoma
    b. Buphthalmos
    c. Open angle glaucoma
    d. Acute iridocyclitis

20. Increased intraocular pressure along with enlarged and thick cornea and large eyeball may suggest: *(CET JUNE 2017)*
    a. Congenital glaucoma
    b. Angle closure glaucoma
    c. Phacomorphic glaucoma
    d. Phacolytic glaucoma

Glaucoma

21. Which of the following does not cause hazy cornea in a newborn? *(AIPG)*
    a. Endothelial dystrophy
    b. Mucoplysaccharidosis
    c. Sclerocornea
    d. Droplet keratopathy

Primary Angle Closure Glaucoma (PACG)

22. Shallow anterior chamber is seen in all except: *(TNPG 2013)*
    a. Old age
    b. Hypermetropia
    c. Steroid induced glaucoma
    d. Angle closure glaucoma

23. Which statements regarding depth of anterior chamber is/are false: *(PGI)*
    a. Depth is less in women than men
    b. Depth corresponds to the volume of aqueous humour
    c. Depth increases with age
    d. Depth is less in hypermetropes
    e. Depth is more in myopes

24. All of the following predispose to angle closure glaucoma except: *(AIIMS 2000)*
    a. Small cornea
    b. Flat cornea
    c. Shallow anterior chamber
    d. Short axial length of the eyeball

25. True about PACG is/are: *(PGI)*
    a. More common in females
    b. Shallow anterior chamber is a risk factor
    c. Deep anterior chamber is a risk factor
    d. Small diameter of the cornea is a risk factor
    e. More common in myopes

26. A 36-year-old female develops pain in the eyes after prone dark room test. Which of the drugs should be avoided? *(AIIMS 2013)*
    a. Acetazolamide
    b. Pilocarpine
    c. Atropine
    d. Timolol

27. All are true about angle closure glaucoma except: *(NEET 2016)*
    a. Vertically oval mid-dilated pupil
    b. Oedematous and hyperemic optic disc
    c. Oedematous cornea
    d. Multiple iris nodules

28. A 50-year-old female presents with acute painful red eye and vertically oval mid-dilated pupil. Most likely diagnosis is: *(AIIMS/ AIPG 2002)*
    a. Acute retrobulbar neuritis
    b. Acute angle closure glaucoma
    c. Acute anterior uveitis
    d. Severe keratoconjunctivitis

29. A 60-year-old male presents with coloured haloes. On Fincham's test, the haloes split and then reunite. The most probable diagnosis is: *(AIIMS 2000)*
    a. Acute congestive glaucoma
    b. Open angle glaucoma
    c. Senile immature cataract
    d. Mucopurulent conjunctivitis

30. A 32-year-old female presents with sudden onset severe pain in the left eye after watching a movie. The pain is severe and there is progressive loss of vision. The ophthalmic surgeon notices ciliary injection and a shallow anterior chamber. Pupil is semi dilated and corneal appears oedematous. The probable diagnosis is: *(CET JUNE 2017)*
    a. Open angle glaucoma
    b. CRAO
    c. Acute angle closure glaucoma
    d. CRVO

31. A 55-year-old female comes to the casualty with history of severe eye pain, redness and diminution of vision. On examination the visual acuity is 6/60, there is circumcorneal congestion, corneal oedema and a shallow anterior chamber. Which is the drug of choice? *(AIIMS 2005)*
    a. Atropine ointment
    b. Intravenous Mannitol
    c. Ciprofloxacin eye drops
    d. Betamethasone eye drops

32. First drug to be given in acute angle closure glaucoma: *(AIIMS)*
    a. Acetazolamide
    b. Atropine
    c. Pilocarpine
    d. Timolol

33. Drug of choice for acute angle closure glaucoma: *(AIIMS/ AIPG/ DNB 2010)*
    a. Pilocarpine
    b. Atropine
    c. Timolol
    d. Acetazolamide

34. Treatment of choice for acute angle closure glaucoma: *(AIPG 2000)*
    a. Pilocarpine
    b. Laser iridotomy
    c. Timolol
    d. Trabeculoplasty

35. Drugs used in acute congestive glaucoma are all except: *(PGI)*
    a. Atropine
    b. Pilocarpine
    c. Acetazolamide
    d. Mannitol
    e. Timolol

36. Treatment of choice of fellow eye in acute congestive glaucoma: *(AIIMS/ PGI 2000)*
    a. Pilocarpine
    b. Nd: YAG iridotomy
    c. Peripheral iridectomy
    d. Careful follow up

37. Miotics are the drug of choice for: *(DNB 2015)*
    a. Angle closure glaucoma
    b. Open angle glaucoma
    c. Congenital glaucoma
    d. Sympathetic ophthalmia

38. Treatment of choice for absolute glaucoma: *(APPG 2013)*
    a. Cyclocryotherapy
    b. Acetazolamide
    c. Trabeculectomy
    d. Timolol

Primary Open Angle Glaucoma (POAG)

39. Open angle glaucoma causes: *(COMEDK 2009)*
    a. Sudden loss of vision
    b. Difficulty in dark adaptation
    c. Amaurosis fugax
    d. Uniocular diplopia

Self Assessment and Review of Ophthalmology

40. In POAG, which of the following is not seen? *(PGI)*
    a. Vertical cupping
    b. Horizontal cupping
    c. Bayonetting of vessels
    d. Dot sign

41. Earliest field defect in primary open angle glaucoma: *(AIIMS/ UPPG 2008)*
    a. Paracentral scotoma
    b. Ring scotoma
    c. Seidel scotoma
    d. Arcuate scotoma

42. A 70-year-old patient presents with progressive deterioration of vision. On examination, the pupillary reaction is sluggish and the IOP is normal. Fundoscopy shows a large and deep cup. Visual field reveals paracentral scotoma. What is the probable diagnosis? *(AIPG)*
    a. Primary angle closure glaucoma
    b. Normal tension glaucoma
    c. Neovascular glaucoma
    d. Absolute glaucoma

Secondary Glaucoma

43. A male patient with history of hypermature cataract presents with sudden onset pain, redness, photophobia in the right eye. On examination, there is a deep anterior chamber with raised IOP. The left eye is normal. What is the likely diagnosis? *(AIIMS 2001)*
    a. Phacomorphic glaucoma
    b. Phacolytic glaucoma
    c. Phacotoxic glaucoma
    d. Phacoanaphylactic uveitis

44. Iridocorneoendothelial syndrome is associated with: *(AIIMS 2008)*
    a. Progressive iris atrophy
    b. Bilateral stromal oedema of cornea
    c. Deposition of collagen in the Descemet's membrane
    d. Deposition of glycosaminoglycans in the Descemet's membrane

45. Malignant glaucoma is seen in: *(PGI)*
    a. After intraocular surgery
    b. Intraocular malignancy
    c. Trauma
    d. Thrombosis

46. Malignant glaucoma, correct statements is/are: *(PGI)*
    a. Anterior chamber is normal
    b. Misdirected aqueous flow
    c. Pilocarpine is the drug of choice
    d. Management is medical only
    e. Atropine is the drug of choice

47. Neovascularization of iris is seen in all except: *(MPPG 2009)*
    a. CRVO
    b. Diabetic retinopathy
    c. Fuch's heterochromic iridocyclitis
    d. Congenital cataract

48. The laser procedure used for treating rubeosis iridis is: *(AIIMS 2006)*
    a. Goniophotocoagulation
    b. Panretinal photocoagulation
    c. Laser trabeculoplasty
    d. Laser iridotomy

49. A 25-year-old patient presents with painless red eye with an IOP of 60 mm Hg. What is the most likely diagnosis? *(AIIMS 2014)*
    a. Chronic papilloedema
    b. Acute angle closure glaucoma
    c. Glaucomatocyclitic crisis
    d. Acute anterior uveitis

50. Krukenberg spindle is seen in: *(DNB 2013)*
    a. Pigmentary glaucoma
    b. Sympathetic ophthalmitis
    c. Retinitis pigmentosa
    d. Chalazion

51. Krukenberg spindle is seen in: *(APPG 2014)*
    a. Corneal endothelium
    b. Retina
    c. Lens
    d. Conjunctiva

Anti-glaucoma Drugs

52. Which carbonic anhydrase inhibitor is used topically as anti-glaucoma medication? *(NEET 2016)*
    a. Acetazolamide
    b. Brinzolamide
    c. Methazolamide
    d. Dichlorphenamide

53. Which of the following drugs is not used topically for the treatment of glaucoma? *(AIPG 2001)*
    a. Timolol
    b. Latanoprost
    c. Acetazolamide
    d. Dorzolamide

54. Contraindications for topical beta-blockers are: *(PGI 2004)*
    a. Hypertension
    b. Asthma
    c. Tachycardia
    d. Hypotension
    e. Depression

55. Which of the following anti-glaucoma medications can cause drowsiness? *(AIPG)*
    a. Latanoprost
    b. Brimonidine
    c. Timolol
    d. Dorzolamide

56. Which anti-glaucoma medication is unsafe in infants? *(DPG 2009/NEET 2016)*
    a. Timolol
    b. Brimonidine
    c. Dorzolamide
    d. Latanoprost

57. Latanoprost acts in glaucoma by: *(AIPG 2004)*
    a. Decreasing aqueous humour production
    b. Increasing uveoscleral outflow
    c. Increasing trabecular outflow
    d. Releasing pupillary block

58. Uveoscleral outflow is increased by: *(DNB 2015)*
    a. Timolol
    b. Bimatoprost
    c. Mannitol
    d. Dorzolamide

59. Which of the following topical drugs causes heterochromia iridis? *(AIIMS 2015)*
    a. Latanoprost
    b. Prednisolone
    c. Olopatadine
    d. Timolol

60. Which anti-glaucoma drug causes pigmentation of eyelids? *(DNB 2015)*
    a. Brimonidine
    b. Timolol
    c. Latanoprost
    d. Dorzolamide

Glaucoma

61. Which of the following drugs is not used in a patient of acute congestive glaucoma having a history of sulfa allergy? *(AIIMS 2005)*
    a. Glycerol
    b. Acetazolamide
    c. Mannitol
    d. Latanoprost

62. Black deposits on conjunctiva in a patient of glaucoma are seen with the use of: *(May AIIMS 2016)*
    a. Epinephrine
    b. Carbonic anhydrase inhibitors
    c. Prostaglandin analogues
    d. B-Blockers

63. Hyperosmotic agents act by: *(APPG 2008)*
    a. Increasing aqueous outflow
    b. Decreasing aqueous production
    c. Decreasing vitreous volume
    d. Increasing uveoscleral outflow

64. Which drug is contraindicated in uveitic glaucoma? *(DNB)*
    a. Beta blockers
    b. Mydriatic
    c. Miotics
    d. Carbonic anhydrase inhibitors

65. Antiglaucoma drug that should be avoided in hypertensives is: *(DNB 2015)*
    a. Timolol
    b. Apraclonidine
    c. Dipivefrine
    d. Dorzolamide

66. Which of these drug combinations is not generally used in glaucoma? *(DNB 2014)*
    a. Timolol + Latanoprost
    b. Timolol + Brimonidine
    c. Timolol + Pilocarpine
    d. Pilocarpine + Latanoprost

67. Which anti glaucoma drug is contraindicated in uveitis: *(DNB 2016)*
    a. Pilocarpine
    b. Timolol
    c. Brimonidine
    d. Latanoprost

68. True about pilocarpine is: *(DNB 2015)*
    a. It acts by decreasing secretion from the ciliary epithelium
    b. It is the drug of choice in angle closure glaucoma
    c. It is a hyperosmotic agent
    d. Side effects include bitter taste and renal calculi

Glaucoma Surgeries and Procedures

69. Laser trabeculoplasty in indicated in: *(AIIMS 2014)*
    a. Neovascular glaucoma
    b. Pseudoexfoliation glaucoma
    c. Chronic angle closure glaucoma
    d. Uveitic glaucoma

70. Glaucoma drainage devices: *(DNB 2015)*
    a. Drain aqueous humour to the posterior segment
    b. Drain aqueous humour to an external device
    c. Decrease the secretion of aqueous humour from the ciliary epithelium
    d. Open up the trabecular meshwork

71. Express shunt in glaucoma is made up of: *(AIIMS 2014)*
    a. Silicon
    b. Titanium
    c. Gold
    d. Stainless steel

72. Laser trabeculoplasty is indicated in the treatment of: *(NEET 2016)*
    a. Open angle glaucoma
    b. Angle closure glaucoma
    c. Buphthalmos
    d. Malignant glaucoma

73. Treatment options for glaucoma are all except: *(PGI)*
    a. Trabeculotomy
    b. Trabeculectomy
    c. Visco canalostomy
    d. Vitrectomy
    e. Iridectomy

74. Triple procedure in glaucoma includes all the following except: *(DNB 2015)*
    a. Trabeculectomy
    b. PCIOL implantation
    c. Extracapsular cataract extraction
    d. Insertion of glaucoma drainage device

75. Hypersecretory glaucoma is seen in: *(AIPG)*
    a. Epidemic dropsy
    b. Marfan's syndrome
    c. Hypertension
    d. Diabetes

ANSWERS AND EXPLANATIONS

1. c. **Ganglion cells.**
   The axons of the ganglion cells of the retina form the nerve fibre layer which continues as the optic nerve. Hence glaucoma is associated with ganglion cell loss *(Ref: Yanoff & Duker 4th edition, p 1016)*
2. c. **Carbonic anhydrase** *(Ref: Yanoff & Duker 4th edition, p 1014)*
3. a. **It is secreted at the rate of 2-3 microlitres per minute. b. secreted by ciliary processes. c. Has less protein than plasma. d. Provides nutrition**
   The normal IOP is 10-21mm Hg *(Ref: Yanoff & Duker 4th edition, p 1012-1014)*
4. b. **Rebound tonometer** *(Ref: Yanoff & Duker 4th edition, p 1020-1021)*
5. a. **Mackay- Marg tonometer** *(Ref: Yanoff & Duker 4th edition, p 1020-1021)*
6. a. **Maklakov tonometer** *(Ref: Yanoff & Duker 4th edition, p 1020-1021)*
7. a. **Applanation tonometer** *(Ref: Yanoff & Duker 4th edition, p 1020-1021)*
8. a. **46 degrees** *(Ref: Yanoff & Duker 4th edition, p 1024)*
9. a. **Gonioscopy** *(Ref: Yanoff & Duker 4th edition, p 1024-1025)*
10. a. **The posterior limit of the Descemet's membrane** *(Ref: Yanoff & Duker 4th edition, p 1024)*
11. b. **Termination of Descemet's membrane of cornea** *(Ref: Yanoff & Duker 4th edition, p 1024)*
12. b. **Glaucoma** *(Ref: Yanoff & Duker 4th edition, p 1029)*
13. b. **The facility of aqueous outflow**
14. a. **Large cornea c. Haab's striae d. High IOP.** *(Ref: Yanoff & Duker 4th edition, p 1102-1103)*
15. d. **Anterior chamber is shallow** *(Ref: Yanoff & Duker 4th edition, p 1102-1103)*
16. a. **Congenital glaucoma** *(Ref: Yanoff & Duker 4th edition, p 1102-1103)*
17. c. **Trabeculotomy with trabeculectomy** *(Ref: Yanoff & Duker 4th edition, p 1105)*
18. a. **Corneal oedema with watering** *(Ref: Yanoff & Duker 4th edition, p 1102-1103)*
19. b. **Buphthalmos** *(Ref: Yanoff & Duker 4th edition, p 1102-1103)*
20. a. **Congenital glaucoma** *(Ref: Yanoff & Duker 4th edition, p 1102-1103)*
21. d. **Droplet keratopathy.** *(Ref: Yanoff & Duker 4th edition, p 1104)*

> **Causes of Hazy cornea in a child (STUMPED)**
> - S- Sclerocornea
> - T- Trauma during birth
> - U- Ulcer
> - M- Mucoplysaccharidosis
> - P- Peter's anomaly
> - E- Endothelial dystrophy
> - D- Dermoid (limbal)
>
> Also Congenital glaucoma

22. c. **Steroid induced glaucoma** *(Ref: Yanoff & Duker 4th edition, p 1080)*
23. b. **Depth corresponds to the volume of aqueous humour c. Depth increases with age** *(Ref: Yanoff & Duker 4th edition, p 1060)*
24. b. **Flat cornea** *(Ref: Yanoff & Duker 4th edition, p 1060)*
25. a. **More common in females b. Shallow anterior chamber is a risk factor. d. Small diameter of the cornea is a risk factor** *(Ref: Yanoff & Duker 4th edition, p 1060)*
26. c. **Atropine** *(Ref: Yanoff & Duker 4th edition, p 1060)*
    Pain after dark room test indicates that the patient has occludable angles. Hence atropine is contraindicated because it is a long acting mydriatic and may precipitate angle closure
27. d. **Multiple iris nodules** *(Ref: Yanoff & Duker 4th edition, p 1064)*
28. b. **Acute angle closure glaucoma** *(Ref: Yanoff & Duker 4th edition, p 1064)*

Glaucoma

29. c. Senile immature cataract

Fincham's test helps to differentiate between coloured haloes in immature cataract and acute congestive glaucoma. When viewed through a stenopaeic slit, the haloes of an immature cataract are broken up into segments but the halo in ACG remains intact.

30. c. Acute angle closure glaucoma *(Ref: Yanoff & Duker 4th edition, p 1064)*

31. b. Intravenous Mannitol *(Ref: Yanoff & Duker 4th edition, p 1065-1066)*

The first drug to be administered in a case of Acute ACG is intravenous Mannitol or oral Acetazolamide. This helps to reduce the IOP by dehydrating and reducing the vitreous volume

Following this Pilocarpine eye drops are used to constrict the pupil and break the acute attack. Thus pilocarpine is the definitive drug for Acute ACG.

Finally, when the corneal oedema has resolved, the patient has to undergo laser iridotomy to prevent such attacks in future. Laser has to be done in the fellow eye also as the disease is bilateral. Hence laser iridotomy is the definitive management of Acute ACG

32. a. Acetazolamide *(Ref: Yanoff & Duker 4th edition, p 1065-1066)*
33. a. Pilocarpine *(Ref: Yanoff & Duker 4th edition, p 1065-1066)*
34. b. Laser iridotomy *(Ref: Yanoff & Duker 4th edition, p 1065-1067)*
35. a. Atropine *(Ref: Yanoff & Duker 4th edition, p 1065-1066)*
36. b. Nd: YAG iridotomy *(Ref: Yanoff & Duker 4th edition, p 1065-1066)*
37. a. Angle closure glaucoma *(Ref: Yanoff & Duker 4th edition, p 1065-1066)*
38. a. Cyclocryotherapy *(Ref: Yanoff & Duker 4th edition, p 1069)*
39. b. Difficulty in dark adaptation
40. b. Horizontal cupping *(Ref: Yanoff & Duker 4th edition, p 1041)*
41. a. Paracentral scotoma *(Ref: Yanoff & Duker 4th edition, p 1030)*
42. b. Normal tension glaucoma *(Ref: Yanoff & Duker 4th edition, p 1057)*

The question describes a patient with normal IOP but optic disc changes and visual field changes suggestive of glaucoma. Hence the answer is normal tension glaucoma.

43. b. Phacolytic glaucoma *(Ref: Yanoff & Duker 4th edition, p 1088)*

Cataract with glaucoma with shallow anterior chamber: Phacomorphic glaucoma
Cataract with glaucoma with normal or deep anterior chamber: Phacolytic glaucoma

44. a. Progressive iris atrophy *(Ref: Yanoff & Duker 4th edition, p 1095)*
45. a. After intraocular surgery *(Ref: Yanoff & Duker 4th edition, p 1092)*
46. b. Misdirected aqueous flow e. Atropine is the drug of choice *(Ref: Yanoff & Duker 4th edition, p 1092)*
47. d. Congenital cataract *(Ref: Yanoff & Duker 4th edition, p 1076)*
48. b. Panretinal photocoagulation *(Ref: Yanoff & Duker 4th edition, p 1078)*
49. c. Glaucomatocyclitic crisis *(Ref: Yanoff & Duker 4th edition, p 1083)*
50. a. Pigmentary glaucoma *(Ref: Yanoff & Duker 4th edition, p 1074)*
51. a. Corneal endothelium *(Ref: Yanoff & Duker 4th edition, p 1074)*
52. b. Brinzolamide *(Ref: Yanoff & Duker 4th edition, p 1118)*

The carbonic anhydrase inhibitors used in glaucoma are Acetazolamide, Dorzolamide and Brinzolamide, of which Acetazolamide is used orally and the other two are used topically

53. c. Acetazolamide *(Ref: Yanoff & Duker 4th edition, p 1118)*

It is used orally.

54. b. Asthma d. Hypotension *(Ref: Yanoff & Duker 4th edition, p 1114-1115)*
55. b. Brimonidine *(Ref: Yanoff & Duker 4th edition, p 1114-1115)*
56. b. Brimonidine *(Ref: Yanoff & Duker 4th edition, p 1114-1115)*

Brimonidine causes CNS depression and drowsiness and hence is contraindicated in children

57. b. Increasing uveoscleral outflow *(Ref: Yanoff & Duker 4th edition, p 1117)*
58. b. Bimatoprost *(Ref: Yanoff & Duker 4th edition, p 1117)*
59. a. Latanoprost. *(Ref: Yanoff & Duker 4th edition, p 1117-1118)*

It causes iris pigmentation and may lead to heterochromia iridis when given unilaterally

Self Assessment and Review of Ophthalmology

Causes of heterochromia iridis
• Iris naevus, iris melanoma
• Ocular melanosis
• Fuch's heterochromic iridocyclitis[Q]
• Siderosis bulbi[Q]
• Congenital Horner's syndrome
• Sturge Weber syndrome[Q]
• Waardenberg syndrome
• Latanoprost[Q]

60. c. **Latanoprost** *(Ref: Yanoff & Duker 4th edition, p 1117-1118)*
    Latanoprost mainly causes iris pigmentation but it may also cause periocular pigmentation.

61. b. **Acetazolamide** *(Ref: Yanoff & Duker 4th edition, p 1116)*
    It has the potential to cause SJS in patients of sulfa allergy

62. a. **Epinephrine** *(Ref: Smolin and Thoft: The Cornea, p 504)*
    Adrenochrome deposits are seen in the conjunctiva after prolonged use of epinephrine. These are products of oxidation and polymerization of epinephrine. However, Epinephrine is not used in glaucoma nowadays

63. c. **Decreasing vitreous volume**

64. c. **Miotics** *(Ref: Yanoff & Duker 4th edition, p 1082)*
    Miotics should not be given in uveitis as they increase the ciliary spasm

65. c. **Dipivefrine**
    Not used nowadays. It must be avoided in hypertensives because it gets converted to adrenaline that may aggravate the hypertension.

66. d. **Pilocarpine+ Latanoprost** *(Ref: Yanoff & Duker 4th edition, p 1082)*
    Both these drugs increase intraocular inflammation and hence the combination is avoided

67. a. **Pilocarpine** *(Ref: Yanoff & Duker 4th edition, p 1082)*
    Actually both Pilocarpine and Latanoprost are contraindicated in uveitis because they increase intraocular inflammation. But Pilocarpine also causes miosis and ciliary spasm which might aggravate pain in uveitis. Hence it may be the better option.

68. b. **It is the drug of choice in angle closure glaucoma** *(Ref: Yanoff & Duker 4th edition, p 1116)*

69. b. **Pseudoexfoliation glaucoma** *(Ref: Yanoff & Duker 4th edition, p 1120)*

70. b. **Drain aqueous humour to an external device** *(Ref: Yanoff & Duker 4th edition, p 1159)*

71. d. **Stainless steel**

72. a. **Open angle glaucoma** *(Ref: Yanoff & Duker 4th edition, p 1129)*

73. d. **Vitrectomy** *(Ref: Yanoff & Duker 4th edition, p 1129-1145)*
    Though vitrectomy is a treatment modality for malignant glaucoma, it is the best choice among the available options

74. d. **Insertion of glaucoma drainage device** *(Ref: Yanoff & Duker 4th edition, p 1146-1147)*
    Triple procedure in glaucoma is a combination of cataract surgery with IOL implantation along with trabeculectomy

75. a. **Epidemic dropsy** *(Ref: Sachdev et al .Pathogenesis of epidemic dropsy glaucoma. Arch Ophthalmol 1988;106:1221-3.)*
    Epidemic dropsy is a rare condition seen due to Argemone mexicana poisoning. It is an example where glaucoma is due to excessive production of aqueous humour.

IMAGE BASED QUESTIONS

1. Identify the test shown in the photograph:

   (AIIMS 2017)

   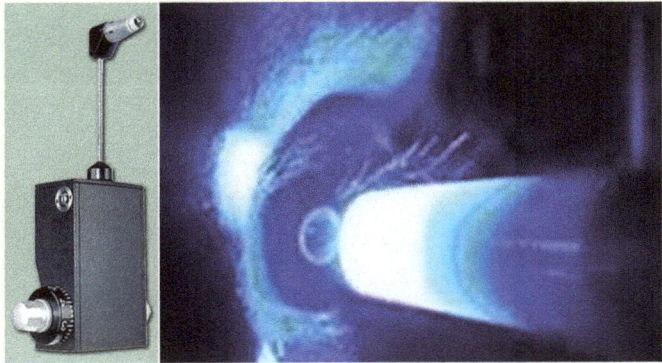

   a. Tonometry
   b. Pachymetry
   c. Laser Interferometry
   d. Refraction

2. Identify the test shown in the photograph:

   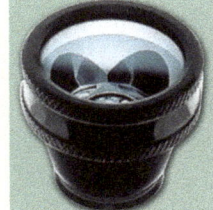 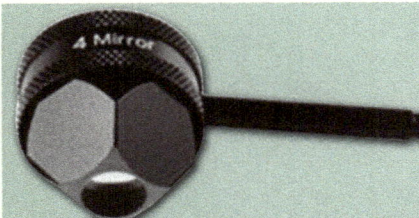

   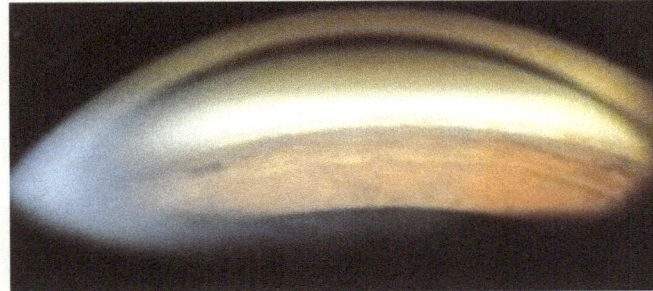

   a. Tonometry
   b. Pachymetry
   c. Gonioscopy
   d. Laser interferometry

3. This is the fundus photo of a 55-year-old male who presented with complaints of headache, eye pain and fatigue. What are the investigations to be done in this patient?

   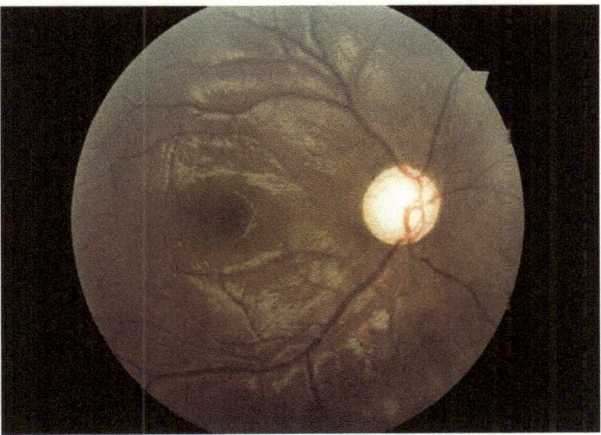

   a. Fundus Fluorescein angiography and OCT
   b. Gonioscopy, Tonometry and Visual fields
   c. Retinoscopy and refraction
   d. Indirect ophthalmoscopy

4. A 65-year-old female patient presents with sudden onset pain and redness in the eye associated with decreased vision. The clinical photograph is given. The IOP is 50 mm Hg. What is the probable diagnosis?

   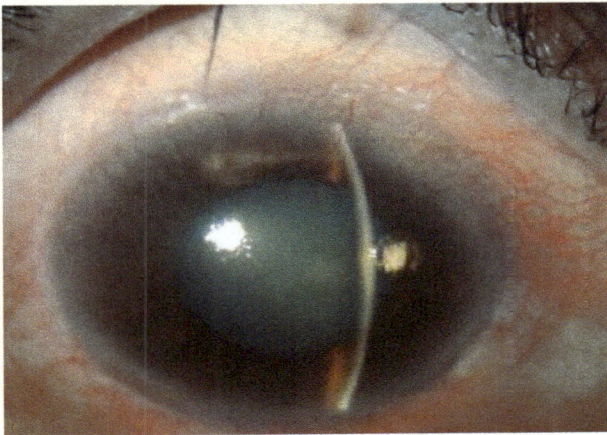

   a. Primary open angle glaucoma
   b. Lens-induced glaucoma
   c. Acute angle closure glaucoma
   d. Pseudo-exfoliation glaucoma

Answer Key: 1. a 2. c 3. b 4. c

5. The clinical photograph of a patient who has undergone a certain glaucoma procedure has been given. What is the laser used?

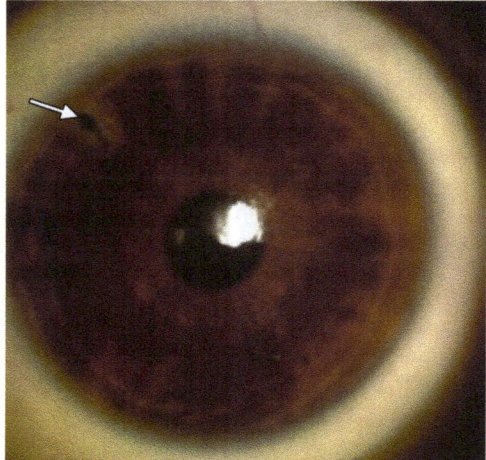

a. Nd: YAG laser
b. Double frequency Nd: YAG laser
c. Femtosecond laser
d. Argon laser

6. Identify the investigation modality whose print out is given in the question:

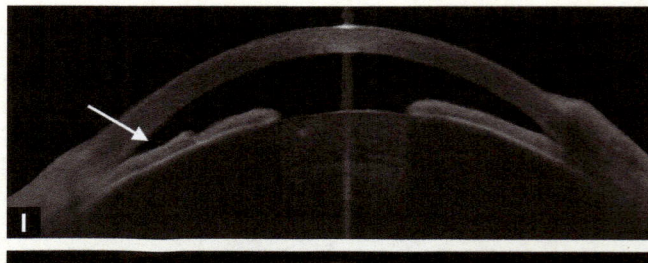

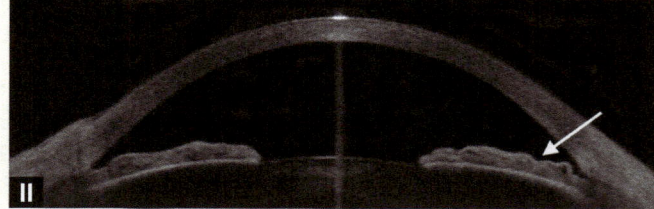

a. Perimetry
b. USG B-Scan
c. Anterior Segment Optical Coherence Tomography (AS-OCT)
d. Fluorescein Angiography

7. From the perimetry printout, what can be the likely diagnosis of the patient?

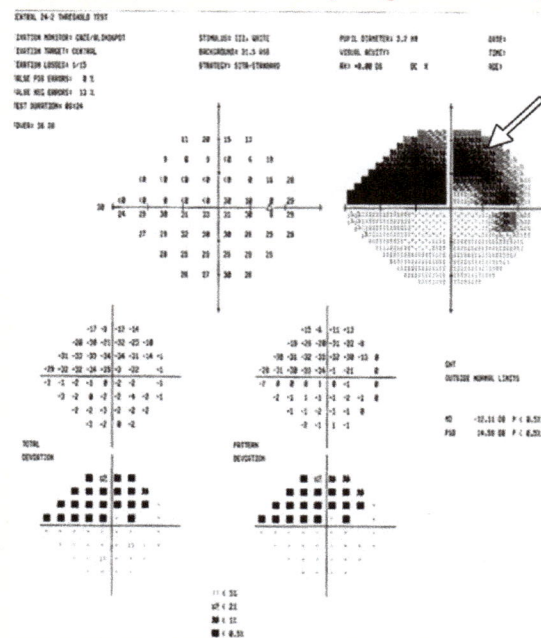

a. Optic chiasma compression
b. Advanced glaucoma
c. Occipital infarct
d. Optic tract lesion

Answer Key: 5. a   6. c   7. b

8. Identify the investigation modality whose print-out is given in the question:

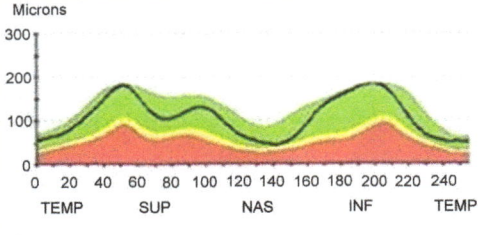
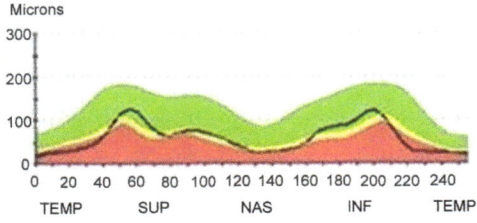
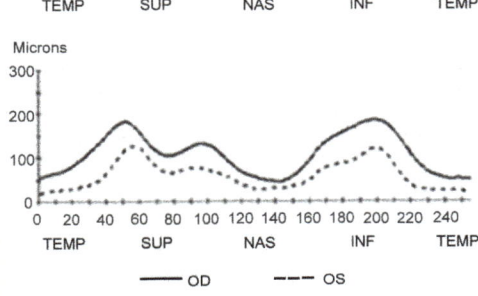
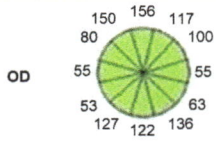
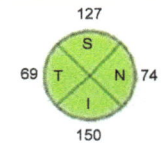
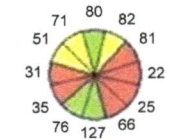
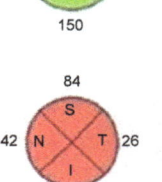
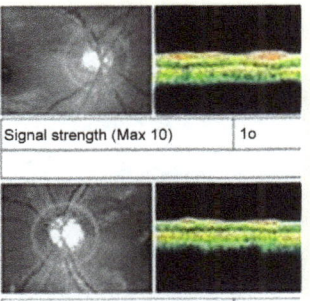

a. Perimetry
b. Anterior segment Optical Coherence Tomography (AS-OCT)
c. Optical coherence tomography for optic disc and retinal nerve fibre layer thickness
d. USG B-Scan

9. An infant presents with epiphora and photophobia. The corneal diameter appears large and the clinical picture is given below. What is the next line of management?

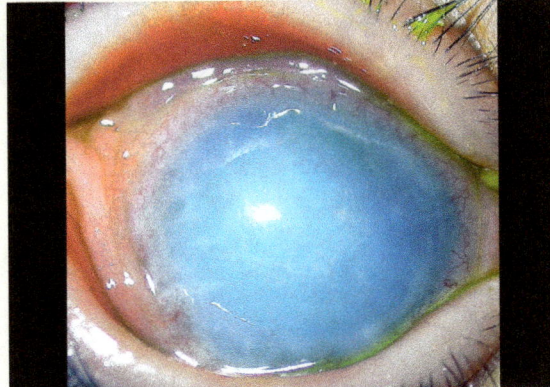

a. Penetrating keratoplasty
b. Wait and watch
c. Examination under anaesthesia to evaluate corneal diameter and IOP
d. Syringing and probing

10. A patient presents with increased IOP, cataract and poorly dilating pupil in the right eye. The clinical picture is given. What is the possible diagnosis?

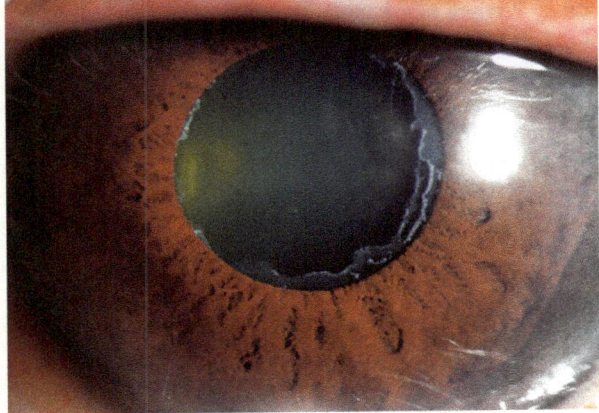

a. Primary angle closure glaucoma
b. Primary open angle glaucoma
c. Pigmentary glaucoma
d. Pseudoexfoliation glaucoma

Answer Key: 8. c 9. c 10. d

Self Assessment and Review of Ophthalmology

11. A 30-year-old male myopic patient presents with increased IOP in both eyes. The clinical picture is given. What is the possible diagnosis?

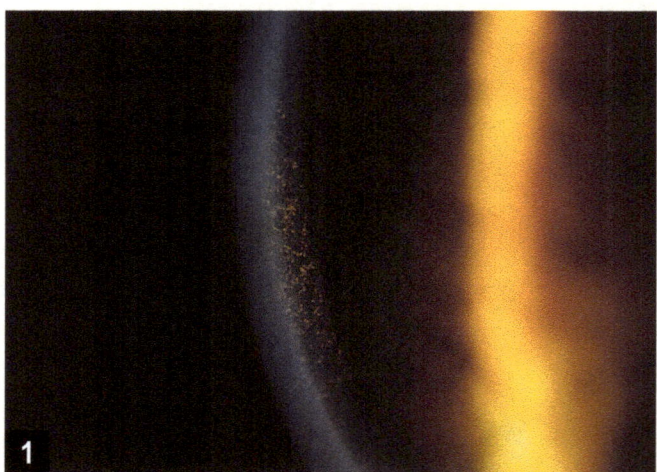

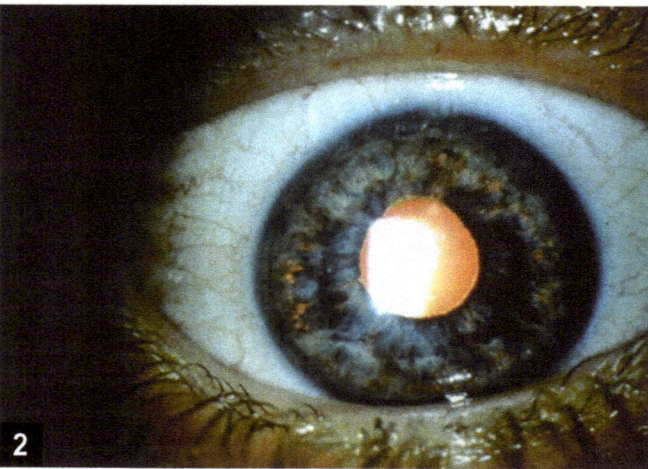

a. Primary open angle glaucoma
b. Primary angle closure glaucoma
c. Pigmentary glaucoma
d. Pseudoexfoliation glaucoma

12. A 60-year-old patient with uncontrolled diabetes and past history of central retinal vein occlusion presents with high IOP in the right eye. The clinical picture of the anterior segment is given. What is the possible diagnosis?

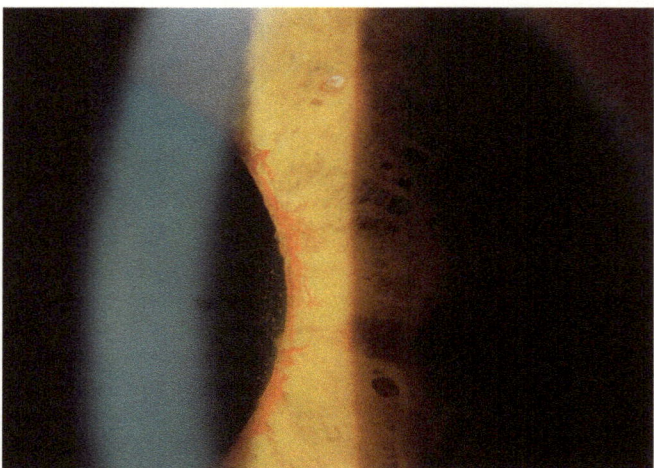

a. Primary open angle glaucoma
b. Pigmentary glaucoma
c. Malignant glaucoma
d. Neovascular glaucoma

13. A patient presents with cataract and high IOP. The clinical picture is given. What is the possible diagnosis?

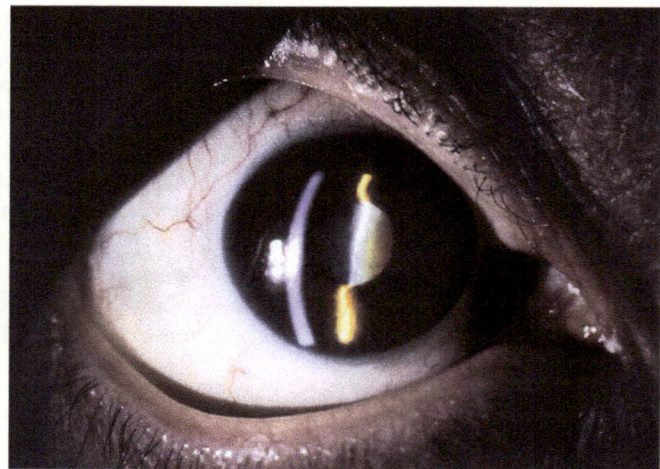

a. Phacolytic glaucoma
b. Phacotoxic glaucoma
c. Primary angle closure glaucoma
d. Malignant glaucoma

Answer Key:　11　c　　　12.　d　　　13.　a

Glaucoma

14. What is the surgery that has been performed in this patient?

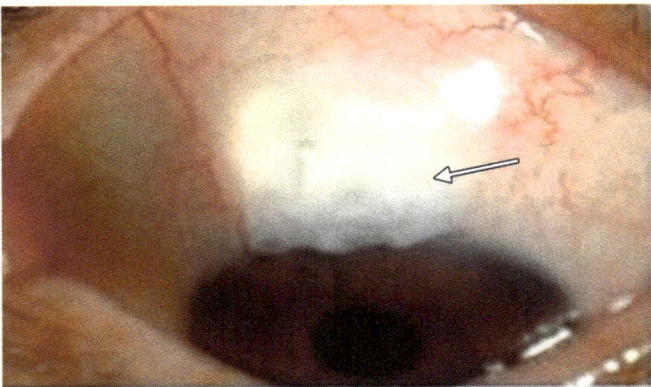

a. Penetrating keratoplasty
b. Trabeculectomy
c. Glaucoma valve surgery
d. Scleral buckling surgery

15. What is the surgery that has been shown in the diagram?

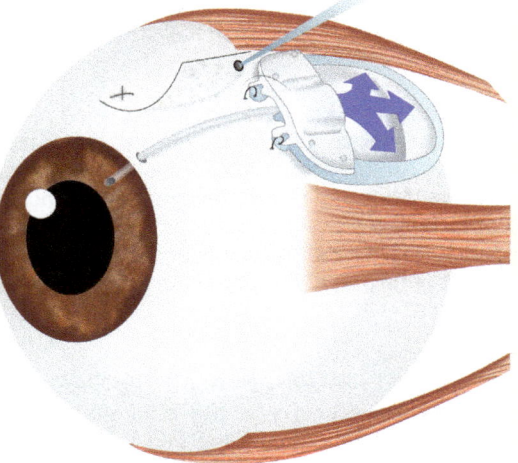

a. Penetrating keratoplasty
b. Trabeculectomy
c. Glaucoma valve surgery
d. Scleral buckling surgery

Answer Key: 14. b   15. c

ANSWERS AND EXPLANATIONS

1. **Answer: a. Tonometry** *(Ref: Kanski 8th edition p 309)*
   The instrument shown in the picture is **Goldmann Applanation Tonometer**. After instilling topical anaesthetic eye drops and **fluorescein** in the conjunctival sac, the applanation biprism is made to touch the apex of the cornea. Examination is done under **cobalt blue filter** of the slit-lamp and IOP is noted from the dial on the instrument

2. **Answer: c. Gonioscopy**
   (Ref: Yanoff & Duker 4th edition p 1040-1041, 1047)
   The question shows pictures of two different types of gonioscopes and the structures visualised at the angle of anterior chamber.

3. **Answer: b. Gonioscopy, Tonometry, Visual fields**
   (Ref: Yanoff & Duker 4th edition p 1040-1041, 1047)
   The depression at the centre of the optic disc is called the optic cup. The normal ratio of the area of the cup to the disc is 0.3:1. Here, the fundus picture shows an increased cup:disc ratio with thinning of the surrounding neuroretinal rim. (C: D ratio is roughly 0.7:1). This, along with symptoms of headache and eye strain is suggestive of glaucoma. Hence the answer.

4. **Answer: c. Acute angle closure glaucoma**
   (Ref: Peyman's Principles and Practice of Ophthalmology 2nd edition, p 1112-13)
   The photograph shows a congested eye with mid-dilated pupil and shallow anterior chamber (space between cornea and iris is decreased). In a 65 year old female, these findings with high IOP suggest acute angle closure glaucoma.

5. **Answer: a. Nd: YAG laser**
   The procedure that the patient has undergone is **laser peripheral iridotomy**. It is done with **Nd: YAG laser.**

6. **Answer: c. Anterior Segment Optical Coherence Tomography**
   AS-OCT is an optical scan of the anterior segment using infra-red light. Its utility in glaucoma is mainly to evaluate the angle of anterior chamber.
   Picture No 1 shows narrow angle (indicated by arrow) whereas Picture No 2 shows normal angle. (indicated by arrow)

7. **Answer: b. Advanced glaucoma**
   The perimetry print out shows a superior **arcuate scotoma**^{Q} (indicated by arrow) which is the characteristic field defect in glaucoma.

8. **Answer: c. Optical coherence tomography for optic disc and retinal nerve fibre layer thickness**
   Optical Coherence Tomography (OCT) is an imaging modality with infra-red light that uses the principle of low-coherence **interferometry** to obtain high resolution images of ocular tissues in both anterior and posterior segment.
   Its utility in glaucoma is to evaluate the optic disc and retinal nerve fibre layer thickness in the peripapillary area. In serial scans, progression of glaucoma over time can be assessed.

9. **Answer: c. Examination under anaesthesia to evaluate corneal diameter and IOP**
   (Ref: Peyman's Principles and Practice of Ophthalmology 2nd edition, p 1226-27)
   The photograph shows large corneal with severe corneal haze. An infant presenting with this clinical picture and associated complains of watering and photophobia suggests a diagnosis of congenital glaucoma and should be evaluated for the same.

10. **Answer: d. Pseudoexfoliation glaucoma**
    (Ref: Peyman's Principles and Practice of Ophthalmology 2nd edition, p 1058-59)
    The picture shows a whitish ring on the anterior lens capsule. This is pseudoexfoliative material and hence the answer is Pseudoexfoliation glaucoma.

    Pseudoexfoliation syndrome (PXF)
    - It is a condition where abnormal fibrillar extracellular pseudoexfoliative material is produced and deposited in the anterior segment of the eye.
    - Structures where PXF material is found are anterior lens capsule, pupillary margin, angle of anterior chamber and ciliary zonules.
    - The clinical features are:
      - Weak zonules leading to subluxated cataract^Q or late subluxation of capsular bag with IOL after cataract surgery.
      - Poorly dilating pupils
      - Wavy pigmented line anterior to the Schwalbe's line is seen on gonioscopy. This is called Sampaolesi line.^{Q}
      - Secondary open angle glaucoma due to blockage of trabecular meshwork

11. **Answer: c. Pigmentary glaucoma**
    (Ref: Peyman's Principles and Practice of Ophthalmology 2nd edition, p 1139-1140)
    Picture 1 shows pigment deposits on the corneal endothelium known as Krukenberg spindle. Picture 2 shows transillumination defects in the iris due to loss of iris pigments. Both these are characteristic of **Pigment Dispersion Syndrome (PDS)** which leads to pigmentary glaucoma.

> **Pigment Dispersion Syndrome (PDS)**
> - It is a condition commonly seen in male patients around 30-50 years of age
> - It is associated with **myopic refractive error**
> - Backward bowing of the iris with rubbing of the iris epithelium and zonules leads to loss of iris pigments. These pigments get deposited in various anterior segment structures.
> - The classical triad is
>   - Krukenberg spindle[Q] (Iris pigments on corneal endothelium)
>   - Iris transillumination defects[Q] (Loss of iris pigments)
>   - Pigmented trabecular meshwork
> - **Secondary open angle glaucoma** occurs due to blockage of the trabecular meshwork by pigments

12. **Answer: d. Neovascular glaucoma**
    (Ref: Peyman's Principles and Practice of Ophthalmology 2nd edition, p 1143-1145)
    The picture shows new vessels at the pupillary margin suggestive of neovascularisation of iris and subsequently the angle. Hence the answer is neovascular glaucoma.

    ### Neovascular glaucoma (NVG)
    - It is a form of **secondary glaucoma** caused by retinal ischaemia.
    - Causes are
      - **Proliferative diabetic retinopathy**[Q]
      - **Central retinal vein occlusion**[Q]
      - **Retinopathy of prematurity**[Q]
      - Eales' disease
      - Ocular ischaemic syndrome
    - Up regulation of proangiogenic factors like **Vascular Endothelial Growth Factor (VEGF)** occurs secondary to retinal ischaemia resulting in neovascularisation of retina, iris and angle of anterior chamber. Fibrovascular proliferation at the angle leads to blockage of aqueous outflow resulting in glaucoma. This is called **neovascular glaucoma.**

13. **Answer: a. Phacolytic glaucoma**
    (Ref: Peyman's Principles and Practice of Ophthalmology 2nd edition, pg 1152--53)
    The picture shows a hypermature cataract. Hypermature cataract causes **phacolytic glaucoma** due to leakage of the liquefied lens proteins into the anterior chamber and subsequent blockage of the trabecular meshwork. It is a type of **secondary open angle glaucoma.**

14. **Answer: b. Trabeculectomy**
    (Ref: Peyman's Principles and Practice of Ophthalmology 2nd edition, pg 1157--58)
    Trabeculectomy is a surgical technique to lower the IOP by draining the aqueous humour via a partial thickness scleral flap into the subconjunctival space and subsequently to the conjunctival vessels.
    The picture shows an elevated area superorly which the area of filtration of the aqueous humour through the scleral flap into the subconjunctival space. This is called the **trabeculectomy bleb.** (indicated by arrow)

15. **Answer: c. Glaucoma valve surgery**
    The picture shows a valve placed in the subconjunctival space with its tube in the anterior chamber to facilitate the outflow of aqueous humour.

10

Neuro-Ophthalmology

VISUAL PATHWAY

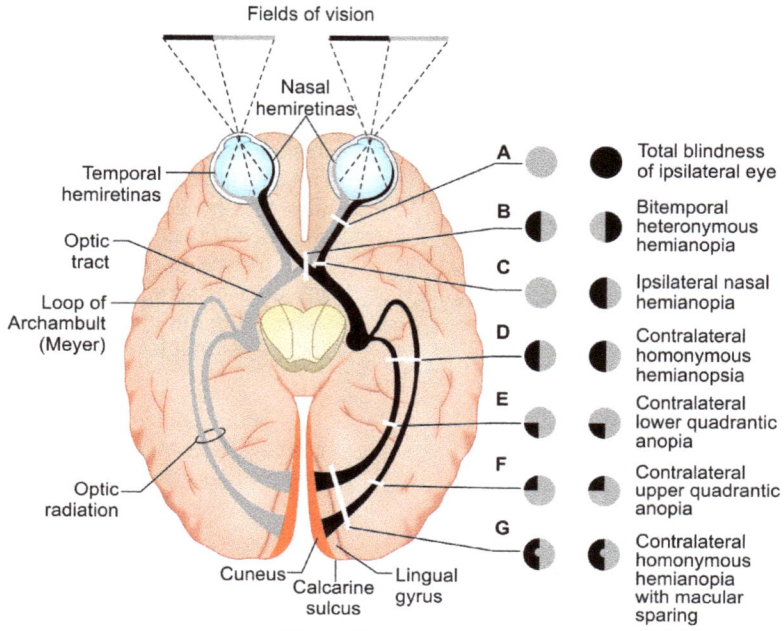

Fig. 1: Visual pathway

The diagram shows the anatomy of the visual pathway. Note that the nasal hemiretina visualizes the temporal field and the temporal hemiretina visualizes the nasal field. Thus, lesions involving the nasal fibers of a particular eye affect the temporal field whereas lesions involving the temporal fibers affect the nasal field.

The structures in the visual pathway, from anterior to posterior are
Optic nerve → Optic chiasma → Optic tract → Lateral geniculate body → Optic radiation → Occipital cortex[Q]

First order neuron	Bipolar cells in retina[Q]
Second order neuron	Ganglion cells in the retina[Q]
Third order neuron	Lateral geniculate body[Q]

A school of thought believes that the first order neurons are the photoreceptors but the concept is still under review.

- The visual impulse travels from the **rods and cones of the retina** via the **bipolar cells, ganglion cells and nerve fiber layer** to the **optic nerve.** Beyond the optic nerve lies the **optic chiasma.**
- At the level of the chiasma, the fibers from the **nasal part of the retina cross over to the other side whereas the temporal fibers continue on the same side.**
- Beyond the optic chiasma is the **optic tract**. Thus, the optic tract contains the temporal fibers from the same side and the nasal fibers which have crossed over from the opposite side.
- Beyond the optic tract, the fibers pass through the **lateral geniculate body** and the **optic radiation**. The optic radiation thus contains the same fibers as the optic tract.
- Finally the fibers reach the **occipital lobe** of the brain where the **primary visual area (area no 17)**[Q] and the accessory visual areas (18 and 19) are located.

Neuro-Ophthalmology

OPTIC NERVE

The optic nerve is about 50 mm long from the globe to the optic chiasma and is divided into the following parts:

- Intraocular – 1 mm
- Intraorbital – 30 mm
- Intracanalicular – 6 mm
- Intracranial – 10 mm

Sheaths are continuous with brain meninges.
Nerve fibres proximal to optic disc are myelinated.

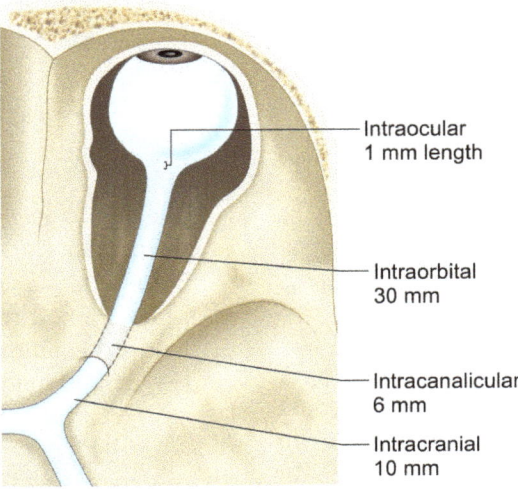

Fig. 2: Parts of the optic nerve

Assessment of optic nerve function

Visual evoked potential (VEP)
- This is an **electrophysiological test** which helps in the assessment of the visual pathway from the optic nerve to the occipital cortex. It mainly used for evaluating optic nerve function. Electrodes are placed on the occipital cortex and the electrical activity elicited in response to a visual stimulus is recorded.
- A most important wave of the VEP is the positive wave known as **P-100** whose peak is seen 100 ms after the stimulus is given.
- **Increase in latency and decrease in amplitude** of P-100 wave is seen in optic nerve disease[Q]

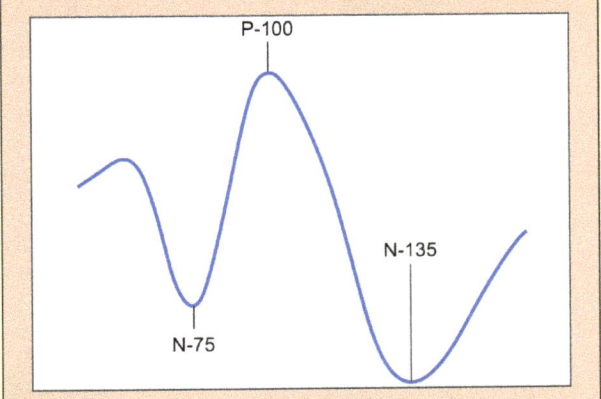

Color vision
- Impaired red-green color vision is seen in all optic nerve diseases except glaucoma where blue-yellow defect is seen

Visual field
- Central, Centrocecal or Altitudinal scotoma are seen in different optic nerve diseases

OPTIC CHIASMA

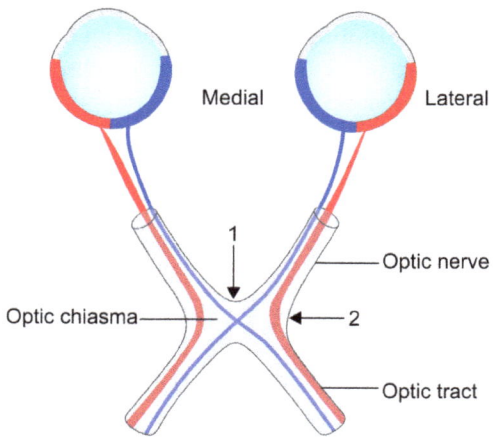

Fig. 3: Optic chiasma: Crossing of fibers of nasal hemiretina to the optic tract of opposite side

At the level of the optic chiasma, the fibers from the nasal hemiretina (represented in blue) cross over to the optic tract of the opposite side whereas the fibers from the temporal hemiretina (represented in red) continue to the optic tract of the same side.

- Lesions involving the **central part of the optic chiasma (Arrow 1)** affect the nasal fibers of both sides resulting in loss of the **temporal field of vision** in both eyes. This is known as **Bitemporal Hemianopia[Q] or Heteronymous Hemianopia[Q]**

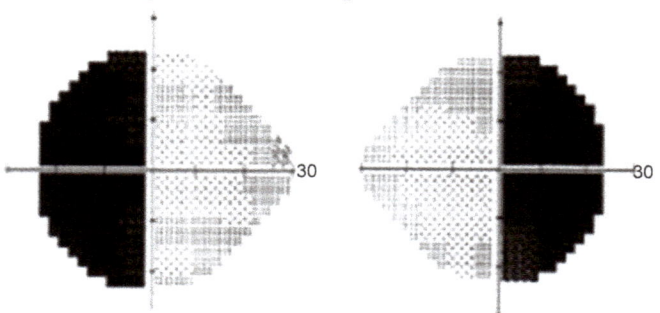

Fig. 4: Bitemporal hemianopia

- Lesions involving the central part of the chiasma are **Pituitary adenoma** and **Craniopharyngioma**.
- In pituitary adenoma, the bitemporal hemianopia starts superiorly and descends downwards. Hence it is called **descending bitemporal hemianopia.[Q]**
- In Craniopharyngioma, the bitemporal hemianopia starts inferiorly and ascends upwards. Hence it is called **ascending bitemporal hemianopia.[Q]**
- Lesions involving the peripheral part of the chiasma (Arrow 2) are rare. They affect the fibers from the temporal hemiretina resulting in loss of nasal field of vision of one or both sides. This is called **Binasal Hemianopia.[Q]**

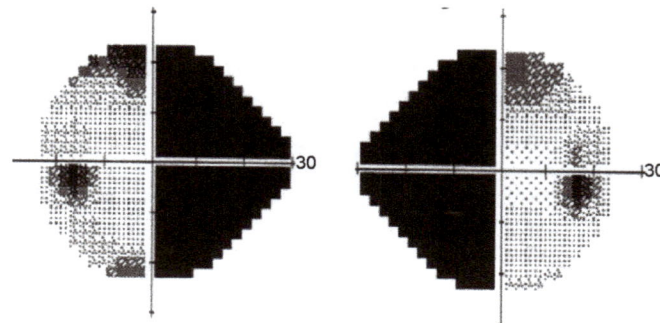

Fig. 5: Binasal hemianopia

OPTIC TRACT

- The optic tract contains the crossed nasal fibers from the opposite side and the uncrossed temporal fibers from the same side.
- Lesions involving the optic tract result in loss of nasal field of the same side and temporal field of the opposite side or contralateral **Homonymous Hemianopia.[Q]**

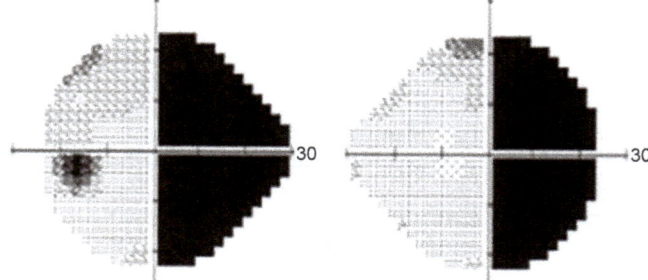

Fig. 6: Right homonymous hemianopia due to left optic tract lesion

OPTIC RADIATION

- The fibers from the optic tract relay into the lateral geniculate body and then continue into the optic radiation. Hence, lesions involving the optic radiation also result in **Homonymous Hemianopia.**
- However the fibers responsible for the superior visual field course initially into the temporal lobe before proceeding posteriorly to reach the occipital lobe (**Meyer's Loop**). Hence, lesions involving the **temporal lobe** produce contralateral homonymous field defect involving only the superior field. This is known as **Superior Quadrantopia** or **Pie in the Sky[Q]**.

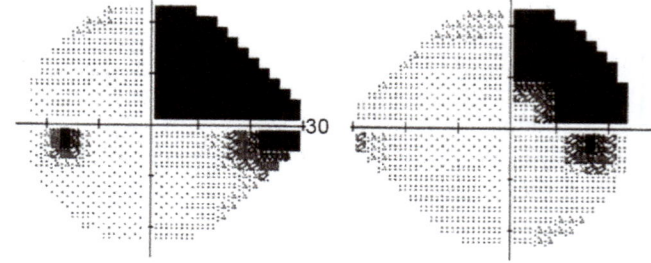

Fig. 7: Pie in the sky

Neuro-Ophthalmology

➤ The fibers responsible for the inferior visual field course through the **parietal lobe** and subsequently to the occipital lobe. Hence lesions of the parietal lobe result in contralateral homonymous field defect involving only the inferior field. This is known as **Inferior Quadrantopia** or **Pie on the Floor**[Q].

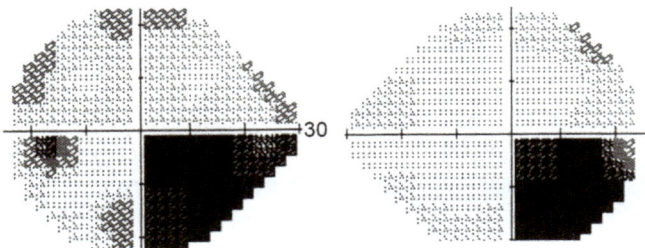

Fig. 8: Pie on the floor

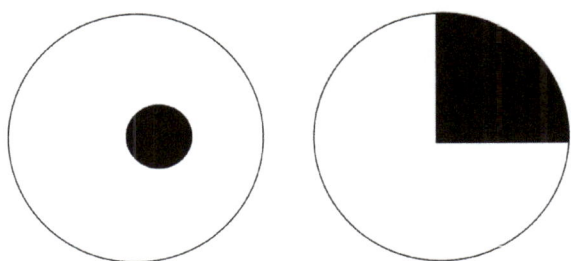

Fig. 10: Junctional scotoma

OCCIPITAL CORTEX

➤ The occipital lobe is the final destination for the visual pathway and the axons are arranged along the margins of the **calcarine sulcus**.

➤ The most common lesion affecting the occipital cortex is ischemic injury or infarct due to occlusion of the posterior cerebral artery which forms the major source of blood supply. However, a branch of the middle cerebral artery provides additional perfusion to the area where the central field is represented. Hence, in infarct due to occlusion of posterior cerebral artery (PCA), this small central field is often spared.

➤ **Occipital cortex lesion** (infarct due to PCA occlusion) results in contralateral **Homonymous Hemianopia with central sparing**[Q].

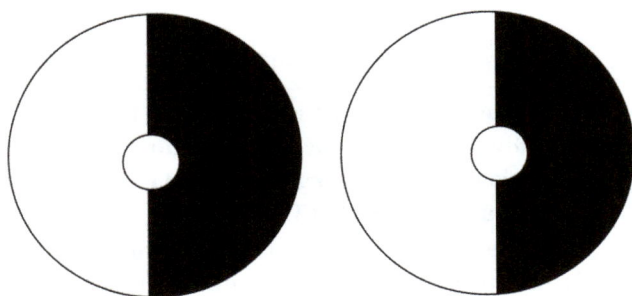

Fig. 9: Homonymous hemianopia with central sparing

JUNCTIONAL SCOTOMA OF TRAQUAIR

➤ Lesion affecting the **proximal part of the optic nerve**[Q] results in a rare type of visual field defect consisting of **ipsilateral central/centrocecal scotoma and contralateral upper temporal hemianopia**.[Q] This is called **junctional scotoma of Traquair.**

> ### Lesions in the visual pathway
>
> Lesions in the visual pathway are associated with typical defects of the visual field depending upon the fibers present in that part of the pathway.
> (Note: Lesions involving the nasal fibers result in temporal field defect. Lesions involving the temporal fibers result in nasal field defect)
>
> • *Optic nerve*: **Central scotoma, Centrocecal scotoma, Altitudinal scotoma**[Q]
> • *Optic chiasma*:
>   • *Central lesion*: **Bitemporal hemianopia**[Q]
>   • *Peripheral lesion*: **Binasal hemianopia**[Q]
> • *Optic tract*: **Incongruous homonymous hemianopia**[Q]
> • *Optic radiation*: **Congruous homonymous hemianopia**[Q]
> • *Occipital cortex*: **Congruous homonymous hemianopia with central sparing**[Q]
> • *Lesion in temporal lobe*: **Superior quadrantopia or Pie in the sky**[Q]
> • *Lesion in the parietal lobe*: **Inferior quadrantopia or Pie on the floor**[Q]
> • *Proximal part of the optic nerve*: **Junctional scotoma of Traquair**[Q]

DEVELOPMENTAL ANOMALIES AND MALFORMATIONS OF OPTIC NERVE

Optic Disc Pit

➤ Optic disc is larger than normal
➤ Contains a pit of variable size in the inferotemporal quadrant
➤ Serous detachment of macula is a common complication.

Optic Disc Coloboma

➤ Autosomal dominant
➤ Discrete white excavation located inferiorly in the disc producing a superior field defect

- Serous detachment of macula is an association
- CHARGE syndrome (Coloboma, Heart defects, choanal Atresia, Retarded growth, Genital, Ear anomalies) is an association.

Morning Glory Syndrome

- Rare unilateral condition
- Large funnel shaped excavation of the disc surrounded by an annulus of chorioretinal disturbance
- **The blood vessels emerge from the disc like the spokes of a wheel**[Q]
- Frontonasal dysplasia, NF-2, PHACE syndrome are associations.

Optic Nerve Hypoplasia

- Usually unilateral
- Small disc surrounded by concentric chorioretinal atrophy (double-ring sign)
- Associated with midline defects of the brain
- de Morsier syndrome associated with absence of septum pellucidum, agenesis of corpus callosum, is seen in 10% cases.

DISEASES OF THE OPTIC NERVE

OPTIC NEURITIS

Inflammatory: Infective or demyelinating disorder affecting the optic nerve.

Etiology

- **Demyelinating diseases like Multiple Sclerosis**[Q]
- Viral infections like Measles, Mumps, and Chickenpox in children
- Granulomatous inflammation like Sarcoidosis, TB, and Syphilis
- Infection of adjacent structures like meninges, sinuses, orbit.

Anatomically it is classified into
- *Papillitis*: Inflammation of the optic disc
- *Neuroretinitis*: Inflammation of the optic disc and surrounding retina
- *Retrobulbar neuritis*: Inflammation of the optic nerve behind the globe.

Symptoms

- *Visual loss*: It is **unilateral and sudden**[Q]
- It may be preceded by pain. Painful ocular movements are seen in retrobulbar neuritis
- *Uthoff's phenomenon*: Impairment of vision increases with increase in body temperature like a hot bath

Signs

- Decrease in visual acuity and contrast sensitivity
- Impairment of red green color vision[Q]
- Pupil shows RAPD[Q]
- *Fundus*: The fundus picture depends upon the anatomical type.

Papillitis	Retrobulbar neuritis	Neuroretinitis
Hyperemia and swelling of optic disc with **blurring of the disc margins** is seen. Dilatation and tortuosity of the vessels is also seen.	Fundus is normal[Q].	Features of papillitis are seen with a ring of exudates around the macula. This is called **macular star**

Investigations

- *Visual field*: **Centrocecal scotoma**[Q]
- *VEP*: Increase in the latency of response is seen
- *MRI brain and orbit*: It helps to rule out multiple sclerosis and decide the further course of management.

Clinical Course

There is spontaneous visual recovery in 90% patients over a period of 4–6 weeks. Only about 10% patients may go on to develop chronic optic neuritis. Prognosis is very good.

> **Treatment of optic neuritis by the Optic Neuritis Treatment Trial (ONTT)**
>
> - **High dose IV Methyl Prednisolone (1 g daily in two divided doses) for 3 days followed by oral Prednisolone (1 mg/kg/day) for 11 days. Total duration of therapy is 14 days**[Q]
> - The role of steroids is to make the visual recovery faster but there is no significant difference in the final visual outcome with spontaneous recovery and steroids[Q]
> - Oral steroids alone increase the rate of recurrence[Q]
> - The visual acuity may return to normal but permanent residual defects may remain in color vision and contrast sensitivity[Q]

Neuro-Ophthalmology

Leber's Hereditary Optic Neuropathy (LHON)

- **Maternally inherited mitochondrial DNA mutation**[Q]
- Seen in males between 15 and 35 years of age
- **Presentation is just like a unilateral case of papillitis but the other eye becomes affected in a few weeks**[Q]
- The disc is hyperemic and edematous with blurred margins. Dilated vessels extend from the disc to the surrounding retina. This is called **telangiectatic microangiopathy**[Q] and is a distinctive feature of LHON
- Minimal response to steroids is seen with subsequent development of optic atrophy
- Prognosis is very poor
- Vitamin B_{12} injections along with steroids is given.

ANTERIOR ISCHEMIC OPTIC NEUROPATHY (AION)

AION is an important cause of visual loss in the middle age and elderly. It is caused by partial or total infarction of the optic nerve due to occlusion of the **short posterior ciliary arteries**[Q]. It is of two main types
- Non-arteritic AION
- Arteritic AION

	Arteritic AION	Non-Arteritic AION
Age	>65 years	>50 years
Predisposing factors	Giant cell arteritis (GCA)	Atherosclerosis **Hypertension Hypercholesterolemia Migraine SLE, PAN**
Symptoms	Sudden loss of vision **Periocular pain** Unilateral	Sudden loss of vision **Painless** Unilateral
Premonitory symptoms	**Amaurosis fugax**[Q] Associated features of GCA **Headache, Jaw Claudication, Polymyalgia rheumatica**[Q]	None
Visual acuity	Severely impaired	Impaired
Pupillary reaction	RAPD	RAPD
Fundus	Severe disc edema with pallor Splinter hemorrhages around disc	Disc edema with pallor
VEP	May be unrecordable or severely extinguished	**Shows increased latency and decreased amplitude**
Visual Field	May not be possible due to poor visual acuity	**Altitudinal scotoma**[Q]
Systemic investigations	**ESR : Very High > 100 mm/hr C-Reactive protein is raised Temporal artery biopsy: It is the confirmatory test for diagnosis**	Hypertension Hypercholesterolemia cANCA and pANCA
Treatment	**IV Methyl Prednisolone (1 g daily for 3 days) followed by oral Prednisolone (60–80 mg/day). It is tapered by 10 mg weekly** Maintenance dose of 5–10 mg may be required indefinitely	No effective treatment is known

Toxic optic neuropathy

- It is a bilateral optic neuropathy occurring in response to different drugs and toxins
- The important toxins and drugs associated are
    - Tobacco
    - Ethyl alcohol, Methyl alcohol
    - Ethambutol[Q]
    - INH[Q]
    - Quinine
    - Digoxin
- Presentation is bilateral impairment of visual acuity and color vision. In early stages the disc may be clinically normal but later shows pallor
- Visual fields show **bilateral centrocecal scotoma**[Q]

PAPILLEDEMA

It is a passive swelling of the optic nerve head secondary to raised intracranial pressure. It is bilateral but may be asymmetrical.

Pathogenesis

- The meningeal sheaths of the optic nerve are continuous with the meninges of the brain. So when the ICT increases, there is transmission of pressure to the optic nerve head
- As a result, there is impairment of axoplasmic flow from the optic nerve towards the brain
- There is also associated venous stasis.

Causes

- Intracranial tumors
- Intracranial abscess
- Subarachnoid hemorrhage
- Aneurysm
- Benign intracranial hypertension
- Malignant hypertension.

Symptoms

- Headache, worse on coughing and straining, associated with vomiting
- Transient obscuration of vision (Amaurosis fugax). **No definitive visual loss**[Q] except in long-standing cases
- Sometimes diplopia may be present due to sixth nerve palsy seen as a consequence of raised ICT.

Signs

- Visual acuity and color vision are normal
- Pupillary reflexes are normal
- Fundus:
    - In the early stage, there is **blurring of nasal, superior, inferior and then temporal disc margins**[Q]. **Loss of venous pulsation is also seen**[Q].
    - In the established stage, there is hyperemia with severe disc edema and obliteration of the physiological cup. Veins are dilated, tortuous and engorged. Multiple flame shaped hemorrhages, cotton wool spots are seen in the peripapillary region. Hard exudates are seen at the fovea.

Investigations

- Visual field: May be normal or **enlargement of the blind spot may be seen**[Q].

Treatment is lowering of ICT by medical, surgical intervention.

Foster Kennedy syndrome[q]

- Unilateral papilledema
- Seen in olfactory lobe tumors
- Ipsilateral optic atrophy due to compression by the tumor
- Contralateral papilledema due to raised ICT

Idiopathic Intracranial Hypertension (IIH)

- It is defined as a condition where raised ICT is seen in the **absence of intracranial space occupying lesion**[Q]. Normal sized ventricles and normal CSF composition is seen
- It is commonly associated with
    - **Steroid withdrawal**
    - **Oral contraceptive pills**[Q]
    - **Vitamin A toxicity**[Q]
    - **Amiodarone**
    - **Outdated tetracyclines**
- May also be seen in certain endocrine disorders like hypothyroidism, hypoparathyroidism, Addison's disease, etc.
- Ophthalmic presentation is with **papilledema.**

Optic atrophy

Optic atrophy refers to degeneration of the fibers of the optic nerve. It is classified into four types:

- *Primary optic atrophy*: It is defined as optic atrophy without preceding swelling of the optic disc. The disc is pale with clearly defined disc margins. Causes are
    - **Hereditary optic neuropathy**
    - **Traumatic optic neuropathy**
    - **Toxic optic neuropathy**
    - **Recurrent retrobulbar neuritis**
    - **Compressive optic neuropathy**
- *Secondary optic atrophy*: It is optic atrophy with preceding edema of the optic disc. The disc is pale and dirty looking with ill-defined gliotic margins. Causes are:
    - **Papillitis**[Q]
    - **AION**[Q]
    - **Chronic papilledema**[Q]
- *Consecutive optic atrophy*: It is secondary to retinal diseases like **Retinitis Pigmentosa**[Q], **CRAO**[Q]
- *Glaucomatous optic atrophy*: It is associated with glaucoma and is called as **cavernous optic atrophy**[Q]

PUPIL

There are two important reflexes involving the pupil

- *Light reflex*: Constriction of bilateral pupils occurs when light is shown on one eye. The eye on which light falls, shows **direct reflex** whereas the other eye shows **consensual reflex**

Neuro-Ophthalmology

- *Near reflex*: This has three components namely **constriction of the pupil, convergence and accommodation.**

Light Reflex

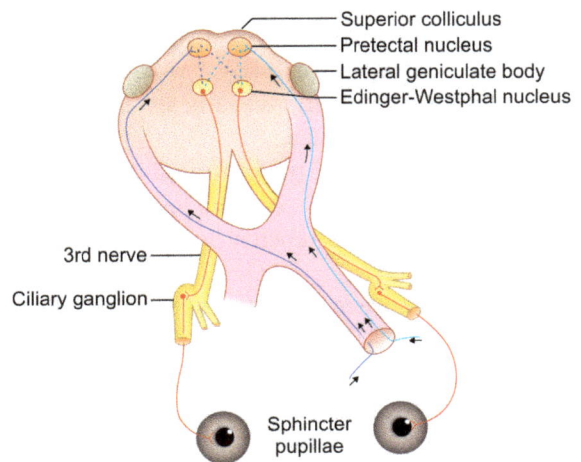

Fig. 11: Anatomical pathway of light reflex

- The impulse from the retina travels via the **optic nerve, optic chiasma and optic tract**^{Q} to reach the **pretectal nucleus**^{Q} in the **dorsal midbrain**^{Q}, which is the center for the reflex. At the level of the chiasma, the fibers from the nasal retina cross over to the other side but the temporal fibers remain on the same side.
- From the pretectal nucleus, the internuncial neurons connect to the **Edinger-Westphal nucleus (parasympathetic nucleus of Oculomotor nerve)**^{Q} of both sides.
- The efferent impulse travels via the **Oculomotor** nerve of both sides up to the **ciliary ganglion.**
- Beyond the ciliary ganglion, these parasympathetic fibers are carried by the **short ciliary nerves**^{Q} which supply the **sphincter pupillae**^{Q} to produce pupillary constriction.

Near Reflex

- The afferent pathway for the near reflex is not clearly understood. The impulse travels from the optic nerve to the occipital cortex. From the cortex it connects to a centre in the **ventral midbrain**^{Q}
- The internuncial neurons connect this centre to the **Edinger-Westphal** nucleus of both sides.
- The efferent impulse travels via the **Oculomotor nerve** to the **ciliary ganglion.** Beyond the ciliary ganglion, **the short ciliary nerves** carry the parasympathetic fibers to the **sphincter pupillae and ciliary muscle.**

ABNORMAL PUPILLARY REACTIONS

	Marcus Gunn pupil (RAPD)	Light-near dissociation	Wernicke's pupil	Adie's tonic pupil
Site of lesion	Optic nerve (unilateral or asymmetrical)	Pretectal nucleus^Q	Optic tract^Q	Post-ganglionic supply to the sphincter pupillae and ciliary muscle
Clinical feature	Tested by **Swinging Flash Light Test**^{Q} When light is swung to the normal eye, both pupils constrict When light is swung to the abnormal eye, both pupils dilate^Q	Light reflex is absent Near reflex is present	Impaired pupillary constriction when light is shown on the nasal half of same side and temporal half of the other side	**Both light reflex and near reflex are impaired** **Anisocoria**^{Q} is seen due to large dilated pupil on the affected side **Denervation hypersensitivity**- Constriction of affected pupil by 0.125% pilocarpine

Light near dissociation

Light reflex is absent but near reflex is present^Q.
The important examples are
- *Argyll-Robertson pupil*^{Q}: Damage to the pretectal nucleus in Neurosyphilis^Q
- *Perinaud's syndrome*: Lesion in the dorsal midbrain
  - Light near dissociation
  - Vertical gaze palsy (Upgaze palsy with normal downgaze)
  - Lid retraction (Collier's sign)
  - Convergence retraction nystagmus

Horner's Syndrome

It is due to disturbance of the sympathetic nerve supply to the dilator pupillae muscle. The sympathetic pathway starts from the **posterior hypothalamus**. The descending fibers reach the **Cilio-spinal Centre of Budge** in the spinal cord. From here, the fibers travel to the **superior cervical ganglion** in the neck. The post-ganglionic fibers join the **ophthalmic branch of Trigeminal nerve**^{Q} and reach the dilator pupillae via **the long ciliary nerves**^{Q}. Along with the dilator pupillae, these nerves also supply the **Muller's muscle** of the lids and the **sweat gland.**

Self Assessment and Review of Ophthalmology

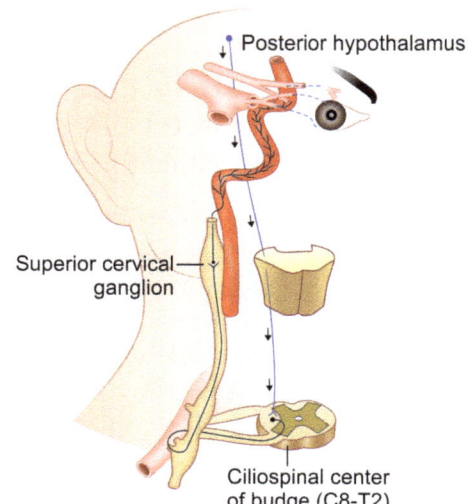

Fig. 12: Anatomical pathway of sympathetic nerve supply

Clinical Features of Horner's Syndrome

- Mild ptosis due to paralysis of Muller's muscle^Q
- Apparent enophthalmos
- **Miosis**^Q
- *Diminished sweating or anhydrosis*^Q: This is seen in pre-ganglionic cases. (Lesion in the pathway prior to the superior cervical ganglion)
- **Heterochromia iridis** in long standing and pediatric cases.

Pharmacological Tests

Cocaine test: Confirms Horner's syndrome^Q. On instillation of the drug, normal pupil dilates but Horner's pupil does not

Hydroxy-amphetamine test: Confirms pre-ganglionic Horner's syndrome. On instillation of the drug, the pupil dilates in preganglionic Horner's syndrome but it does not dilate in post-ganglionic cases.

Adrenaline test: Confirms postganglionic Horner's syndrome. On instillation of adrenaline, the dilatation is very prominent and quick in post-ganglionic cases due to denervation hypersensitivity.

CRANIAL NERVE PALSIES

Oculomotor (Third) Nerve Palsy

Anatomy: The course of the nerve from the midbrain to the muscles can be divided into the following parts.
- *Nucleus*: The nuclear complex is located in the **midbrain** at level of superior colliculus. It has both unpaired and paired sub-nuclei.
  - An **unpaired sub-nucleus**^Q supplies the **bilateral levator muscles**^Q.
  - The **paired superior rectus** sub-nucleus controls the **contralateral muscle**^Q.
  - **Paired sub-nuclei of medial rectus, inferior rectus and inferior oblique control the ipsilateral muscles.**
  - **The Edinger-Westphal nucleus** supplies parasympathetic input to the **sphincter pupillae and ciliary muscles.**
- *Fasciculus*: The fibers pass through the red nucleus and medial aspect of cerebral peduncle. It is also associated with the cerebellar peduncle. Lesion of the fasciculus leads to:

	Features	Site of lesion
Benedict syndrome^Q	Ipsilateral third nerve palsy with contralateral flapping tremors^Q	Dorsal part of fasciculus as it passes through the **red nucleus**^Q
Weber syndrome^Q	Ipsilateral third nerve palsy with contralateral hemiplegia^Q	Ventral part of fasciculus as it passes through the **cerebral peduncle**
Nothnagel syndrome^Q	Ipsilateral third nerve palsy with ataxia^Q	Fasciculus in association with **cerebellar peduncle**
Claude syndrome	Combination of **Benedict** and **Nothnagel** syndromes	

- *Basilar part*: It starts as a series of rootlets, which join to form a trunk which traverses the subarachnoid space unaccompanied by cranial nerves. So, **isolated III N palsy is usually basilar in origin**^Q. This part of the nerve is closely associated with **the posterior communicating artery.**
- *Intracavernous part*: The nerve enters the cavernous sinus and lies in lateral wall above the fourth nerve. In the anterior part of the cavernous sinus, the nerve divides into superior and inferior divisions which enter the orbit through the superior orbital fissure
- *Intra-orbital part*: The superior division supplies the levator and superior rectus. Inferior division supplies the medial, inferior recti and inferior oblique. It also contains parasympathetic fibers to sphincter pupillae and ciliary muscle.

Pupillomotor fibers which lie in the superficial part of the nerve are supplied by pial blood vessels while main trunk of the nerve is supplied by vasa nervorum. Hence vascular causes of third nerve palsy which affect the vasa nervorum are pupil sparing^Q.

Neuro-Ophthalmology

Causes of Third Nerve Palsy

- **Vascular** causes like hypertension, diabetes (**most common cause in adults**)^Q
- **Trauma (most common cause in children)**^{Q}
- Tumors
- Aneurysm of posterior communicating artery

Clinical Features of third nerve palsy

- **Ptosis**^{Q} due to involvement of levator palpebrae superioris muscle
- The eye is positioned **down and out**^{Q} due to the action of the unaffected muscles, superior oblique and lateral rectus
- Fixed dilated pupil due to involvement of the sphincter pupillae
- Weakness of accommodation due to ciliary muscle involvement

TROCHLEAR (FOURTH NERVE PALSY)

Anatomy: The course of the nerve from the midbrain to the muscle is divided into the following parts:

- *Nucleus*: Located in the midbrain at the level of the inferior colliculus. It controls the **contralateral superior oblique muscle.**
- *Fasciculus*: The fibers decussate in the anterior medullary velum.
- *Basilar part*: It leaves the brainstem **from the dorsal aspect**^{Q}. It curves around the brainstem, passes beneath the tentorial edge, pierces the dura and enters the cavernous sinus.
- *Intracavernous part*: It lies in the lateral wall of the cavernous sinus between the third nerve and ophthalmic nerve. It passes through the superior orbital fissure to enter the orbit.
- *Orbital part*: It innervates the superior oblique **from the orbital surface**^{Q}.

Causes of fourth nerve palsy: Trauma (most common)^Q

Clinical features of fourth nerve palsy

- Vertical/torsional diplopia^Q
- **Diplopia is maximum in downgaze** (direction of action of superior oblique muscle)^Q
- Eye is **deviated upwards** due to underaction of superior oblique (depressor). This is called **hypertropia**^{Q}
- **Hypertropia and diplopia worsen in opposite gaze and head tilt to same side**^{Q}
- **Compensatory head posture is head tilt to opposite side**^{Q}
- *Clinical test for superior oblique palsy*: **Bielschowsky test**^{Q} **and Park's three step test**^{Q}

Abducens (Sixth) Nerve Palsy

Anatomy: The course of the nerve from the pons to the muscle is divided into the following parts:

- *Nucleus*: It lies in the mid portion of **pons** and is closely related to the **facial nerve**.
- *Fasciculus*: It passes ventrally and leaves the brainstem at the ponto-medullary junction, lateral to the pyramidal prominence. It is also closely related to the seventh nerve. Lesion in the fasciculus causes:
  - *Millard–Gubler syndrome*^{Q}: Lesion involving the fasciculus and pyramidal tract. Features are **ipsilateral sixth and seventh nerve palsy with contralateral hemiplegia**^{Q}
- *Basilar part*: It leaves the brainstem at the ponto-medullary junction. This part of the nerve comes in contact with important structures like the tip of the petrous bone and inferior petrosal sinus, before it enters the cavernous sinus. Lesions affecting this part are:
  - Raised intracranial pressure: In posterior fossa tumors or pseudotumor cerebri, there is herniation of the brainstem. As a result, the sixth nerves of both sides are stretched over the petrous tip leading to **bilateral sixth nerve palsy (false localizing sign).**
  - *Gradenigo syndrome*^{Q}: Inflammation of the petrous apex leads to involvement of fifth, sixth, seventh and eighth cranial nerves.
- *Intracavernous part*: It lies in the substance of the cavernous sinus in close association with the internal carotid artery and the sympathetic plexus.
- *Intraorbital part*: It enters the orbit through the superior orbital fissure and supplies the lateral rectus.

Causes of Sixth Nerve Palsy

- **Vascular** causes like diabetes (**most common cause in adults**)^Q
- **Trauma (most common cause in children)**^{Q}
- Tumors
- Petrositis, mastoiditis.

Clinical features of sixth nerve palsy

- **Horizontal uncrossed diplopia**^{Q}
- Diplopia is maximum on lateral gaze to the affected side (direction of action of the muscle)^Q
- Medial deviation of eyeball or **esotropia**^{Q}
- **Face turn to the same side is the compensatory posture**^{Q}

Self Assessment and Review of Ophthalmology

ANISOCORIA (FLOWCHART 1)

Anisocoria is defined as pupillary inequality of 0.4 mm or more. The causes of anisocoria are
- Physiological
- Pharmacological
- Third cranial nerve palsy
- Adie's tonic pupil
- Horner's syndrome

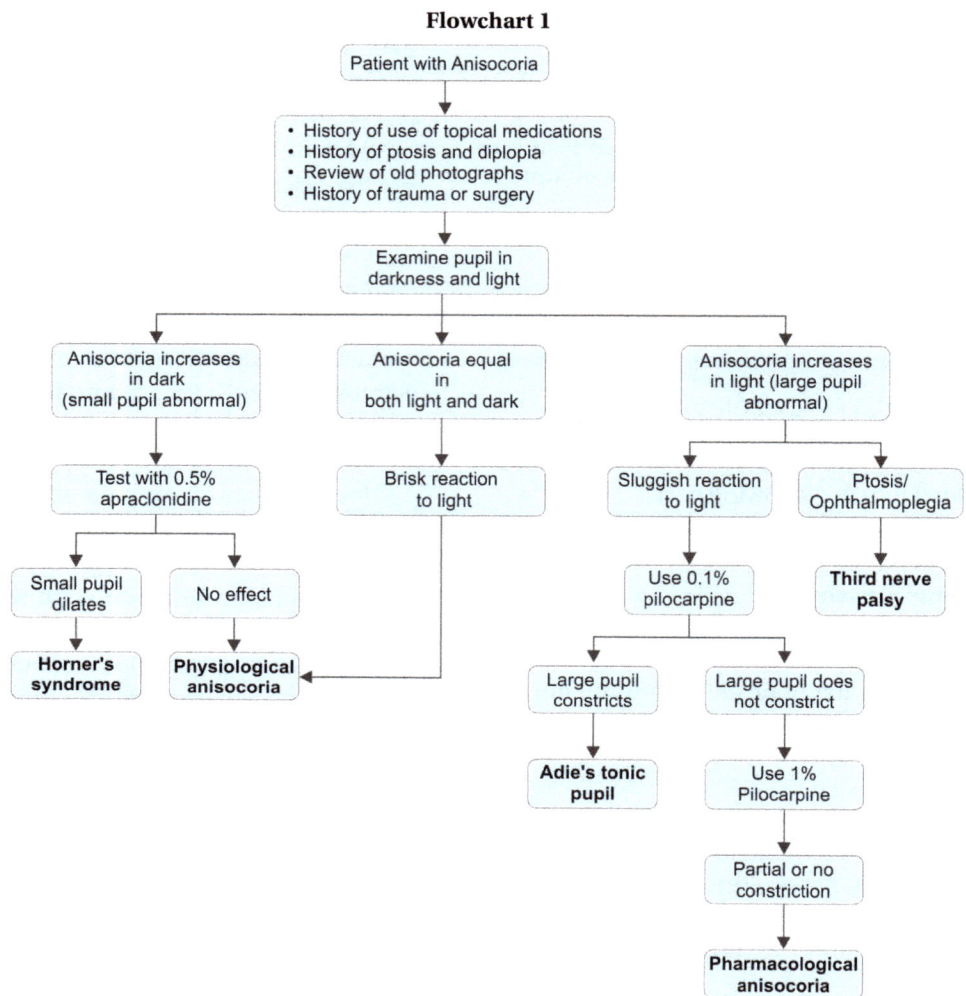

SUPRANUCLEAR CONTROL OF OCULAR MOVEMENTS

CONJUGATE EYE MOVEMENTS

- They are **binocular** movements where both eyes move synchronously in the same direction.
- They are called **versions** and are controlled at the cerebral and brainstem levels.
- **Supranuclear disturbances produce gaze palsies characterised by absence of diplopia.**

The important types of conjugate movements are

Saccades	Pursuits
Fast movements	**Slow** movements
Move the eye from one object to another	Following movement to maintain fixation on an object of interest
Controlled by **contralateral frontal lobe**[Q]	Controlled by **ipsilateral occipital lobe**[Q]

Neuro-Ophthalmology

HORIZONTAL GAZE PATHWAY

- Horizontal gaze involves two muscles namely, **the ipsilateral lateral rectus** and the **contralateral medial rectus.**
- The center for the horizontal gaze is the **PPRF (parapontine reticular formation)**^{Q}.
- From PPRF, the neurons connect to the **ipsilateral sixth nerve nucleus.**
- From sixth nerve nucleus, the neurons pass through the **medial longitudinal fasciculus (MLF)** to the **contralateral medial rectus subnucleus.**

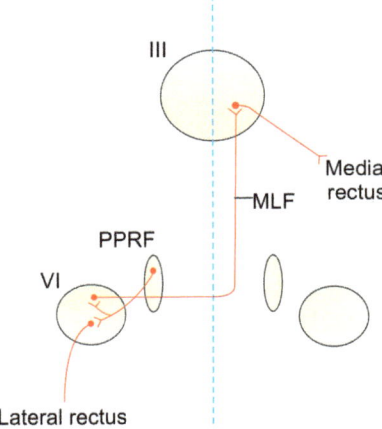

Fig. 13: Horizontal gaze pathway

Lesions of horizontal gaze pathway

- *Horizontal gaze palsy*: This is caused due to lesion in the **PPRF of the same side** ^{Q}
- *Internuclear ophthalmoplegia (INO)*: This is caused by lesion in the **MLF** ^{Q}
- *One and a half syndrome*: This is caused by lesion in both **PPRF and MLF of the same side**^{Q}.

Vertical Gaze Pathway

The centre for the vertical gaze is the **rostral interstitial nucleus of the dorsal midbrain** (riMLF)^Q.

The important types of vertical gaze palsy are
- **Perinaud's syndrome:** Upgaze palsy
- **Steel Richardson syndrome:** Downgaze palsy

Nystagmus

Involuntary, regular, repetitive, rhythmic to-and-fro oscillation of the eyes.

Clinical Types

- Physiological nystagmus
  - *End point nystagmus*: It is seen in extremes of gaze
  - *Optokinetic nystagmus*: It is a jerk nystagmus induced by repetitive moving stimuli like an optokinetic drum (Catford drum)
  - *Vestibular nystagmus*: It is seen when the external auditory canal is stimulated by cold or warm water. It is a jerk nystagmus where the direction of the fast component is remembered by the mnemonic **COWS** meaning "cold opposite warm same".
- *Sensory deprivation nystagmus*: It is seen due to poor vision since early childhood usually less than 2 years of age. Causes are congenital cataract, macular hypoplasia, albinism, etc.
- *Motor imbalance nystagmus*: The important types are
  - *Ataxic Nystagmus*: It occurs in the abducting eye in **Inter Nuclear Ophthalmoplegia (INO)**^{Q}
  - *Down Beat Nystagmus*: It is seen in lesions at cervico-medullary junction^Q
  - *Upbeat Nystagmus*: It is seen in phenytoin intoxication and posterior fossa lesions
  - *Sea-Saw Nystagmus of Maddox*: It is a special type of nystagmus where one eye elevates and intorts whereas the other eye depresses and extorts. It is seen in **optic chiasma lesions**^{Q}.

? Must Remember

- *Bitemporal hemianopia*: Lesion in optic chiasma
- *Pie in the sky*: Lesion in temporal lobe/Meyer's loop
- *Weber syndrome*: Ipsilateral third nerve palsy with contralateral hemiplegia
- *Millard-Gubler syndrome*: Ipsilateral sixth and seventh nerve palsy with contralateral hemiplegia
- *Horizontal gaze palsy*: Lesion in Para-pontine Reticular Formation (PPRF)
- *Internuclear ophthalmoplegia*: Lesion in Medial Longitudinal Fasciculus (MLF)

QUESTIONS

Visual Pathway

1. Optic nerve is: *(DPG)*
   a. First order neuron
   b. Second order neuron
   c. Third order neuron
   d. Fourth order neuron

2. The visual pathway consists of all except: *(PGI)*
   a. Optic tract
   b. Geniculocalcarine tract
   c. Inferior colliculus
   d. Lateral geniculate body
   e. Pretectal nucleus

3. Bitemporal hemianopia is characteristic of: *(AIIMS 2006)*
   a. Glaucoma
   b. Optic neuritis
   c. Pituitary tumor
   d. Retinal detachment

4. Visual pathway lesion at the level of the optic chiasma will result in: *(May AIIMS 2017)*
   a. Binasal hemianopia
   b. Bitemporal hemianopia
   c. Central scotoma
   d. Homonymous hemianopia

5. Homonymous hemianopia is seen in lesion of: *(PGI 2012)*
   a. Optic tract
   b. Optic nerve
   c. Optic radiation
   d. Optic chiasma
   e. Occipital cortex

6. Visual field defect in optic chiasma lesions is/are: *(PGI 2014)*
   a. Bitemporal hemianopia
   b. Binasal hemianopia
   c. Homonymous upper temporal hemianopia
   d. Heteronymous upper temporal hemianopia
   e. Homonymous upper nasal hemianopia

7. A homonymous upper quadrantic field defect is due to lesion of: *(AIIMS 2000)*
   a. Parietal lobe
   b. Temporal lobe
   c. Occipital lobe
   d. Optic chiasma

8. A lesion of the optic radiation involving the Meyer's loop causes: *(AIIMS 2002)*
   a. Homonymous hemianopia
   b. Centrocecal scotoma
   c. Superior quadrantopia
   d. Inferior quadrantopia

9. Macular sparing is a feature of lesion in: *(JIPMER 2001)*
   a. Optic nerve
   b. Optic tract
   c. Optic radiation
   d. Occipital cortex

10. Optic radiation arises from: *(CET 2017)*
    a. Lateral geniculate body
    b. Medial geniculate body
    c. Superior colliculus
    d. Inferior colliculus

11. The primary visual cortex is located in: *(COMEDK 2013)*
    a. Parieto-occipital sulcus
    b. Superior temporal sulcus
    c. Posterior part of calcarine sulcus
    d. Central sulcus

12. True about cortical blindness is: *(AIIMS)*
    a. Direct and consensual reflexes are present in both eyes
    b. Direct and consensual reflexes are absent in both eyes
    c. Direct reflex is present but consensual reflex is absent on the normal side
    d. Direct reflex is absent but consensual reflex is present on the normal side

13. A patient presents with headache and difficulty in vision. On perimetry, right eye shows superotemporal quadrantopia and left eye shows centrocecal scotoma. Likely site of lesion is: *(AIPG 2009)*
    a. Left optic nerve and chiasma
    b. Left optic tract and chiasma
    c. Right optic nerve and chiasma
    d. Right optic tract and chiasma

14. A female patient presents with loss of vision in both eyes. On examination normal pupillary responses are seen with normal fundus. VER shows extinguished response. The most likely diagnosis is: *(AIIMS)*
    a. Hysteria
    b. Retrobulbar neuritis
    c. Cortical blindness
    d. Retinal detachment

Pupillary Reflexes

15. Which of the following is not a part of the pupillary reflex pathway? *(DNB 2015)*
    a. Edinger-Westphal nucleus
    b. Medial geniculate body
    c. Pretectal nucleus
    d. Ganglion cells in the retina

16. Components of the pupillary light reflex are: *(PGI)*
    a. Retina
    b. Pretectal nucleus
    c. Lateral geniculate body
    d. Edinger-Westphal nucleus
    e. Calcarine sulcus

17. Marcus Gunn pupil is due to: *(Maharashtra PG 2005)*
    a. Defect anterior to chiasma
    b. Defect at the optic chiasma
    c. Defect posterior to the chiasma
    d. Defect in the ciliary muscle

18. Marcus Gunn pupil is seen in lesion of: *(NEET 2016)*
    a. Retinal detachment
    b. Optic neuritis
    c. Retinitis pigmentosa
    d. Diabetic retinopathy

Neuro-Ophthalmology

19. In RAPD, when light is moved from normal to affected eye, there is: *(AIPG)*
    a. Dilatation of both pupils
    b. Constriction of both pupils
    c. Dilatation in affected eye and constriction in normal eye
    d. Dilatation in normal eye and constriction in affected eye

20. Wernicke's hemianopic pupil is due to lesion in: *(AIPG/ DNB 2015)*
    a. Optic tract
    b. Optic radiation
    c. Optic chiasma
    d. Lateral geniculate body

21. Pupil which responds to convergence but not light is: *(DPG 2008)*
    a. Adie's pupil
    b. Argyll- Robertson pupil
    c. Hutchison pupil
    d. Myotonic pupil

22. All of the following are true regarding Argyll-Robertson pupil except: *(AIPG 2011)*
    a. Near reflex is normal
    b. Direct light reflex is absent
    c. Consensual light reflex is present
    d. Visual acuity is normal

23. Argyll-Robertson pupil is seen in: *(DNB 2014)*
    a. Multiple sclerosis
    b. Midbrain tumour
    c. Neurosyphilis
    d. All of the above

24. Dilator pupillae is supplied by: *(WBPG 2013)*
    a. Cholinergic fibers of Oculomotor nerve
    b. Adrenergic fibers of Oculomotor nerve
    c. Trigeminal nerve
    d. Facial nerve

25. Which of the following is seen in Horner's syndrome? *(DNB 2014)*
    a. Anhydrosis
    b. Conjunctivitis
    c. Blepharitis
    d. Optic neuritis

26. Anisocoria in Horner's syndrome is due to: *(CET June 2017)*
    a. Oculosympathetic palsy
    b. Oculoparasympathetic palsy
    c. Oculomotor nerve palsy
    d. Abducens nerve palsy

27. Horner's syndrome causes all except: *(DNB 2014)*
    a. Enophthalmos
    b. Mydriasis
    c. Anhydrosis
    d. Narrow palpebral aperture

28. Anisocoria with ptosis is seen in: *(DNB 2015)*
    a. Horner's syndrome
    b. CHARGE syndrome
    c. Usher syndrome
    d. Sixth cranial nerve palsy

29. Anisocoria means: *(DNB 2016)*
    a. Unequal size of the pupils
    b. Differential perception of object size by the two eyes
    c. Differential perception of object shape by the two eyes
    d. Difference in corneal thickness

Optic Neuritis

30. All of the following are true regarding optic neuritis except: *(AIPG 2001)*
    a. Decreased visual acuity
    b. Decreased pupillary reaction
    c. Abnormal electroretinogram
    d. Abnormal visual evoked potential

31. Which of the following statements regarding optic neuritis is false: *(DNB 2015)*
    a. Oral steroid therapy alone is contraindicated
    b. MRI brain and orbit helps to decide treatment
    c. Steroids may help to decrease the duration of vision loss but do not affect the final visual outcome
    d. Color vision recovers faster than visual acuity

32. Optic neuritis is characterized by all of the following except: *(APPG 2014)*
    a. Strongly associated with demyelinating disease
    b. Subacute unilateral vision loss
    c. Pain in exacerbated by ocular movements
    d. Optic disc is always abnormal in the acute stage

33. Investigation of choice in optic neuritis is: *(NEET 2016)*
    a. MRI brain and orbit
    b. CT Scan brain and orbit
    c. Vitreous biopsy
    d. Electroretinogram

34. A child presents with sudden loss of vision in the right eye with painful ocular movements. There are no obvious signs on ophthalmoscopy. The most likely diagnosis is: *(AIPG)*
    a. Optic nerve glioma
    b. Retrobulbar neuritis
    c. Craniopharyngioma
    d. Papillitis

35. A young male patient presents with blurring of vision in the right eye followed by the left eye after 3 months. The disc is hyperemic and edematous with circumpapillary telangiectasia. Perimetry shows centrocecal scotoma. The likely diagnosis is: *(AIIMS 2009)*
    a. Optic neuritis
    b. Acute papilledema
    c. Toxic optic neuropathy
    d. Leber's hereditary optic neuropathy (LHON)

36. The most common inherited blindness due to mitochondrial anomaly is: *(AIPG 2004)*
    a. Retinitis pigmentosa
    b. Leber's congenital amaurosis
    c. Leber's hereditary optic neuropathy (LHON)
    d. Retinopathy of prematurity

37. Leber's hereditary optic neuropathy (LHON). True is: *(Manipal 2009)*
    a. Typically presents in the fourth decade
    b. Males do not transmit the disease
    c. Is inherited in X-linked fashion
    d. The optic nerve becomes pale early in the disease

Papilledema

38. **Earliest sign in papilledema is:** *(DNB 2015)*
    a. Blurring of disc margins
    b. Loss of venous pulsation
    c. Hyperemia of disc
    d. Cotton wool spots

39. **All of the following are true about papilledema except:** *(AIPG 2007)*
    a. Collection of extracellular fluid
    b. Disruption of neurofilaments
    c. Stasis of axoplasmic transport
    d. Swelling of the axons

40. **Fundoscopic features of papilledema include all of the following except:** *(AIPG 2008)*
    a. Ill-defined disc margins
    b. Deep physiological cup
    c. Absent venous pulsations
    d. Bending of the blood vessels

41. **All of the following are true regarding papilledema except:** *(AIPG)*
    a. It is a non-inflammatory phenomenon
    b. Transient loss of vision occurs
    c. First sign is blurring of nasal disc margin
    d. Sudden loss of vision with painful ocular movements is seen

42. **Papilledema is characterized by all of the following except:** *(AIIMS)*
    a. Loss of venous pulsations
    b. Transient obscuration of vision
    c. Sudden painless loss of vision
    d. Disc edema

43. **Which of the following is/are seen in papilledema?** *(PGI 2013)*
    a. Normal blind spot
    b. Normal visual acuity even in the last stage
    c. Loss of venous pulsations at the disc
    d. Sluggish pupillary reaction
    e. Normal color vision

44. **Unilateral papilledema with optic atrophy on the other side is a feature of:** *(DPG 2010)*
    a. Foster Kennedy syndrome
    b. Fischer syndrome
    c. Vogt-Koyanagi Harada disease
    d. WAGR syndrome

45. **Which of these ophthalmic manifestations is least likely due to acute meningococcal meningitis?** *(DNB 2015)*
    a. Papilledema
    b. Cranial nerve palsy
    c. Optic neuritis
    d. Glaucoma

46. **A 40-year-old lady presents with headache and papilledema. CT scan of brain shows normal ventricles. Diagnosis is:** *(AIPG)*
    a. Benign intracranial hypertension
    b. Malignant hypertension
    c. Papillitis
    d. Raised intraocular pressure

47. **Disc edema is seen in:** *(DNB 2014)*
    a. CRVO
    b. CRAO
    c. BRVO
    d. BRAO

48. **Papilledema is seen in all except:** *(DNB 2013)*
    a. Pseudotumor cerebri
    b. CRVO
    c. Raised ICT
    d. Hypervitaminosis B

49. **Altitudinal field defect is seen in:** *(DNB 2013)*
    a. Ischemic optic neuropathy
    b. CRVO
    c. CRAO
    d. Papilledema

50. **Enlargement of the blind spot is seen in:** *(AIPG 2000)*
    a. Papillitis
    b. Papilledema
    c. Avulsion of the optic nerve
    d. Retinal detachment

Optic Neuropathy

51. **A patient with right brow injury due to RTA presents with sudden loss of vision in the right eye. The pupil shows absent direct reflex but normal consensual reflex in the right eye. The fundus is normal. The treatment of choice is:** *(AIPG)*
    a. Intensive intravenous corticosteroids as prescribed for spinal injuries to be instituted within six hours
    b. Pulse methyl prednisolone 250 mg four times a day for three days
    c. Oral prednisolone 1.5 mg/kg body weight
    d. Emergency optic canal decompression

52. **All of the following drugs can cause optic neuropathy except:** *(AIPG 2011)*
    a. Rifampicin
    b. Digoxin
    c. Chloroquine
    d. Ethambutol

53. **Vitamin B_{12} deficiency causes:** *(AIPG 2001)*
    a. Bitemporal hemianopia
    b. Binasal hemianopia
    c. Heteronymous hemianopia
    d. Centrocecal scotoma

54. **Optic atrophy is not seen in:** *(AIIMS 2013)*
    a. Retinitis pigmentosa
    b. Methanol poisoning
    c. Central retinal artery occlusion
    d. Polypoidal choroidal vasculopathy

55. **Consecutive optic atrophy is seen in:** *(UPPG 2014)*
    a. Papilledema
    b. Papillitis
    c. Retinal detachment
    d. Retinitis pigmentosa

56. **A 15-year-old boy has bilateral optic atrophy with diabetes mellitus and diabetes insipidus. The likely diagnosis is:** *(AIPG 2000)*
    a. Kjer syndrome
    b. Behr syndrome
    c. Wolfram syndrome
    d. Leber's congenital amaurosis

57. **Wolfram syndrome is characterized by all except:** *(DNB 2016)*
    a. Optic atrophy
    b. Diabetes mellitus
    c. Diabetes insipidus
    d. Parathyroid hyperplasia

Neuro-Ophthalmology

Cranial Nerve Palsy

58. Which of the following can cause third nerve palsy: *(PGI)*
    a. Posterior communicating artery aneurysm
    b. Tolosa- Hunt syndrome
    c. Midbrain infarct
    d. Pons infarct
    e. Lateral medullary syndrome

59. Inferior division of oculomotor nerve enters the orbit through: *(CET June 2017)*
    a. Inferior orbital fissure
    b. Superior orbital fissure
    c. Foramen rotundum
    d. Foramen lacerum

60. Oculomotor nerve palsy causes all except: *(AIIMS 2011)*
    a. Miosis
    b. Ptosis
    c. Outward deviation of eyeball
    d. Diplopia

61. All of the following are seen in oculomotor nerve palsy except: *(NEET 2016)*
    a. Ptosis
    b. Paralysis of accommodation
    c. Lateral gaze is affected
    d. Upward gaze is affected

62. Isolated third nerve palsy with pupillary sparing is seen in: *(AIPG 2007)*
    a. Aneurysmal rupture
    b. Trauma
    c. Diabetes
    d. Raised ICT

63. The frequent cause of isolated IIIrd, IVth and VIth cranial nerve palsies in adults is: *(COMEDK 2015)*
    a. Microvascular ischemia
    b. Oligodendroglioma
    c. Posterior cerebral artery aneurysm
    d. Brainstem infarction

64. A 72-year-old patient presents with diplopia. Which of the following features is suggestive of IIIrd nerve palsy due to posterior communicating artery aneurysm? *(JIPMER 2015)*
    a. Convergent squint
    b. Pupil not reacting to light
    c. Constricted pupil
    d. Exophthalmos

65. Lateral rectus palsy is characterized by: *(AIPG 2000)*
    a. Crossed diplopia
    b. Uncrossed diplopia
    c. Downward deviation of the eyeball
    d. Upward deviation of the eyeball

66. In right lateral rectus palsy, all are true except: *(AIIMS 2000)*
    a. Face turn to left
    b. Medial convergent squint
    c. Inability to abduct right eye
    d. Horizontal diplopia

67. Feature of left sided sixth nerve palsy: *(AIIMS 2008)*
    a. Accommodative paresis of left eye
    b. Ptosis of left eye
    c. Adduction weakness of left eye
    d. Diplopia in left gaze

68. A patient presents with head tilted to the right side. On examination, he has left hypertropia which increases on looking to the right side. The muscle most likely to be paralyzed is: *(AIIMS 2008)*
    a. Left superior oblique
    b. Left inferior oblique
    c. Right superior oblique
    d. Right inferior oblique

69. Diplopia in superior oblique palsy is described as: *(AIPG 2011)*
    a. Vertical on looking down
    b. Vertical on looking up
    c. Horizontal on looking in
    d. Horizontal on looking out

70. A patient has moderate ptosis with restriction of ocular movements in all directions but no squint or diplopia. The diagnosis is: *(AIIMS 2009)*
    a. Thyroid ophthalmopathy
    b. Chronic progressive external ophthalmoplegia
    c. Myasthenia gravis
    d. Multiple cranial nerve palsies

Gaze Palsy

71. Left sided lateral gaze is affected in lesion of: *(AIPG)*
    a. Left frontal lobe
    b. Left occipital lobe
    c. Right frontal lobe
    d. Right occipital lobe

72. Horizontal gaze palsy is due to lesion in: *(PGI)*
    a. Parapontine reticular formation
    b. Pretectal nucleus
    c. Medial longitudinal fasciculus
    d. Occipital lobe

73. Internuclear ophthalmoplegia is due to lesion in: *(AIIMS 2002)*
    a. Occipital lobe
    b. Pretectal nucleus
    c. Medial longitudinal fasciculus
    d. Parapontine reticular formation

74. One and a half syndrome is due to lesion in: *(Jipmer 2011)*
    a. Parapontine reticular formation (PPRF)
    b. Medial longitudinal fasciculus (MLF)
    c. Both PPRF and MLF
    d. Occipital lobe

75. A patient presents with diplopia. On examination, adduction deficit is seen in one eye and abducting saccades in the other eye. Convergence is preserved. What is the likely diagnosis? *(AIIMS 2009)*
    a. Partial third nerve palsy
    b. Internuclear ophthalmoplegia
    c. Duane's retraction syndrome
    d. Absence of medial rectus muscle

Miscellaneous

76. Downbeat nystagmus is a feature of: *(PGI 2013)*
    a. Cerebellar lesion
    b. Arnold-Chiari malformation
    c. Pontine lesion
    d. Optic neuritis

77. A patient has right homonymous hemianopia with defective optokinetic nystagmus. The lesion is most likely to be in: *(AIIMS 2005)*
    a. Frontal lobe
    b. Occipital lobe
    c. Parietal lobe
    d. Temporal lobe

78. **Ophthalmoplegic migraine means:** *(AIPG/ AIIMS 2003)*
    a. Headache with irreversible loss of optic nerve function
    b. Recurrent third nerve palsy associated with headache
    c. Headache associated with third, fourth and sixth nerve palsy
    d. Headache associated with optic neuritis

79. **Lamina cribrosa is absent in:** *(AIPG 2006)*
    a. Morning glory syndrome
    b. Nanophthalmos
    c. Coloboma of retina
    d. Optic nerve agenesis

80. **CHARGE syndrome includes all except:** *(DNB 2016)*
    a. Coloboma
    b. Heart defects
    c. Urogenital anomalies
    d. Esophageal atresia

81. A patient was suffering from ptosis with hypotropia. After injection of a certain drug, considerable improvement is seen in both ptosis and squint. What is the possible diagnosis? *(AIIMS Nov 2017)*
    a. Sixth cranial nerve palsy
    b. Myasthenia gravis
    c. Third cranial nerve palsy
    d. Tolosa-Hunt syndrome

Neuro-Ophthalmology

ANSWERS AND EXPLANATIONS

1. **b. Second order neuron** *(Ref: Yanoff & Duker 4th edition, p 866-867)*
   The second order neurons of the visual pathway are the ganglion cells. The optic nerve is formed by the axons of the ganglion cells, hence the answer.
2. **c. Inferior colliculus, e. Pretectal nucleus** *(Ref: Kanski 6th edition, p 812-815)*
3. **c. Pituitary tumor** *(Ref: Yanoff & Duker 4th edition, p 904-905)*
4. **b. Bitemporal hemianopia** *(Ref: Yanoff & Duker 4th edition, p 904-905)*
5. **a. Optic tract, c. Optic radiation, e. Occipital cortex**
6. **a. Bitemporal hemianopia, b. Binasal hemianopia, d. Heteronymous upper temporal hemianopia**
   (Ref: Yanoff & Duker 4th edition, p 904-905)
   - At the centre of the optic chiasma, the fibers from the nasal retina of both eyes cross over to the other side. Hence any lesion affecting the centre of the chiasma will cause Bitemporal hemianopia or Heteronymous hemianopia
   - Sometimes, in early cases the hemianopia may be incomplete either heteronymous upper temporal or lower temporal
   - In the periphery of the chiasma are the fibers from the temporal retina of both eyes. Thus a peripheral lesion may lead to Binasal hemianopia. (rare)
7. **b. Temporal lobe** *(Ref: Yanoff & Duker 4th edition, p 910)*
8. **c. Superior quadrantopia** *(Ref: Yanoff & Duker 4th edition, p 910)*
9. **d. Occipital cortex** *(Ref: Yanoff & Duker 4th edition, p 910-911)*
10. **a. Lateral geniculate body** *(Ref: Yanoff & Duker 4th edition, p 910-911)*
11. **c. Posterior part of calcarine sulcus** *(Ref: Yanoff & Duker 4th edition, p 910-911)*
    The primary visual area (Area no 17) is located in the calcarine sulcus in the occipital lobe of the brain. The accessory visual areas are Area 18 and Area 19
12. **a. Direct and consensual reflexes are present in both eyes**
    Cortical blindness means loss of vision due to lesion in occipital cortex. Since the center for the pupillary reflex is located in the pretectal nucleus in the midbrain, this reflex remains unaffected in cortical blindness
13. **a. Left optic nerve and chiasma** *(Ref: Yanoff & Duker 4th edition, p 904-905)*
    This is a slightly tricky question. The question says that the patient has left centrocecal scotoma. So the left optic nerve is affected. The patient also has an upper temporal field defect on the right side probably due to an early chiasma lesion
14. **c. Cortical blindness** *(Ref: Yanoff & Duker 4th edition, p 911-913)*
    Cortical Blindness means loss of vision due to lesion in the occipital cortex like infarct, hemorrhage etc. The features are
    - Sudden painless loss of vision
    - Normal pupillary reflex
    - Normal fundus
    So, in order to rule out hysteria or malingering, VEP is done. In cortical blindness, VEP will show a decreased or extinguished response whereas it will be normal in hysteria or malingering
15. **b. Medial geniculate body** *(Ref: Yanoff & Duker 4th edition, p 960, Kanski 6th edition, p 802)*
16. **a. Retina, b. Pretectal nucleus, d. Edinger-Westphal nucleus**
    (Ref: Yanoff & Duker 4th edition, p 960, Kanski 6th edition, p 802)
17. **a. Defect anterior to chiasma** *(Ref: Yanoff & Duker 4th edition, p 958-959)*
18. **b. Optic neuritis** *(Ref: Yanoff & Duker 4th edition, p 958-959)*
19. **a. Dilatation of both pupils** *(Ref: Yanoff & Duker 4th edition, p 958-959)*
20. **a. Optic tract** *(Ref: Kanski 6th edition, p 813)*
21. **b. Argyll- Robertson pupil** *(Ref: Kanski 6th edition, p 803)*
22. **c. Consensual light reflex is present** *(Ref: Kanski 6th edition, p 803)*
23. **c. Neurosyphilis** *(Ref: Kanski 6th edition, p 803)*
24. **c. Trigeminal nerve** *(Ref: Kanski 6th edition, p 804)*
25. **a. Anhydrosis** *(Ref: Kanski 6th edition, p 805)*

Self Assessment and Review of Ophthalmology

26. a. Oculosympathetic palsy (Ref: Kanski 6th edition, p 805)
27. b. Mydriasis (Ref: Kanski 6th edition, p 805)
28. a. Horner's syndrome (Ref: Kanski 6th edition, p 805)
29. a. Unequal size of the pupils (Ref: Yanoff & Duker 4th edition, p 960)
30. c. Abnormal electroretinogram (Ref: Yanoff & Duker 4th edition, p 879-880)
31. d. Color vision recovers faster than visual acuity (Ref: Yanoff & Duker 4th edition, p 883)
32. d. Optic disc is always abnormal in the acute stage (Ref: Yanoff & Duker 4th edition, p 879)
    In retrobulbar neuritis, the optic disc is normal in the acute stage
33. a. MRI brain and orbit (Ref: Yanoff & Duker 4th edition, p 879)
    MRI brain and orbit helps to rule out demyelinating disorders which are the most common cause of optic neuritis
34. b. Retrobulbar neuritis (Ref: Yanoff & Duker 4th edition, p 879)
35. d. Leber's Hereditary Optic Neuropathy (LHON) (Ref: Yanoff & Duker 4th edition, p 891)
36. c. Leber's Hereditary Optic Neuropathy (LHON) (Ref: Yanoff & Duker 4th edition, p 891)
37. b. Males do not transmit the disease (Ref: Yanoff & Duker 4th edition, p 890)
38. a. Blurring of disc margins (Ref: Yanoff & Duker 4th edition, p 875)
39. b. Disruption of neurofilament (Ref: Yanoff & Duker 4th edition, p 875-876)
    In papilledema, there is back transmission of the subarachnoid pressure to the optic nerve. This leads to axonal stasis and swelling. There is also impaired venous drainage. But there is no disruption of any neuronal fibers in papilledema
40. b. Deep physiological cup (Ref: Yanoff & Duker 4th edition, p 875)
    There is obliteration of the physiological cup due to disc swelling
41. d. Sudden loss of vision with painful ocular movements is seen (Ref: Yanoff & Duker 4th edition, p 876)
    In papilledema, transient obscuration of vision or Amaurosis fugax may be seen but there is no significant vision loss
42. c. Sudden painless loss of vision (Ref: Yanoff & Duker 4th edition, p 876)
43. c. Loss of venous pulsations at the disc, e. Normal color vision (Ref: Kanski 6th edition, p 801)
    Visual acuity is usually normal but in chronic end stage papilledema, it may be decreased
44. a. Foster Kennedy syndrome
45. d. Glaucoma
    All the others may be possible due to meningitis and raised intracranial pressure
46. a. Benign intracranial hypertension (Ref: Yanoff & Duker 4th edition, p 875)
    The condition is presently called Idiopathic Intracranial Hypertension (IIH)
47. a. CRVO (Ref: Yanoff & Duker 4th edition, p 877)
    Causes of disc edema are: (unilateral)
    * Papillitis
    * CRVO
    * Optic nerve head drusen
    * Foster Kennedy syndrome
48. d. Hypervitaminosis B (Ref: Yanoff & Duker 4th edition, p 875)
    Hypervitaminosis A leads to Idiopathic Intracranial Hypertension (IIH)
49. a. Ischemic optic neuropathy (Ref: Yanoff & Duker 4th edition, p 885)
50. b. Papilledema (Ref: Yanoff & Duker 4th edition, p 876)
51. a. Intensive intravenous corticosteroids as prescribed for spinal injuries to be instituted within six hours
    (Ref: Yanoff & Duker 4th edition, p 899)
    The case described is of Traumatic Optic Neuropathy. The treatment is high dose intravenous corticosteroids in the same regimen prescribed for spinal injuries
52. a. Rifampicin (Ref: Yanoff & Duker 4th edition, p 890)
53. d. Centrocecal scotoma (Ref: Yanoff & Duker 4th edition, p 890)
    Vitamin B_{12} deficiency is an important cause of nutritional optic neuropathy
54. d. Polypoidal choroidal vasculopathy (Ref: Kanski 6th edition, p 788)
    Polypoidal choroidal vasculopathy is a variant of ARMD and is not associated with the optic nerve
55. d. Retinitis pigmentosa
56. c. Wolfram syndrome (Ref: Kanski 6th edition, p 798)

Neuro-Ophthalmology

The important types of hereditary optic neuropathies are
- Leber's hereditary optic neuropathy (LHON)
- Kjer's optic neuropathy- It is an autosomal dominant optic atrophy which presents with vision loss in early childhood. It has no significant systemic features
- Wolfram syndrome-It is an autosomal recessive disorder described by the eponym DIDMOAD meaning Diabetes Insipidus, Diabetes Mellitus, Optic Atrophy, Deafness
- Behr syndrome- It is an autosomal recessive disorder with features of optic atrophy, pyramidal tract signs, ataxia, mental retardation, urinary incontinence, pes cavus

57. d. **Parathyroid hyperplasia** (Ref: Kanski 6th edition, p 798)
58. a. **Posterior communicating artery aneurysm, b. Tolosa-Hunt syndrome, c. Midbrain infarct**
(Ref: Yanoff & Duker 4th edition, p 929)
59. b. **Superior orbital fissure** (Ref: Yanoff & Duker 4th edition, p 929)
Both divisions of Oculomotor nerve enter the orbit through the superior orbital fissure
60. a. **Miosis** (Ref: Yanoff & Duker 4th edition, p 929)
61. c. **Lateral gaze is affected** (Ref: Yanoff & Duker 4th edition, p 929)
62. c. **Diabetes** (Ref: Yanoff & Duker 4th edition, p 929)
63. a. **Microvascular ischemia** (Ref: Yanoff & Duker 4th edition, p 929)
Microvascular ischemia due to diabetes, hypertension, etc. frequently causes isolated nerve palsies
64. b. **Pupil not reacting to light** (Ref: Yanoff & Duker 4th edition, p 929)
65. b. **Uncrossed diplopia** (Ref: Yanoff & Duker 4th edition, p 928)
66. a. **Face turn to the left** (Ref: Kanski 6th edition, p 824)
67. d. **Diplopia in left gaze** (Ref: Kanski 6th edition, p 824)
68. a. **Left superior oblique** (Ref: Yanoff & Duker 4th edition, p 929)
69. a. **Vertical on looking down** (Ref: Yanoff & Duker 4th edition, p 929)
70. b. **Chronic progressive external ophthalmoplegia**
(Ref: Yanoff & Duker 4th edition, p 943, Kanski 6th edition, p 827-828)

Chronic progressive external ophthalmoplegia (CPEO) is a condition which presents with gradually progressive bilateral ptosis and involvement of multiple extraocular muscles. Clinically there is minimal squint and no diplopia. The possible causes are
- Kearne Sayre syndrome Q
- Oculopharyngeal dystrophy
- Myotonic dystrophy Q
- Vitamin E deficiency

Episodic ophthalmoplegia is seen in
- Myasthenia gravis
- Eaten Lambert syndrome
- Botulism
- Organophosphorous poisoning
- Snake bite
- Familial periodic paralysis

71. c. **Right frontal lobe** (Ref: Yanoff & Duker 4th edition, p 915)
The center for the lateral gaze is the ipsilateral PPRF. But the PPRF is under the control of the contralateral frontal lobe. Hence for the left gaze, the center is the left PPRF which is controlled by the right frontal lobe
72. a. **Parapontine reticular formation** (Ref: Yanoff & Duker 4th edition, p 915, 918)
73. c. **Medial longitudinal fasciculus** (Ref: Yanoff & Duker 4th edition, p 915, 918)
74. c. **Both PPRF and MLF** (Ref: Yanoff & Duker 4th edition, p 919)
75. b. **Internuclear ophthalmoplegia** (Ref: Yanoff & Duker 4th edition, p 919)

Please refer to the text on pathway of horizontal gaze

The pathway for horizontal gaze may be summarized as

Parapontine reticular formation (PPRF)
↓
Sixth nerve nucleus of the same side
↓ MLF
Third nerve nucleus of the opposite side

Internuclear ophthalmoplegia (INO) is a defect of the horizontal gaze which is caused due to lesion in the medial longitudinal fasciculus (MLF). The MLF connects the sixth nerve nucleus to the third nerve nucleus of the opposite side. Thus, in INO, during lateral gaze the following features are seen
- The adducting eye fails to move because the third nerve nucleus does not receive any input
- The abducting eye moves laterally but suffers from abducting saccades
- Convergence is normal as the pathway for convergence is completely different

76. b. **Arnold-Chiari malformation** *(Ref: Kanski 6th edition, p 833)*

Downbeat nystagmus is due to lesion at cervico-medullary junction. Arnold- Chiari malformation is one such condition

77. c. **Parietal lobe** *(Ref: Kanski 6th edition, p 832)*

Lesion in parietal lobe leads to Pie on the floor or Inferior quadrantopia (incomplete homonymous hemianopia). Parietal lobe lesion also leads to defective optokinetic nystagmus. Hence the answer.

78. c. **Headache with third, fourth and sixth cranial nerve palsies**
- Ophthalmoplegic migraine is defined as headache with migranous characteristics accompanied or followed within 4 days by paresis of one or more ocular nerves namely third, fourth and sixth. (Most commonly the third cranial nerve). At least two attacks meeting the criterion are required for diagnosis
- Posterior fossa, parasellar and orbital lesions should have been ruled out by appropriate investigations

79. a. **Morning glory syndrome** *(Ref: Yanoff & Duker 4th edition, p 871)*
80. d. **Esophageal atresia** *(Ref: Yanoff & Duker 4th edition, p 872)*
81. b. **Myasthenia gravis** *(Ref: Kanski 8th edition p 838-840)*

Myasthenia gravis is an autoimmune disease in which antibodies mediate damage and destruction of acetylcholine receptors in striated muscle. The disease is more common in **females**[Q]. It may be generalized, bulbar or ocular.

Ocular myasthenia gravis

Ocular involvement is seen in **90%** cases and is the presenting feature in **60%** cases
- Ptosis is **bilateral**[Q] but **asymmetrical**[Q]. It is typically worse at the **end of the day**. It worsens on **prolonged upgaze** due to fatigue.
- Diplopia is seen when one or more extraocular muscles are affected
- Nystagmoid movements may be seen in extremes of gaze
- *Ice pack test*[Q]: Application of ice pack on the ptotic lid for 2 minutes results in improvement of ptosis. Cold inhibits the breakdown of acetylcholine by acetylcholinesterase. It is about 75% sensitive
- *Edrophonium/Neostigmine test*[Q]: Injection of a short-acting anticholinesterase results in a transient improvement in muscle weakness in myasthenia gravis. It is about **85%** sensitive in ocular myasthenia gravis. (This is shown in the picture in the question)
- *Antibody testing*[Q]: It confirms the diagnosis of myasthenia gravis
- *Electromyography and muscle biopsy:* These are other tests used in myasthenia gravis
- *Thoracic imaging (MRI/CT):* This is done to rule out thymoma which may be present in about 10% cases.

IMAGE BASED QUESTIONS

1. Identify this anomaly:

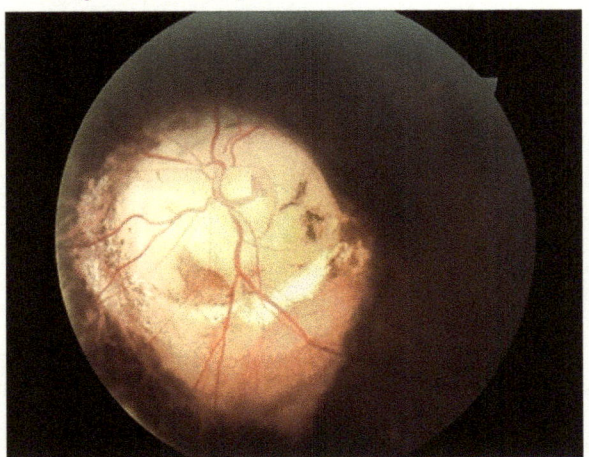

   a. Nanophthalmos
   b. Persistent hyperplastic primary vitreous
   c. Morning glory syndrome
   d. Optic disc hypoplasia

2. From the perimetry picture, identify the most likely diagnosis of the patient:

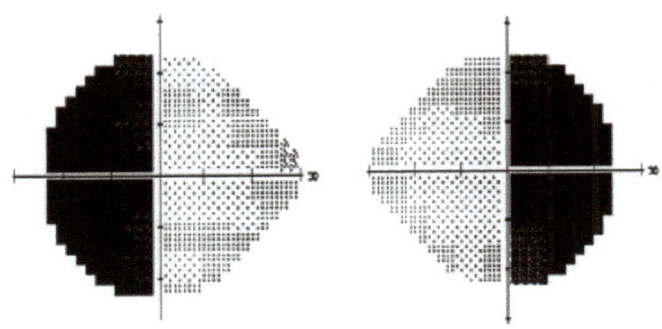

   a. Optic neuritis
   b. Pituitary adenoma
   c. Occipital infarct
   d. Posterior fossa tumor

3. From the perimetry, identify the site of lesion in the brain

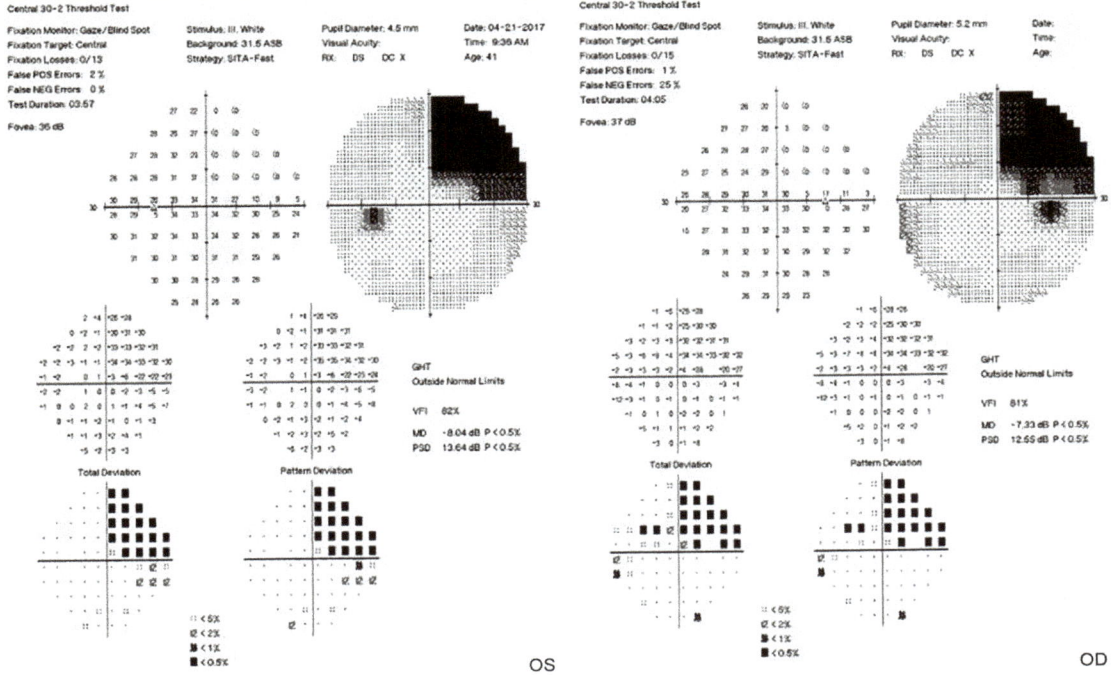

   a. Right optic tract
   b. Left optic tract
   c. Right temporal lobe
   d. Left temporal lobe

Answer Key: 1. c   2. b   3. d

4. From the perimetry, identify the site of lesion in the brain:

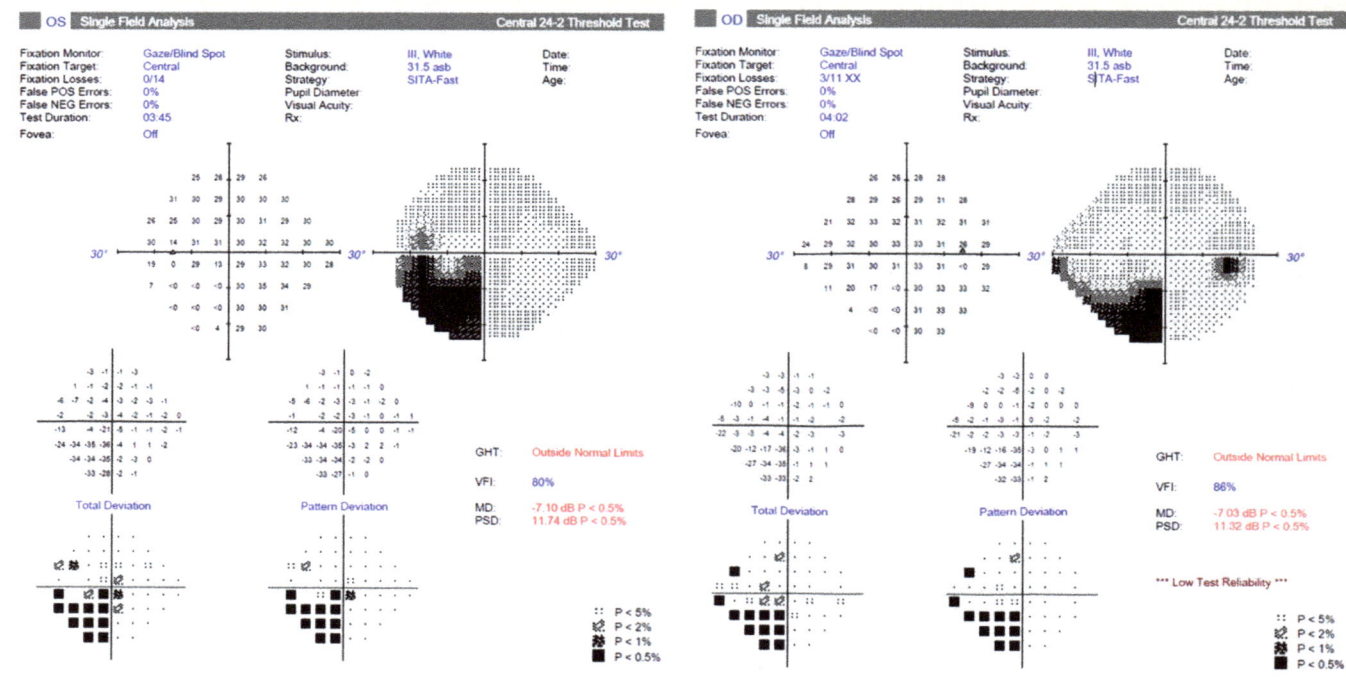

- a. Right optic tract
- b. Left optic tract
- c. Right parietal lobe
- d. Left parietal lobe

5. From the perimetry, identify the site of lesion in the brain:

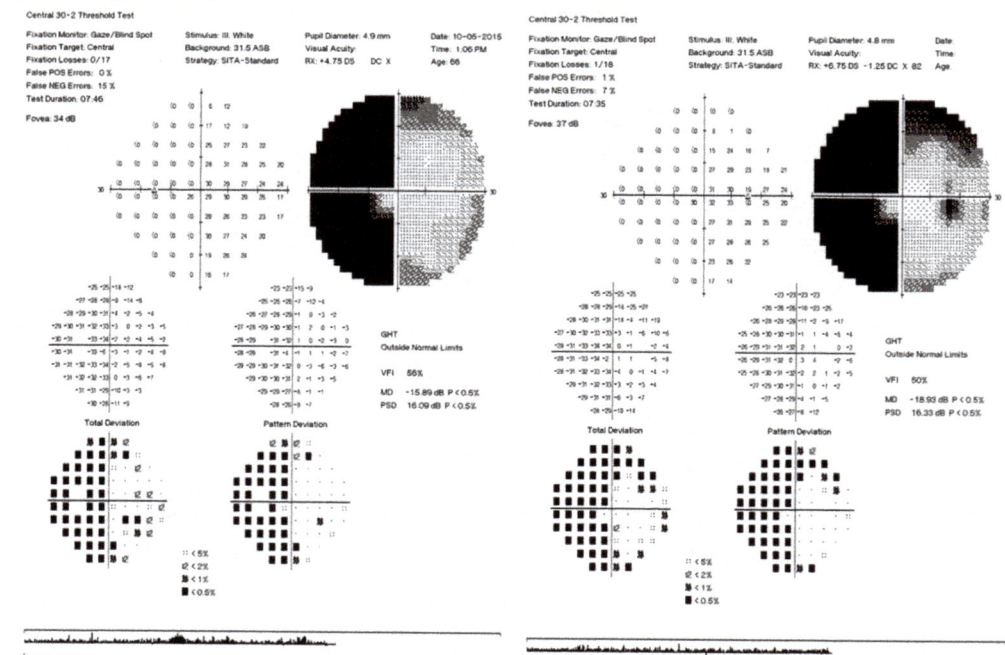

- a. Right temporal lobe
- b. Left occipital lobe
- c. Right occipital lobe
- d. Left temporal lobe

Answer Key: 4. c   5. c

Neuro-Ophthalmology

6. A patient presents with severe headache associated with vomiting. The fundus picture is similar in both eyes. From the clinical photograph, what is the possible diagnosis? *(NEET Pattern)*

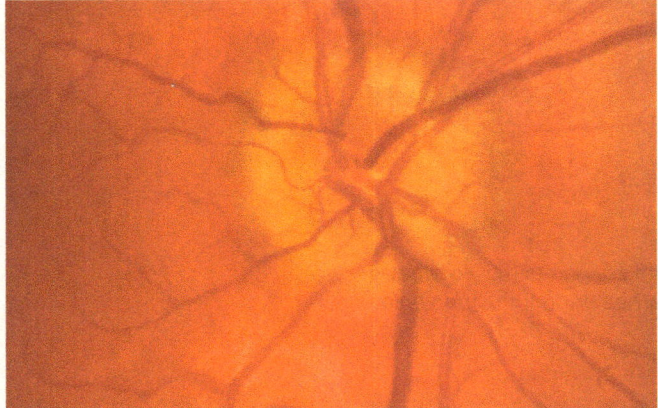

   a. Optic neuritis
   b. Optic atrophy
   c. Papilledema
   d. CRAO

7. A patient presents with sudden painless loss of vision in the right eye. He has history of diabetes and HTN. The fundus photograph is given. What is the possible diagnosis?

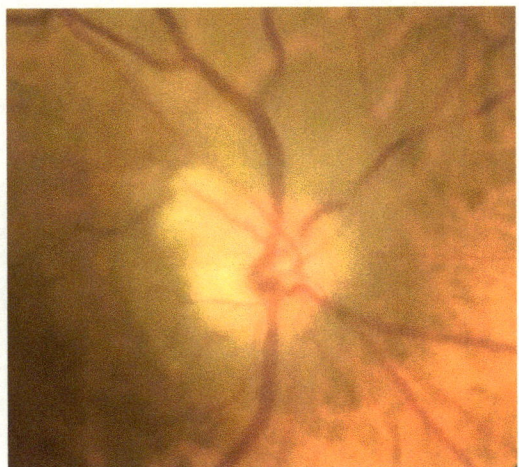

   a. Papilledema
   b. Optic neuritis
   c. Anterior ischemic optic neuropathy (AION)
   d. Hypertensive retinopathy

8. A patient presents to the OPD with complaint of sudden onset diplopia. On examination there is a face turn to the right. From the clinical photograph, identify the likely diagnosis:

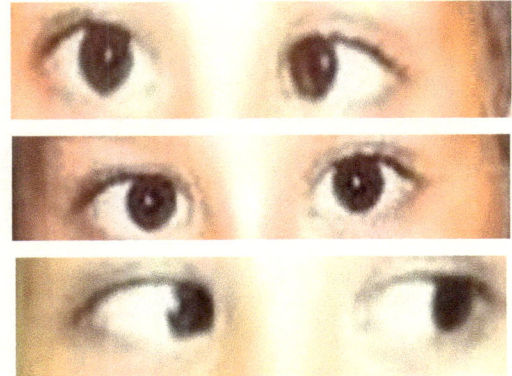

   a. Horizontal gaze palsy
   b. Internuclear ophthalmoplegia
   c. Superior oblique palsy
   d. Lateral rectus palsy

9. The picture in the question is representative of which of the following conditions: *(Nov AIIMS 2016)*

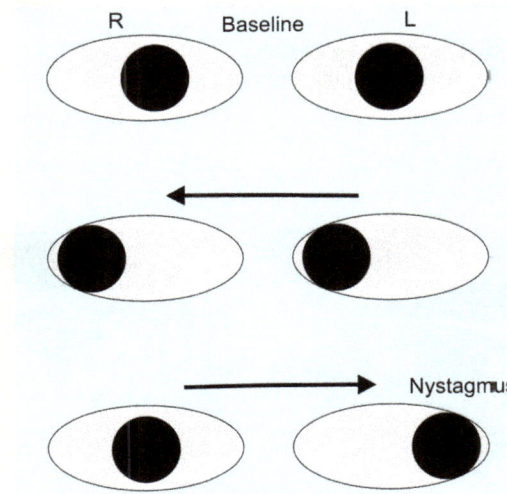

   a. Horizontal gaze palsy
   b. Internuclear ophthalmoplegia
   c. Third nerve palsy
   d. Duane's retraction syndrome

Answer Key: 6. c   7. c   8. d   9. b

Self Assessment and Review of Ophthalmology

10. From the clinical photograph given in the question, what is the diagnosis?

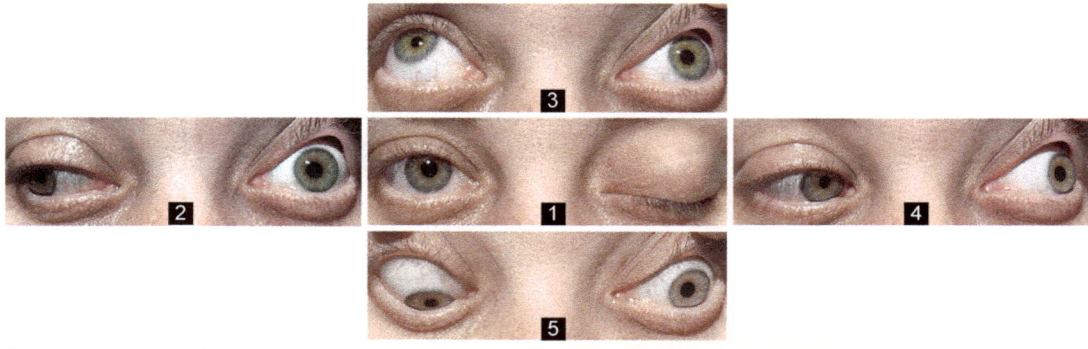

   a. Sixth cranial nerve palsy
   b. Pupil sparing third nerve palsy
   c. Pupil involving third nerve palsy
   d. Internuclear ophthalmoplegia

11. From the clinical photograph given in the question, what is the diagnosis?

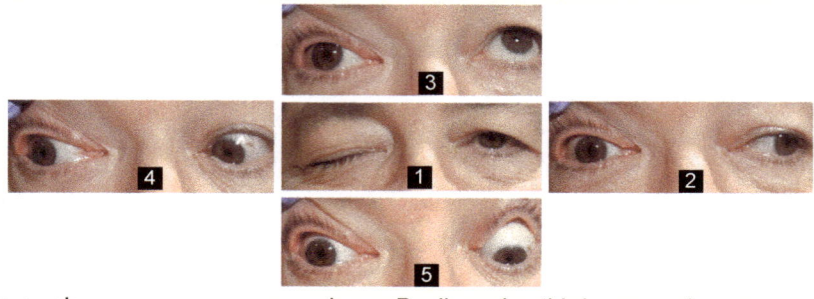

   a. Sixth cranial nerve palsy
   b. Pupil sparing third nerve palsy
   c. Pupil involving third nerve palsy
   d. Internuclear ophthalmoplegia

12. A patient presents with vertical diplopia after trauma. The clinical photograph is given. What is the most probable diagnosis?

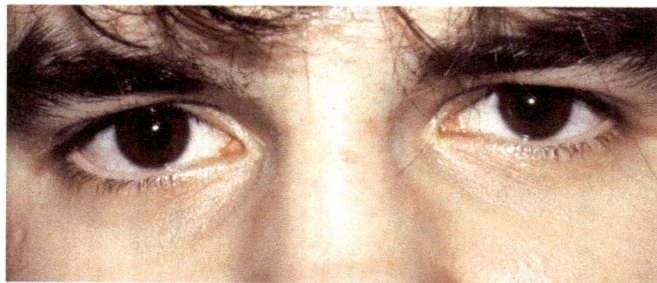

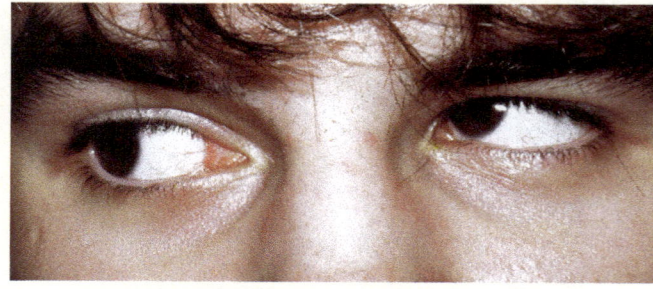

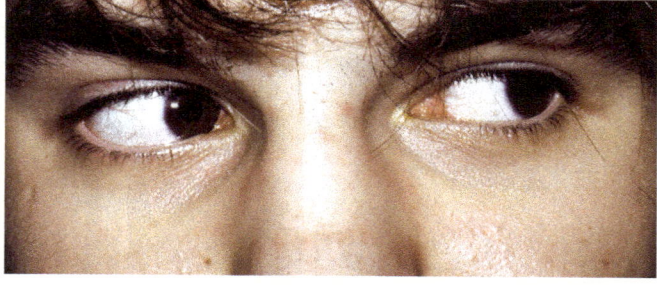

   a. Third nerve palsy
   b. Fourth nerve palsy
   c. Sixth nerve palsy
   d. Internuclear ophthalmoplegia

Answer Key: 10. c   11. b   12. b

13. The clinical photographs of patient are given. The first photograph is under ambient light and the second photograph is after instillation of topical cocaine in both eyes. What is the diagnosis?

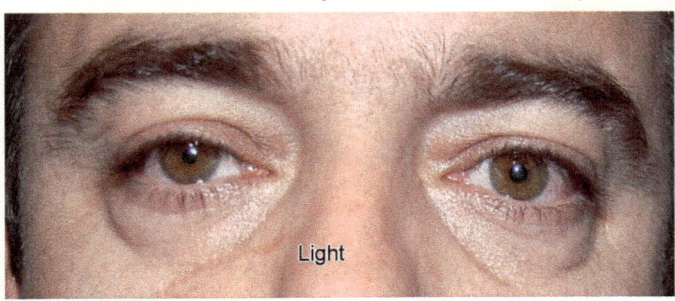
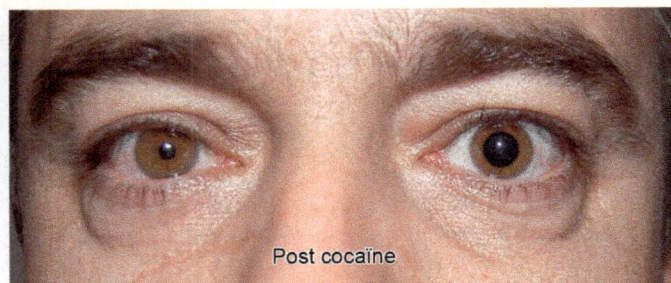

- a. Argyll Robertson pupil
- b. Hutchison's pupil
- c. Horner's syndrome
- d. Light-near dissociation

Answer Key: 13. c

ANSWERS AND EXPLANATIONS

1. **Answer: c. Morning glory syndrome**
   (Ref: Yanoff & Duker 4th edition p 871-872)
   This is an anomaly of the optic disc which is associated with disc excavation and absence of lamina cribrosa. The disc looks large with the vessels emanating from it like the spokes of a wheel.

2. **Answer: b. Pituitary adenoma**
   (Ref: Yanoff & Duker 4th edition p 904-905)
   This is a picture showing the perimetry or visual field analysis of a patient. The field defect here is **Bitemporal Hemianopia** which means that the temporal field of both eyes is affected. This is classically seen in lesions which compress the optic chiasma like pituitary **adenoma**[Q] or **craniopharyngioma**[Q]
   In **pituitary adenoma**, the field defect begins superiorly and progresses downwards, hence it is called **descending bitemporal hemianopia**[Q]
   In **craniopharyngioma**, the field defect begins inferiorly and progresses upwards, hence it is called ascending bitemporal hemianopia[Q]

3. **Answer d. Left temporal lobe**
   (Ref.: Peyman's Principles and Practices of Ophthalmology, 2nd edition, p 1622)
   The perimetry shows **right superior homonymous quadrantopia or "pie in the sky"**. Hence the site of lesion is left temporal lobe.

4. **Answer c. Right parietal lobe**
   (Ref.: Peyman's Principles and Practices of Ophthalmology, 2nd edition, pg 1623)
   The perimetry shows **left inferior homonymous quadrantopia or pie on the floor"**. Hence the site of the lesion is right parietal lobe

5. **Answer c. Right occipital lobe**
   (Ref.: Peyman's Principles and Practices of Ophthalmology, 2nd edition, p 1623)
   The perimetry shows **left homonymous hemianopia with central sparing.** Hence, the site of the lesion is right occipital lobe.

6. **Answer: c. Papilledema**
   (Ref: Kanski 6th edition p 799-801)
   The photograph shows hyperemic disc with blurred margins, suggestive of disc edema. The history is suggestive of raised intracranial pressure. Hence the answer is papilledema

7. **Answer c. Anterior ischemic optic neuropathy (AION)**
   (Ref.: Peyman's Principles and Practices of Ophthalmology, 2nd edition, p 1647)
   The photograph shows a pale disc with blurred margins suggestive of disc edema. In a patient with diabetes and HTN, vision loss with pallid disc edema is suggestive of AION.

8. **Answer: d. Lateral rectus palsy**
   (Ref: Yanoff & Duker 4th edition p 1230-1231)
   The photograph shows the ocular alignment and movements in primary position, right and left gazes. The central photograph (primary position) shows esotropia in the right eye. In right gaze, there is limitation of abduction in the right eye and the left eye is normal. In left gaze, both eyes are normal. Thus the patient has diplopia, face turn to right, esotropia with limitation of abduction in right eye. Thus the diagnosis is right lateral rectus palsy

9. **Answer: b. Internuclear ophthalmoplegia**
   (Ref: Yanoff & Duker 4th edition p 918-919)
   Internuclear ophthalmoplegia is a condition where the medial longitudinal faciculus (MLF) of the brain is affected. (See section on Gaze palsy in chapter on Neurophthalmology). The photograph shows that in primary position, both eyes are straight or orthotropic. On right gaze, the ocular movements are normal. On left gaze, the left eye abducts but the right eye does not adduct. Also the abducting left eye suffers from nystagmus.
   Thus the typical features of **Internuclear Ophthalmoplegia** can be summarized as
   - It is caused due to lesion in **Medial Longitudinal Fasciculus (MLF)**[Q]
   - On lateral gaze, **abduction is normal but adduction of the other eye is affected**[Q].
   - The **abducting eye** shows nystagmus called as **ataxic nystagmus**[Q]
   - **Convergence is normal**[Q]

   Points to Remember

   In **Horizontal gaze palsy**, there is a lesion in the **Parapontine Reticular Formation (PPRF)**. On lateral gaze, **both abduction and adduction are affected**[Q]
   In **Third nerve palsy**, adduction is affected and in primary position there is divergent squint or exotropia. Convergence is also affected
   In **Duanne's retraction syndrome (Type II)**, there is defective adduction with mild exotropia or divergent squint. Retraction of the globe on attempted adduction is also seen.

10. **Answer c. Pupil involving third nerve palsy**
    (Ref.: Peyman's Principles and Practices of Ophthalmology, 2nd edition, p 1647)
    The photograph severe ptosis of the left eye (1) with limitation of adduction (2), elevation (3) and depression (5). Abduction is normal (4). The pupil of the left eye is dilated. Hence, the diagnosis is pupil involving third nerve palsy of the left eye.

11. **Answer b. Pupil sparing third nerve palsy**
    (Ref.: Peyman's Principles and Practices of Ophthalmology, 2nd edition, p 1648)

Neuro-Ophthalmology

The photograph severe ptosis of the right eye (1) with limitation of adduction (2), elevation (3) and depression (5). Abduction is normal (4). The pupil of the right is normal. Hence, the diagnosis is pupil involving third nerve palsy of the right eye.

12. **Answer b. Fourth nerve palsy**

    (Ref.: Peyman's Principles and Practices of Ophthalmology, 2nd edition, p 1346)

    The photograph shows left hypertropia (left eye is slightly elevated as compared to right eye) which increases in right gaze and decreases in left gaze. This is suggestive of left superior oblique palsy or left fourth nerve palsy.

13. **Answer c. Horner's syndrome.**

    (Ref.: Peyman's Principles and Practices of Ophthalmology, 2nd edition, p 1650)

    The first photograph shows mild ptosis in the right eye with anisocoria, the right pupil being slightly smaller than the left. The second photograph shows dilatation of the left pupil with no change in the size of the right pupil after instillation of topical cocaine. Hence, the diagnosis is Horner's syndrome in right eye.

Adnexae and Orbit

LACRIMAL SYSTEM

Anatomy

The lacrimal system consists of the lacrimal glands and the lacrimal drainage system.

- *Main lacrimal gland*: It lies in the **superotemporal part of the orbit**^{Q}. It has two parts which lie above and below the LPS muscle. It is mainly responsible for **reflex tear secretion**^{Q}. The ducts from this gland end in the superior and inferior fornix
- *Accessory lacrimal glands*: They are the glands of **Krause and Wolfring**^{Q} which are concerned with the **basal tear secretion**^{Q}. They are located in the plica, inferior fornix and infra-orbital region
- *Lacrimal drainage system*: The components are:
  - *Puncta*: There are two puncta, upper and lower on the papilla lacrimalis in medial part of the lid
  - *Canaliculi*: From the puncta arises the canaliculus. Each canaliculus has a short **vertical portion (2 mm)** and a long **horizontal portion (8 mm)**. The upper and lower canaliculi join together to form the common canaliculus which leads to the lacrimal sac. It is guarded by the **valve of Rosenmuller**
  - *Lacrimal sac*: It lies in the lacrimal fossa between the anterior and posterior lacrimal crests in medial wall of orbit formed by lacrimal bone and frontal process of maxilla.
  - *Nasolacrimal duct (NLD)*: The NLD connects the lacrimal sac to the **inferior meatus of the nose**^{Q}. It is about 18 mm long of which the upper 12 mm is osseous and the lower 6 mm is membranous. It passes **downwards, backwards and laterally**^{Q}. Its opening at the nose is guarded by the **valve of Hasner**^{Q}.

> **Tear film**
>
> The tear film is made of three layers namely
> - *Outer lipid layer*: This is an oily layer secreted by the **meibomian glands**^{Q} of the eyelid. Its function is to **prevent evaporation**^{Q} of the aqueous layer
> - *Middle aqueous layer*: This is the main layer of the tear film produced by the main and accessory lacrimal glands
> - *Inner mucin layer*: This layer is produced by the **goblet cells**^{Q} of the conjunctiva. This layer converts the hydrophobic corneal surface to a **hydrophilic** surface so that the aqueous layer can spread over it.

Dry Eye Disease

Deficiency of the tear film is referred to as dry eye.
It may be of three types depending upon the layer of the tear film which is deficient

	Evaporative Dry eye	Aqueous layer deficiency dry eye	Mucin layer deficiency dry eye
Causes	Meibomian gland disease **Posterior blepharitis**^{Q} **Lagophthalmos**^{Q} **Proptosis**^{Q} Air-conditioned room	Sjogren's syndrome Collagen vascular diseases like Rheumatoid arthritis, SLE This is also called Keratoconjunctivitis sicca	Chemical burns Thermal burns **Steven Johnson syndrome**^{Q} Ocular cicatricial pemphigoid **Herpes zoster**^{Q} **Trachoma**^{Q}

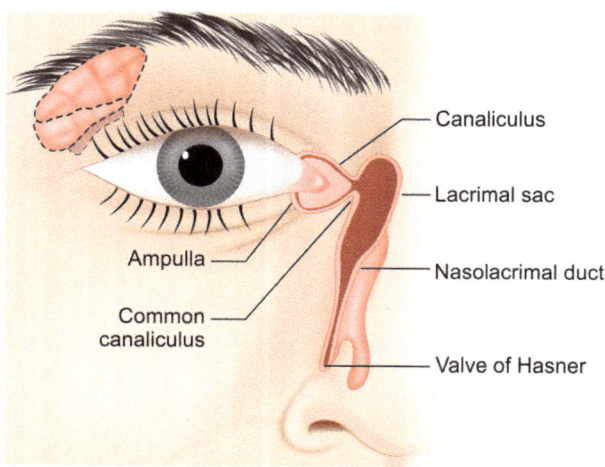

Fig. 1: Anatomy of the lacrimal system

Contd...

Contd...

	Evaporative Dry eye	Aqueous layer deficiency dry eye	Mucin layer deficiency dry eye
	Deficiency of lipid layer or excessive evaporation	Reduced secretion from lacrimal glands	Parenchymatous damage to conjunctiva resulting in decreased mucin secretion

Symptoms

Irritation, burning and foreign body sensation

Signs

- There is a decrease in the height of the marginal tear strip with strands of mucous and debris on the corneal surface
- Punctate epithelial erosions may be seen.

Tests for dry eye

- *Tear film break up time (TBUT)*: Normal value is > 10 seconds
- Schirmer's test^Q
  - Normal 10-25 mm
  - Borderline 5-10 mm
  - Impaired <5 mm
- Phenol red test
- Vital dye staining
  - *Rose Bengal*: It has an affinity for devitalized epithelial cells and mucus
  - *Fluorescein*: It stains the punctuate epithelial erosions
- Conjunctival impression cytology
- Lysozyme assay
- Tear osmolarity assay
- Conjunctival biopsy

Treatment

- Tear conservation by decreasing room temperature, use of humidifiers
- *Tear substitutes*: The common tear substitutes are **polyvinyl alcohol, carboxymethyl cellulose, hydroxypropyl methyl cellulose, and hyaluronic acid**^{Q}
- Mucolytics like acetylcysteine which disperse mucus filaments and plaque
- **Cyclosporine** eye drops for keratoconjunctivitis sicca. Systemic steroids, immunosuppressants may also be used in severe cases
- Reduction of tear drainage by **punctal occlusion.**
- **Tarsorrhaphy**^{Q} is done in cases of lagophthalmos and proptosis
- **Mucous membrane grafting and amniotic membrane grafting**^{Q} are options for parenchymatous conjunctival damage

EPIPHORA

Epiphora means watering. The causes of epiphora may be classified as:

- *Hyperlacrimation*: Conditions which increase reflex tearing like conjunctivitis, keratitis, foreign body etc
- *Inadequate drainage*: This may be due **anatomical obstruction** in the drainage pathway or **functional obstruction due to lacrimal pump failure**^{Q}

Tests for lacrimal drainage

- Syringing and probing
- Jones' dye test
- Fluorescein dye disappearance test
- Dacryocystography (DCG): **Confirmatory test for anatomical obstruction**^{Q}
- *Radionucleotide testing (Dacryoscintigraphy)*: **Confirmatory test for functional obstruction**^{Q}

Congenital Dacryocystitis

- Developmentally, NLD is solid, but becomes hollow or canalized by end of normal gestation. In some children, this process of canalization is delayed and may get completed by the first year of life
- Failure of canalisation of the lower end of NLD leads to congenital dacryocystitis. **The site of obstruction is the valve of Hasner**^{Q}.
- The child is brought with complains of watering and discharge
- Ocular examination is normal. **Regurgitation of mucoid fluid is seen on pressing over the lacrimal sac, suggestive of obstruction in the NLD**
- The treatment options are
  - *Hydrostatic massage (Criggler's massage)*^{Q}: When done properly, NLD obstruction is relieved in more than 90% infants
  - *Syringing and probing*: It is usually done if massage is ineffective after **1 year of age**^{C}
  - Balloon dacryocystoplasty^Q
  - Lacrimal intubation
  - *Dacryocystorhinostomy (DCR)*: **It is usually done after 3 years of age**^{Q}.

Acute Dacryocystitis

- This is an acute suppurative inflammation of the lacrimal sac. The cause is obstruction in the NLD leading to stasis of secretion in the sac and secondary infection
- The patient presents with sudden onset pain and swelling in the area of the sac. It may be associated with systemic features like fever
- Complications
    - Lacrimal abscess
    - Lacrimal fistula
    - **Orbital cellulitis**^{Q}
- Treatment
    - Systemic antibiotics and anti-inflammatory drugs
    - Hot compression and antibiotics are given locally
    - **DCR is done 4–6 weeks after the resolution of the acute episode**^{Q}.

Chronic Dacryocystitis

- This is a low-grade inflammation in the sac due to stasis of secretion as a result of NLD obstruction
- The patient presents with complains of watering and discharge
- **Regurgitation test is positive**^{Q}.
- **Syringing test shows mucoid regurgitation from other punctum suggestive of NLD obstruction.**
- Complications
    - Mucocele
    - Encysted mucocele
    - Pyocele
    - Acute on chronic dacryocystitis
    - Fibrosed sac
- Treatment is DCR

LACRIMAL SURGERIES

Dacryocystorhinostomy (DCR)

Anastomosis made between **lacrimal sac and middle meatus of nose**^{Q}. This bypasses the obstruction of NLD.

Indications

- Chronic dacryocystitis/ NLD block
- Atonic lacrimal sac
- Mucocele
- Lacryolith
- Congenital dacryocystitis, when other measures have failed

Contraindications

- Acute dacryocystitis
- Tuberculosis of sac
- Malignancy of sac
- Obstructive lesions in the nose like nasal polyp, deviated nasal septum, atrophic rhinitis
- Obstruction above the sac like canalicular obstruction
- Very old patients

Dacryocystectomy (DCT)

In this procedure, the lacrimal sac is removed. It is done in old patients where a prolonged surgery like DCR may be difficult.

EYELIDS

Basic Anatomy

The layers of the eyelid from outside inwards are

- Skin and subcutaneous tissue
- *Layer of striated muscle (LPS and orbicularis oculi) Fibrous tissue*: It consists of the **tarsal plate** at the center and the **orbital septum** in the periphery
- *Layer of non-striated muscle (Muller's muscle)*: It arises from the LPS and gets inserted into the tarsus. It is an **accessory lid elevator**^{Q}
- Palpebral conjunctiva

Levator palpebrae superioris (LPS)

- **It is main elevator of the eyelids**^{Q}
- It arises from the **sphenoid** at the apex of the orbit. It passes above the superior rectus along the roof of the orbit to reach the eyelids. It is then converted to a thin aponeurosis.
- LPS aponeurosis splits into two layers. **The superficial layer inserts into the skin of the lid forming the lid crease. The deep layer inserts into the tarsal plate**^{Q}.

Orbicularis oculi

- It is responsible for **lid closure**^{Q}.
- The palpebral part of the muscle arises from the frontal process of maxilla and lacrimal bone and inserts into the lateral palpebral raphe.

Adnexae and Orbit

Glands of the Eyelids

	Meibomian glands	Glands of Zeis	Glands of Moll
Type of gland	Modified sebaceous glands^Q	Modified sebaceous glands^Q	**Modified sweat glands^Q**
Location	Located in the tarsal plate but their ducts open at the lid margin	Located at the **base of the lash follicle^Q**	Located at the lid margin between two lash follicles

Inflammation of Eyelids

- *Seborrheic blepharitis*: It is a chronic inflammation of the anterior lid lamina involving the glands of Zeis and Moll associated with seborrheic dermatitis or dandruff. Treatment is lid hygiene and local antibiotic-steroid.
- *Staphylococcal anterior blepharitis*: It is a chronic inflammation of the anterior lamina of the lids involving the glands of Zeis and Moll. It is associated with scaling and crusting of the lid margin. The crusts on removal may leave small bleeding ulcers on the lid margin. **Long standing cases may lead to madarosis, poliosis, trichiasis and thickening of the lid margins^Q**. Treatment is lid hygiene and local antibiotic steroid.

Inflammation of the Lid Glands

	External Hordeolum/Stye	Internal Hordeolum	Chalazion
Definition	Acute inflammation of **Gland of Zeis^Q**	Acute inflammation of **Meibomian gland^Q**	Chronic granulomatous inflammation of Meibomian gland^Q
Clinical features	Painful lid swelling Point of maximum tenderness is at the **base of the involved lash follicle^Q**	Painful lid swelling Point of maximum tenderness is away from the lid margin	**Painless lid swelling** More common in upper lid
Treatment	Hot compress Antibiotics/ Anti-inflammatory drugs **Epilation of the involved eyelash^Q**	Hot compress Antibiotics/ Anti-inflammatory drugs	**Intralesional steroids^Q** **Incision and currettage^Q**

PTOSIS

Drooping of the eyelid is referred to as ptosis. The causes of ptosis are divided into

Neurogenic	Myogenic	Aponeurotic	Mechanical
Third nerve palsy Horner's syndrome **Marcus-Gunn jaw-winking syndrome^Q**	Simple congenital ptosis Ocular myopathies Myasthenia gravis **Blepharophimosis syndrome^Q**	Involutional Traumatic	Lid tumors

Blepharophimosis syndrome^Q
This is a congenital condition associated with **bilateral ptosis, telecanthus, epicanthus inversus and lateral ectropion^Q**.

Marcus-Gunn jaw-winking syndrome^Q
This is a condition where aberrant communication between the **third nerve and fifth nerve^Q** leads to synchronous movement of the lid with movement of the jaw.

Treatment

- *Fasanella-Servat^Q operation*: Procedure of choice for ptosis due to Horner's syndrome
- *LPS resection^Q*: This may be done through conjunctival route (**Blaskovic's operation**)^Q or cutaneous route (**Everbuch's operation**)^Q. It is done in cases of moderate ptosis with good LPS function.
- *Fascia lata sling/ Frontalis sling^Q*: Procedure of choice for severe ptosis with poor LPS function
- *Procedure of choice for Marcus Gunn jaw-winking syndrome*: **LPS excision with fascia lata sling^Q**

ENTROPION

It is the inward turning of the lid margin leading to rubbing of the eyelashes on the cornea. It is of the following types:
- *Involutional*: It is more common in the lower lid due to thinning of the tarsus, laxity of the canthal tendons, and weakness of the lower lid retractors. The surgeries for correction are
    - Transverse lid sutures
    - Modified Wheeler's operation
    - Weis' procedure
    - *Lester Jones procedure*: For severe, recurrent cases^Q
- *Cicatricial*: It is more common on the upper lid due to scarring of the palpebral conjunctiva. The causes are

trachoma, herpes, Steven Johnson syndrome, ocular cicatricial pemphigoid, chemical and thermal burns. The surgeries for correction are
- Wedge resection of tarso-conjunctiva
- **Tarsal fracture**^{Q}
- Mucous membrane grafting

➤ *Congenital*: It is seen more commonly in the lower lid. It usually resolves spontaneously in 1-2 years

➤ *Acute spastic*: It is due to spasm of the orbicularis in essential blepharospasm.

ECTROPION

It is the outward turning of the lid margin. It causes epiphora. The different types are

➤ *Involutional*: It affects the lower lid and is caused by weakness of orbicularis and laxity of the medial and lateral canthal tendons. The corrective surgeries are
- *Ziegler's cautery*: For medial ectropion
- *Medial conjunctivoplasty*: For medial ectropion
- *Lazy-T procedure*: for medial ectropion
- *Modified Kuhnt-Szymanowsky procedure*^{Q}: For severe cases involving both medial and lateral side of eyelid

➤ *Paralytic ectropion*: This is due to facial nerve palsy and may lead to exposure keratopathy. The treatment is
- Lubricant eye drops and tarsorrhaphy
- **Medial canthoplasty**

TRICHIASIS

➤ Inward turning or misdirection of eyelashes which rub on the surface of the cornea
➤ Treatment is **epilation (temporary), electrolysis or cryotherapy (permanent)**^{Q}

DISTICHIASIS

➤ Presence of a second row of eyelashes along the opening of the meibomian glands
➤ Treatment is required only if the lashes disturb the cornea. Options are the same as trichiasis.

Causes of Trichomegaly (increase in the length of eyelashes)
- *Drug induced*: **Phenytoin**^{Q}, **Topical prostaglandin analogues**^{Q}, Cyclosporine
- Malnutrition
- AIDS
- Porphyria
- Hypothyroidism
- Certain rare congenital conditions like Hermanasky-Pudlak syndrome, Cornelia de Lange syndrome, Oliver McFarlane syndrome

Causes of Madarosis (loss of eyelashes)	Causes of poliosis (whitening of eyelashes)
• Chronic anterior blepharitis^Q	• Chronic anterior blepharitis^Q
• Infiltrating lid tumors	• Sympathetic ophthalmitis
• Burns	• Vitiligo
• Radiotherapy and chemotherapy	• Vogt-Koyanagi Harada's disease^Q
• Leprosy^Q	• Waardenberg syndrome
• Myxoedema^Q	• Tuberous sclerosis
• SLE	• Albinism
• Generalised alopecia, psoriasis	• Marfan's syndrome (rarely)

Causes of lid retraction

- Thyroid eye disease^Q
- Contralateral ptosis
- Upper lid scarring
- Surgical overcorrection of ptosis
- Third nerve misdirection
- Duane's retraction syndrome
- Perinaud's syndrome (Collier's sign)
- Infantile hydrocephalus (Setting sun sign)
- Uremia

ORBIT

ANATOMY

The orbit has four walls, roof, and floor, medial and lateral. The medial walls are parallel whereas the lateral walls make an angle of 90° with each other. The base of the orbit is at the orbital margin and the apex is at the optic foramen. Volume of orbit is 30 cc.

Walls of the Orbit

	Roof	Medial wall	Floor	Lateral wall
1.	Orbital plate of frontal bone	Frontal process of Maxilla	Maxilla	Zygomatic bone
2.	**Lesser wing of sphenoid**^{Q}	Lacrimal bone	Zygomatic bone	**Greater wing of sphenoid**^{Q}
3.		Ethmoid	**Palatine bone**^{Q}	
4.		**Body of sphenoid**^{Q}		

➤ **Floor is the most frequently fractured wall of orbit in trauma**^{Q}

Adnexae and Orbit

- Medial wall is the weakest wall^Q
- Lateral wall is the strongest wall^Q

Optic Canal/Optic Foramen

- It is formed by the **lesser wing and greater wing of sphenoid**^Q.
- It lies between **the roof and medial wall of the orbit**^Q
- Vertically oval. Length 6–11 mm, Diameter 4–6 mm
- It transmits
    - Optic nerve with its coverings^Q
    - Ophthalmic artery^Q
- Best view for imaging optic canal is **Rheese**^Q view.

Superior Orbital Fissure (SOF)

- It lies between **lesser and greater wing of sphenoid**^Q
- It lies between **the roof and lateral wall of the orbit**^Q
- It is situated lateral to optic foramen at the orbital apex
- It is comma shaped, approximately 22 mm long.
- It is divided into three parts by the tendinous ring called the **Annulus of Zinn**^Q.

Structures Passing Through Superior Orbital Fissure

Above annulus of Zinn	Through annulus of zinn	Below annulus of Zinn
Lacrimal nerve^Q Frontal nerve^Q Trochlear nerve^Q Superior ophthalmic vein	Two divisions of oculomotor nerve^Q Abducens nerve^Q Nasociliary nerve^Q	Inferior ophthalmic vein

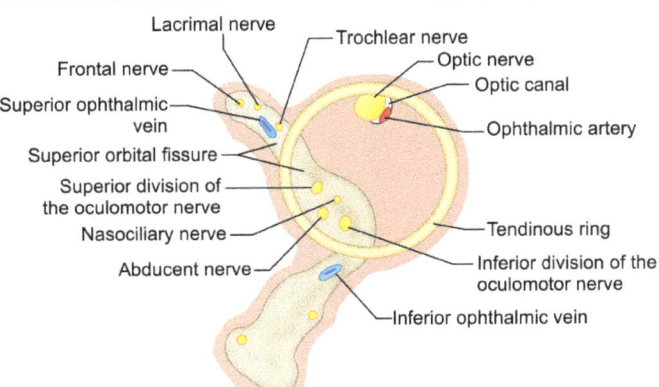

Fig. 2: Superior orbital fissure

Spaces of the orbit

- *Subperiosteal space*: between the orbital wall and the periorbita
- *Extraconal space*: Between the periorbita and the extraocular muscles
- *Intraconal space*: Enclosed on all sides by extraocular muscles

Another structure whose anatomy we must know while studying orbital diseases is the cavernous sinus.

Cavernous Sinus

- It is a venous sinus in the brain. There are two sinuses located on either side of the optic chiasma. Each sinus has valveless communication with the facial veins and so infection in the dangerous area of the face has the potential to reach the cavernous sinus
- It also communicates with the cavernous sinus of the other side, so that involvement is frequently **bilateral**^Q

Structures in the Cavernous Sinus

- Within the cavernous sinus lie
    - **Internal carotid artery and**
    - **VIth cranial nerve**^Q
- In the lateral wall of the sinus lie
    - **IIIrd cranial nerve**^Q
    - **IVth cranial nerve**^Q
    - **Ophthalmic branch of Trigeminal nerve**^Q

- Thus involvement of cavernous sinus presents with
    - Involvement of **IIIrd, IVth, VIth, Ophthalmic and Maxillary nerves**^Q
    - **Proptosis**^Q (due to engorgement of the orbital veins which communicate with the cavernous sinus)
    - Conjunctival congestion and chemosis

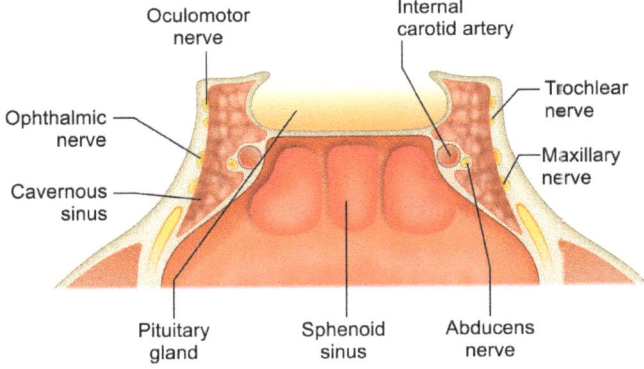

Fig. 3: Cavernous sinus

Proptosis

Protrusion of the eyeball is known as proptosis. An absolute protrusion of > 21 mm or a relative difference of >2 mm between the two eyes is known as proptosis. It may be axial or non-axial (associated with ocular deviation)

Measurement of proptosis is done by **Hertel's exophthalmometer or Luedde's exophthalmometer (in children)**^{Q.}

Causes of axial proptosis	Causes of non-axial proptosis
• *Thyroid ophthalmopathy*^Q	• Lacrimal gland tumor
• *Orbital cellulitis*^Q	• Frontal mucocele
• *Carotido- cavernous fistula*^Q	• Ethmoidal mucocele
• Cavernous sinus thrombosis	• Carcinoma maxillary sinus
• Retinoblastoma	• Encephalocele
• Optic nerve glioma	• Meningomyelocele
• Ophthalmic artery aneurysm	• Rhabdomyosarcoma
• Optic nerve meningioma	• Metastatic neuroblastoma
• Cavernous hemangioma^Q	• Chloroma
• Pseudotumor	• Orbital varix

Causes of pulsatile proptosis	Causes of bilateral proptosis
Carotido-cavernous fistula^Q	*Thyroid ophthalmopathy*^Q
Ophthalmic artery aneurysm	Carotido-cavernous fistula^Q
Encephalocoele^Q	Cavernous sinus thrombosis^Q
Meningomyelocoele^Q	Metastatic neuroblastoma^Q
	Chloroma^Q

Causes of intermittent proptosis	Causes of Pseudoproptosis
Encephalocele	High myopia
Meningomyelocele	Buphthalmos
Orbital varix	Microphthalmos, phthisis in other eye

Important to Remember

- Most common cause of unilateral proptosis in children: **Orbital cellulitis**^Q
- Most common cause of bilateral proptosis in children: **Chloroma**^Q
- Most common cause of unilateral proptosis in adults: **Thyroid ophthalmopathy**^Q
- Most common cause of bilateral proptosis in adults: **Thyroid ophthalmopathy**^Q

Thyroid Ophthalmopathy

This is also known as Ophthalmic Graves' disease (OGD). It is a bilateral condition but it starts unilaterally. The thyroid status of the patient may be **hyperthyroid, euthyroid or hypothyroid,** but it is usually hyperthyroid. Thyroid ophthalmopathy has two stages

- *Active stage*: In this stage, there is infiltration of the orbit with inflammatory cells resulting in orbital soft tissue edema and proliferation. Thus the signs in this stage are due to inflammation and edema
- *Quiescent stage*: In this stage, there is resolution of the orbital edema with secondary fibrosis.

Eyelid signs

- *Dalrymple's sign*^Q: Upper lid retraction (generally the 1st sign to appear)
- *Von Graefe's sign*^Q: Upper lid lag on down gaze
- *Kocher sign*^Q: Staring & frightened look.
- *Rosenbach sign*^Q: Tremor of closed lids.
- *Stellwag sign*^Q: Infrequent blinking
- *Mobius sign*^Q: Poor convergence

Soft Tissue Signs

- Lid edema
- Conjunctival congestion and chemosis
- **Superior limbic keratitis**^Q

Proptosis

Bilateral proptosis, axial, non-pulsatile^Q

Dysthyroid Optic Neuropathy

This is due to direct compression of the optic nerve and its blood supply by raised intraorbital pressure.

Restrictive Thyroid Myopathy

Inferior rectus is the first muscle to be involved^{Q.}

Treatment

- Lubricant eye drops
- Systemic steroids
- Systemic immunosuppressants
- Orbital radiotherapy
- Orbital decompression is done in cases not responding to medical therapy. Indications are
  - Proptosis leading to exposure keratopathy
  - Dysthyroid optic neuropathy

Orbital Cellulitis

- Orbital cellulitis is usually due to spread of infection from nasopharynx, ethmoidal, frontal and maxillary sinuses.
- The causative organisms are *Haemophilus influenzae*, Streptococcus pneumoniae, *Staphylococcus aureus, Streptococcus pyogenes*
- The patient presents with sudden onset pain and swelling of the eye associated with fever.
- **The signs are lid edema, chemosis and proptosis. Proptosis is axial and non-pulsatile. Limitation of ocular movements is seen**^Q
- Complications are subperiosteal abscess, cavernous sinus thrombosis, intracranial spread
- Treatment is systemic antibiotics

Adnexae and Orbit

Carotido-cavernous fistula

- It is an abnormal communication between **the internal carotid artery and the cavernous sinus**[Q]
- It may be **post-traumatic** or spontaneous (due to hypertension, atherosclerosis, aneurysm)
- Patient presents with **bilateral proptosis**[Q] which begins unilaterally. **Proptosis is axial, pulsatile. It is associated with thrill and bruit which may be abolished by pressing on the ipsilateral carotid**[Q]
- It is associated with **congestion and chemosis**[Q] due to dilatation of orbital veins
- It may also lead to **third, fourth and sixth cranial nerve palsy**[Q], usually starting with the sixth nerve
- Treatment is surgical

Cavernous sinus thrombosis

- **Cavernous sinus thrombosis develops due to uncontrolled infection in the dangerous area of the face like orbital cellulitis, dacryocystitis**[Q]
- Patient presents with high fever and headache.
- There is **bilateral proptosis**[Q] which begins unilaterally. **Proptosis is axial and non-pulsatile**[Q].
- Engorgement of orbital veins leads to **conjunctival congestion and chemosis**
- There may also be associated **palsy of third, fourth and sixth cranial nerves**[Q] starting with the sixth nerve
- Treatment is high dose intravenous antibiotics

Blow-out fracture of the orbit

- This is a **fracture of the orbital floor**[Q] without involving the rim of the orbit
- It is associated with blunt trauma like fist injury and cricket ball injury
- The features are
  - Peri-orbital ecchymosis
  - Crepitus on palpation (subcutaneous emphysema)
  - Anesthesia in the area of the cheek due to injury to the infraorbital nerve

Blow-out fracture of the orbit

  - **Enophthalmos**[Q]
  - **Diplopia due to entrapment of the inferior rectus. Diplopia is present both in upgaze and downgaze and it is called double gaze diplopia**[Q]
- Treatment is orbital floor reconstruction

Destructive Ocular Surgeries

There are three main types of destructive ocular surgeries

- *Enucleation*: It is the removal of the eyeball with a part of the optic nerve. So at the end of the procedure a stump of the optic nerve is left behind. Indications are
  - **Intraocular malignancies like retinoblastoma (absolute indication)**[Q]
  - Severely traumatized eye (to prevent sympathetic ophthalmia in the other eye)
  - Microphthalmos, Phthisis bulbi
  - Painful blind eye

Absolute contraindication: **Panophthalmitis**[Q]

- *Evisceration*: In this procedure, a corneal button is removed. The intraocular contents are removed by an evisceration spoon. A frill of sclera attached with the optic nerve is left at the end of the procedure. Indications are
  - **Panophthalmitis (absolute indication)**[Q]
  - Microphthalmos, phthisis bulbi
  - Painful blind eye

Absolute contraindication: **Intraocular malignancies**[Q]

- *Exanteration*: This procedure is rarely done now. It involves removal of the globe, orbital soft tissues, periosteum of the orbital wall, part or whole of the lids. Indications are
  - Orbital malignancies
  - Mucormycosis

QUESTIONS

Inflammation of Lid Glands

1. An elderly female presented with recurrent swelling of the upper eyelid. Histopathological evaluation revealed it to be a chalazion. What would be the histopathological finding? *(AIIMS 2013)*
   a. Lipogranuloma
   b. Suppurative granuloma
   c. Foreign body granuloma
   d. Xanthogranuloma

2. Lipogranulomatous inflammation is seen in: *(AIIMS 2014)*
   a. Fungal infection
   b. Tuberculosis
   c. Chalazion
   d. Viral infection

3. Which of the following are true regarding chalazion? *(PGI)*
   a. Mucous cyst
   b. Sebaceous cyst
   c. It is due to staphylococcal infection
   d. Recurrence may imply malignancy
   e. Occlusion of the meibomian gland

4. Treatment of chalazion: *(PGI)*
   a. Incision and drainage
   b. Intralesional steroid
   c. Curettage
   d. Pressure bandage
   e. Antibiotics

5. A recurrent chalazion should be subjected to histopathological examination to rule out the possibility of: *(AIIMS 2006)*
   a. Squamous cell Ca
   b. Sebaceous cell Ca
   c. Malignant melanoma
   d. Basal cell Ca

Anomalies of Lid Position

6. Which elevator muscle of the eyelid is involuntary? *(NEET 2016)*
   a. Levator palpebrae superioris
   b. Frontalis
   c. Muller's muscle
   d. Orbicularis oculi

7. Fasanella Servat operation is indicated in: *(AIPG 2003)*
   a. Congenital ptosis
   b. Traumatic ptosis
   c. Myasthenia gravis
   d. Horner's syndrome

8. A patient with ptosis presents with retraction of the ptotic eyelid on chewing. This is called: *(AIPG 2010)*
   a. Marcus Gunn jaw winking syndrome
   b. Third nerve misdirection syndrome
   c. Abducens palsy
   d. Oculomotor palsy

9. Bilateral ptosis is not seen in: *(AIPG 2001)*
   a. Marfan's syndrome
   b. Myasthenia gravis
   c. Myotonic dystrophy
   d. Kearne Sayre syndrome

10. The operation of plication of inferior lid retractors is indicated in: *(AIPG 2003)*
    a. Senile ectropion
    b. Senile entropion
    c. Cicatricial entropion
    d. Paralytic ectropion

11. Fibrous attachment of the lid to the eyeball is called : *(WBPG 2008)*
    a. Symblepharon
    b. Entropion
    c. Ectropion
    d. Anklyoblepharon

12. Most common malignant tumour of the eyelids: *(AIIMS 2009)*
    a. Sebaceous cell Ca
    b. Basal cell Ca
    c. Squamous cell Ca
    d. Malignant melanoma

13. Telecanthus means: *(AIIMS)*
    a. Widened interpupillary distance
    b. Widened root of nose with normal interpupillary distance
    c. Widely separated medial orbital wall
    d. Widely separated canthi

14. Distichiasis means: *(DNB 2016)*
    a. Increased number of eyelashes in the lower lid
    b. Second row of eyelashes
    c. Increased thickness of eyelashes
    d. Increased pigmentation of eyelashes

Anatomy of the Orbit

15. Medial wall of the orbit is formed by all except : *(NEET 2016)*
    a. Ethmoid bone
    b. Sphenoid bone
    c. Frontal bone
    d. Lacrimal bone

16. Site of entry of inferior division of Oculomotor nerve into the orbit is: *(CET 2017)*
    a. Inferior orbital fissure
    b. Superior orbital fissure
    c. Foramen lacerum
    d. Foramen rotundum

17. Structures passing through superior orbital fissure are: *(PGI)*
    a. IInd cranial nerve
    b. IIIrd cranial nerve
    c. IVth cranial nerve
    d. VIth cranial nerve
    e. Lacrimal nerve

Proptosis

18. Purulent inflammation of the tissues of the orbit is called: *(Kerala PG 2015)*
    a. Orbital cellulitis
    b. Endophthalmitis
    c. Panophthalmitis
    d. Dacryocystitis

19. Which of the following conditions causes pseudoproptosis? *(CET 2017)*
    a. Hyperthyroidism
    b. Orbital pseudotumour
    c. High myopia
    d. Optic nerve glioma

Adnexae and Orbit

20. Most common cause of unilateral proptosis in adults: (NEET 2016)
    a. Thyroid ophthalmopathy b. Rhabdomyosarcoma
    c. Orbital cellulitis
    d. Orbital blow out fracture

21. Most common cause of unilateral proptosis: (AIIMS/ DNB 2013)
    a. Thyrotoxicosis b. Retinoblastoma
    c. Intraocular haemorrhage d. Raised IOP

22. Commonest cause of bilateral proptosis in children: (AIPG 2011)
    a. Cavernous haemangioma b. Chloroma
    c. Fibrous histiocytoma d. Rhabdomyosarcoma

23. Most common cause of bilateral proptosis in children: (AIIMS 2013)
    a. Rhabdomyosarcoma b. Lymphoma
    c. Retinoblastoma d. Neuroblastoma

24. Kamla, aged 45 years presents with unilateral mild axial proptosis. There is no redness or pain. Investigation of choice is: (AIIMS 2000)
    a. T3 and T4 to rule out thyrotoxicosis
    b. CT scan to rule out meningioma
    c. Doppler to rule out haemangioma
    d. USG to rule out orbital pseudotumour

25. Features of thyroid ophthalmopathy are: (PGI)
    a. External ophthalmoplegia
    b. Internal ophthalmoplegia
    c. Proptosis
    d. Enlargement of extraocular muscle
    e. Lid lag

26. Darlymple sign is seen in: (DNB 2015)
    a. Thyroid ophthalmopathy
    b. Cavernous sinus thrombosis
    c. Orbital cellulitis
    d. Cavernous haemangioma

27. First muscle to be involved in thyroid ophthalmopathy: (AIPG)
    a. Medial rectus b. Inferior rectus
    c. Lateral rectus d. Superior rectus

28. Thyroid ophthalmopathy: All of the following are treatment modalities except: (DNB 2015)
    a. Radiation b. Steroids
    c. B-Blockers d. Orbital decompression

29. Infection from the dangerous area of the face spreads to the cavernous sinus via which of the following veins? (COMEDK 2015)
    a. Maxillary veins b. Retromandibular veins
    c. Superficial temporal vein d. Ophthalmic veins

30. Paralysis of IIIrd, IVth and VIth cranial nerves with involvement of ophthalmic division of the Vth cranial nerve localises the lesion to: (AIPG 2010)
    a. Cavernous sinus b. Apex of the orbit
    c. Brainstem d. Base of the skull

31. A 19-year-old young girl with previous history of repeated pain over medial canthus and chronic use of nasal decongestants presented with abrupt onset of fever and chills and rigor, diplopia on lateral gaze, moderate proptosis and chemosis. On examination, optic disc is congested. Most likely diagnosis is: (AIIMS 2009)
    a. Cavernous sinus thrombosis
    b. Orbital cellulitis
    c. Acute ethmoidal sinusitis
    d. Orbital apex syndrome

32. All of the following could result from infection with right cavernous sinus except: (AIIMS 2003)
    a. Constricted pupil in response to light
    b. Engorgement of retinal veins seen on ophthalmological examination
    c. Ptosis of right eyelid
    d. Right ophthalmoplegia

33. A retrobulbar intraconal mass with well defined capsule presenting with slowly progressive proptosis in the 2nd to 4th decade. Most likely diagnosis: (AIIMS)
    a. Capillary haemangioma
    b. Cavernous haemangioma
    c. Lymphangioma
    d. Haemangiopericytoma

34. A patient presents with unilateral proptosis which is compressible and increases on bending forward. No thrill or bruit is present. MRI shows retrobulbar mass with enhancement. The likely diagnosis is: (AIIMS 2010)
    a. AV malformation b. Orbital varix
    c. Orbital encephalocele d. Neurofibromatosis

35. An 8-year-old boy presents with proptosis in the left eye for 3 months. CT scan reveals intraorbital extraconal mass lesion. Biopsy shows embryonal rhabdomyosarcoma. Metastatic workup is normal. The standard line of management is: (AIIMS 2010)
    a. Chemotherapy
    b. Wide local excision
    c. Chemotherapy and radiotherapy
    d. Enucleation

36. In which side is the globe displaced in lacrimal gland tumour? (NEET 2016)
    a. Superior b. Inferonasal
    c. Inferotemporal d. Nasal

37. Most common type of optic nerve glioma is: (AIIMS)
    a. Gemiocytic b. Fibrous
    c. Protoplasmic d. Pilocytic

38. Optic nerve glioma is associated with: (DNB 2015)
    a. Neurofibromatosis I b. Neurofibromatosis II
    c. Von Hippel Lindau disease d. Sturge Weber syndrome

39. All of the following types of lymphoma may be seen in the orbit except: (AIIMS 2003)
    a. Non-Hodgkin's lymphoma, mixed lymphocytic and histiocytic
    b. Non-Hodgkin's lymphoma, poorly differentiated
    c. Burkitt's lymphoma
    d. Hodgkin's lymphoma

Orbital Fracture

40. Blow out fracture of the orbit involves:
(CET JUNE 2017)
a. Superior wall
b. Postero-medial part of the orbital floor
c. Medial wall
d. Lateral wall

41. Blow out fracture of the orbit involves: *(DNB 2013)*
a. Floor
b. Medial wall
c. Roof
d. Lateral wall

42. True about blow out fracture of the orbit is/are: *(PGI)*
a. Herniates into maxillary antrum
b. Extraocular movements are restricted
c. Looking down is easy
d. Diplopia is present
e. Orbital floor reconstruction is the treatment

43. Most common cause of fracture of roof of orbit is:
(AIIMS 2009)
a. Blow on back of head
b. Blow on the forehead
c. Blow on the parietal bone
d. Blow on upper jaw

Tear Film/Dry Eye/Epiphora

44. Mucin layer deficiency of tear film is seen in:
(AIIMS 2006)
a. Keratoconjunctivitis sicca
b. Lacrimal gland removal
c. Canalicular block
d. Herpes zoster

45. Epiphora means: *(AIPG 2002)*
a. Cerebrospinal fluid running from nose after fracture of anterior cranial fossa
b. A presenting feature of a cerebral tumour
c. An abnormal flow of tears due to obstruction of the lacrimal duct
d. Eversion of lower eyelid following injury

46. A two month old child presents with epiphora and regurgitation: The likely diagnosis is: *(DNB)*
a. Mucopurulent conjunctivitis
b. Congenital dacryocystitis
c. Buphthalmos
d. Encysted mucocele

47. Most common site of obstruction in congenital NLD obstruction: *(PGI 2013)*
a. Upper canaliculus
b. Lower canaliculus
c. Common canaliculus
d. Valve of Hasner
e. Middle turbinate

48. Initial treatment of congenital dacryocystitis is:
(PGI 2005)
a. Massage
b. Probing
c. DCR
d. Antibiotics
e. No treatment is needed

49. Treatment of chronic dacryocystitis is: *(DNB 2014)*
a. Dacryocystorhinostomy
b. Antibiotics
c. Probing
d. Massage

50. A 60-year-old man presents with watering from his right eye since 1 year. Syringing revealed a patent drainage system. Rest of the ocular examination was normal. Provisional diagnosis of lacrimal pump failure was made. Confirmation of diagnosis is done by: *(AIIMS 2002)*
a. Dacryoscintigraphy
b. Dacryocystography
c. Pressure syringing
d. Canaliculus irrigation test

51. Phenol red test for dry eye: True statement is:
(May AIIMS 2016)
a. It requires topical anesthesia
b. It measures the volume of tears as it changes colour on contact with tears
c. If colour changes to blue, it depicts mucin deficiency
d. It requires a pH meter

52. Parasitosis of extraocular muscles is seen in:
(DNB 2015)
a. Trichinosis
b. Amoebiasis
c. Cysticercosis
d. Ascariasis

Adnexae and Orbit

ANSWERS AND EXPLANATIONS

1. **a. Lipogranuloma** *(Ref: Yanoff & Duker 4th edition, p 1304)*
2. **c. Chalazion** *(Ref: Yanoff & Duker 4th edition, p 1304)*
3. **b. Sebaceous cyst, d. Recurrence may imply malignancy, e. Occlusion of the meibomian gland**
   (Ref: Yanoff & Duker 4th edition, p 1304)
4. **b. Intralesional steroid, c. Curettage** *(Ref: Yanoff & Duker 4th edition, p 1304)*
5. **b. Sebaceous cell Ca** *(Ref: Yanoff & Duker 4th edition, p 1304)*
6. **c. Muller's muscle** *(Ref: Yanoff & Duker 4th edition, p 1274)*
7. **d. Horner's syndrome** *(Ref: Yanoff & Duker 4th edition, p 1274)*
8. **a. Marcus Gunn jaw winking syndrome** *(Ref: Yanoff & Duker 4th edition, p 1273)*
9. **a. Marfan's syndrome** *(Ref: Yanoff & Duker 4th edition, p 1272-1274)*

Causes of bilateral ptosis
• Senile/Involutional/ Aponeurotic
• Congenital
• Blepharophimosis syndrome
• Myasthenia gravis[Q]
• Chronic progressive external ophthalmoplegia[Q]
• Ocular myopathies
• Myotonic dystrophy

10. **b. Senile entropion** *(Ref: Yanoff & Duker 4th edition, p 1280)*
11. **a. Symblepharon**
12. **b. Basal cell Ca** *(Ref: Kanski 6th edition, p 109)*
    Most common lid malignancy in recurrent chalazion: Sebaceous cell Ca[Q]
13. **b. Widened root of the nose with normal interpupillary distance**
14. **b. Second row of eyelashes** *(Ref: Kanski 6th edition, p 121)*
15. **c. Frontal bone** *(Ref: Yanoff & Duker 4th edition, p 1260-1261)*
16. **b. Superior orbital fissure** *(Ref: Yanoff & Duker 4th edition, p 1260-1261)*
17. **b. IIIrd cranial nerve, c. IVth cranial nerve, d. VIth cranial nerve, e. Lacrimal nerve**
    (Ref: Yanoff & Duker 4th edition, p 1260-1261)
18. **a. Orbital cellulitis** *(Ref: Yanoff & Duker 4th edition, p 1328)*
19. **c. High myopia**
    Large size of the globe in high myopia gives an impression of proptosis when there is no actual protrusion of the globe, hence called pseudoproptosis.
20. **a. Thyroid ophthalmopathy** *(Ref: Yanoff & Duker 4th edition, p 1327)*
21. **a. Thyrotoxicosis** *(Ref: Yanoff & Duker 4th edition, p 1327)*
22. **b. Chloroma** *(Ref: Update on orbital tumours: American Academy of Ophthalmology;2014)*
23. **d. Neuroblastoma** *(Ref: Update on orbital tumours: American Academy of Ophthalmology; 2014)*
    Since chloroma is not present among the options, we have chosen neuroblastoma as the answer:
24. **a. T3 and T4 to rule out thyrotoxicosis** *(Ref: Yanoff & Duker 4th edition, p 1327)*
    The most common cause of proptosis in adult is thyroid ophthalmopathy, hence investigation should rule out thyroid disease as the first step
25. **c. Proptosis, d. Enlargement of the extraocular muscles, e. Lid lag** *(Ref: Kanski 6th edition, p 170-175)*
    Thyroid orbitopathy leads to intraorbital infiltration of inflammatory cells and orbital soft tissue edema. This leads to enlargement of the extraocular muscles. When this edema resolves, there is secondary fibrosis leading to restriction of ocular movements. This is called restrictive ophthalmopathy not ophthalmoplegia

26.	a.	Thyroid ophthalmopathy	*(Ref: Kanski 6th edition, p170-175)*
27.	b.	Inferior rectus	*(Ref: Kanski 6th edition, p170-175)*
28.	c.	B-Blockers	*(Ref: Kanski 6th edition, p170-175)*
29.	d.	Ophthalmic veins	*(Ref: Yanoff & Duker 4th edition, p 901)*
30.	a.	Cavernous sinus	*(Ref: Yanoff & Duker 4th edition, p 984)*

Involvement of the cavernous sinus presents with
- Proptosis
- Chemosis
- Paralysis of third, fourth and sixth cranial nerves starting with the sixth nerve

31. a. **Cavernous sinus Thrombosis** *(Ref: Yanoff &Duker 4th edition, p 983-984)*

The question describes a patient with sinusitis who develops sudden onset fever, chills associated with proptosis. This may be due to orbital cellulitis or cavernous sinus thrombosis. The question however mentions diplopia in lateral gaze suggestive of involvement of the sixth nerve; hence the more probable answer is cavernous sinus thrombosis.

32. a. **Constricted pupil in response to light** *(Ref: Yanoff &Duker 4th edition, p 983-984)*

Involvement of the cavernous sinus leads to third nerve palsy. Thus the patient will have dilatation and not constriction of the pupil

33. b. **Cavernous haemangioma** *(Ref: Kanski 6th edition, p 192)*

The most common benign orbital tumour in adult is Cavernous haemangioma^Q. It is an intraconal mass presenting with gradually progressive axial proptosis

Most common benign orbital tumour in children: Dermoid^Q

Most common orbital malignancy in adult: Lymphoma^Q

Most common orbital malignancy in children: Rhabdomyosarcoma^Q

34. b. **Orbital varix** *(Ref: Kanski 6th edition, p 181-182)*

Orbital varix is a cause of non-axial proptosis, usually intermittent. The proptosis becomes evident on coughing, straining and bending forward. Orbital encephalocele also has similar features but it is pulsatile and does not show enhancement with contrast. Hence the answer

AV malformation or Carotido-cavernous fistula gives rise to pulsatile, axial proptosis associated with thrill and bruit

35. c. **Chemotherapy and radiotherapy** *(Ref: Kanski 6th edition, p200-201, Yanoff & Duker 4th edition, p 1321-1322)*

Rhabdomyosarcoma is the most common orbital malignancy in children^Q. It presents with non-axial proptosis which is sudden in onset and very rapidly progressive. Hence it is also called **malignant proptosis.**

Most common variety of Rhabdomyosarcoma: Embryonal^Q

Least common variety: Pleomorphic^Q

Best prognosis: Pleomorphic^Q

Worst prognosis: Alveolar^Q

Treatment is chemotherapy with radiotherapy.

Causes of malignant proptosis:
- Rhabdomyosarcoma^Q
- Orbital cellulitis^Q
- Chocolate cyst^Q

36. b. **Inferonasal**

As the lacrimal gland is located in the superotemporal quadrant of the orbit, the displacement of the globe in lacrimal gland enlargement is inferonasal

37. d. **Pilocytic** *(Ref: Kanski 6th edition, p 195-196)*

Features of optic nerve glioma
- It is seen in young girls less than 10 years of age
- It is associated with Neurofibromatosis I^Q
- Commonest histological variety is Pilocytic astrocytoma^Q
- It presents with gradual onset, slowly progressive proptosis which is axial, non-pulsatile
- It is associated with vision loss

38.	a.	Neurofibromatosis I	*(Ref: Kanski 6th edition, p 195-196)*
39.	d.	Hodgkin's lymphoma	*(Ref: Yanoff & Duker 4th edition, p 1325)*
40.	b.	Postero-medial part of the orbital floor	*(Ref: Kanski 6th edition, p 848-849)*
41.	a.	Floor	*(Ref: Kanski 6th edition, p 848-849)*

Adnexae and Orbit

42. a. **Herniates into the maxillary antrum, b. Extraocular movements are restricted, d. Diplopia is present e. Orbital floor reconstruction is the treatment** *(Ref: Kanski 6th edition, p 848-849)*
43. b. **Blow on the forehead** *(Ref: Kanski 6th edition, p 851)*
44. d. **Herpes zoster**
45. c. **An abnormal flow of tears due to obstruction of the lacrimal duct** *(Ref: Yanoff & Duker 4th edition, p 1346)*
46. b. **Congenital dacryocystitis** *(Ref: Yanoff & Duker 4th edition, p 1348)*
47. d. **Valve of Hasner** *(Ref: Yanoff & Duker 4th edition, p 1348)*
48. a. **Massage** *(Ref: Yanoff & Duker 4th edition, p 1349)*
49. a. **Dacryocystorhinostomy** *(Ref: Yanoff & Duker 4th edition, p 1350)*
50. a. **Dacryoscintigraphy** *(Ref: Kanski 6th edition, p 156)*

    Lacrimal pump failure means inability of the lid muscles to push the tears towards the punctum for drainage. It is also called functional obstruction and is confirmed by Dacryoscintigraphy

51. b. **It measures the volume of tear as it changes colour on contact with tears** *(Ref: Yanoff & Duker 4th edition, p 277)*

    It is an obsolete test

52. c. **Cysticercosis**

IMAGE BASED QUESTIONS

1. From the clinical photograph, decide the most appropriate line of management for the patient

   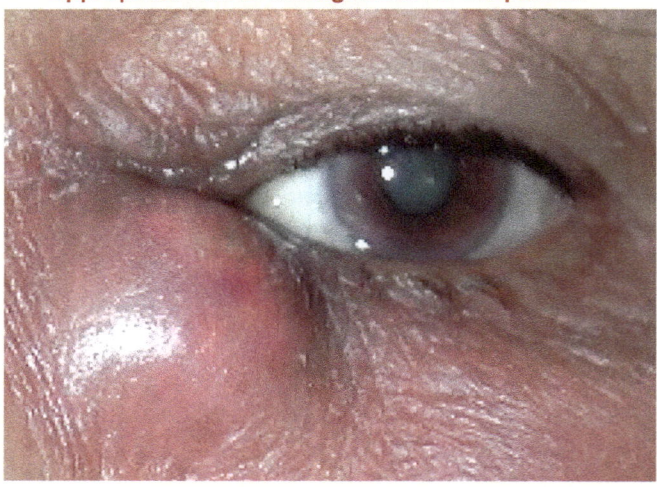

   a. Syringing and probing
   b. Immediate DCR
   c. Antibiotics followed by DCR after 4-6 weeks
   d. Antibiotics only

2. What is the use of the instrument given in the picture?

   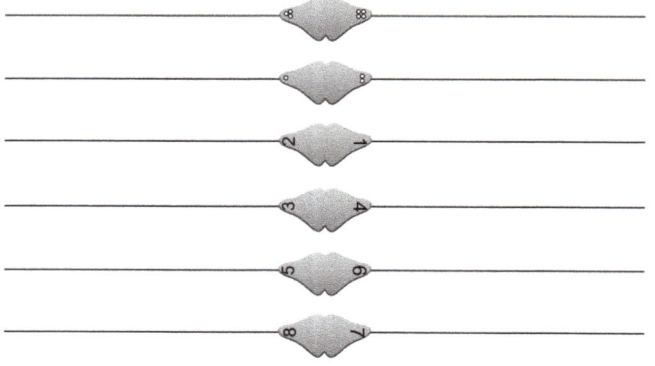

   a. Syringing
   b. Dilatation of the punctum
   c. Probing of the lacrimal drainage pathway
   d. None of the above

3. Name the instrument shown in the picture.

   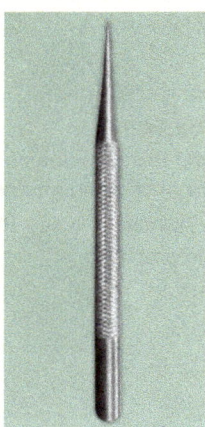

   a. Bowman's probe
   b. Nettleship's punctum dilator
   c. Syringing cannula
   d. Simcoe's cannula

4. A certain procedure is shown in the picture. What is the clinical condition for which this procedure is advised?

   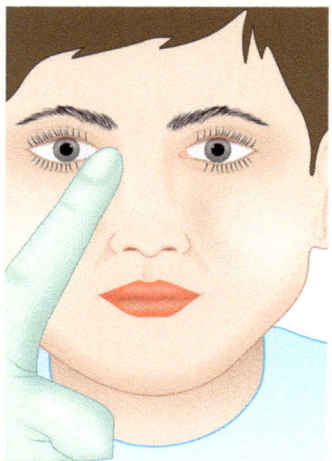

   a. Congenital dacryocystitis
   b. Acute dacryocystitis
   c. Acute dacryoadenitis
   d. Chronic dacryocystitis

Answer Key: 1. c   2. c   3. b   4 a

Adnexae and Orbit

5. A certain test is shown in the picture. What is it used for the evaluation of?

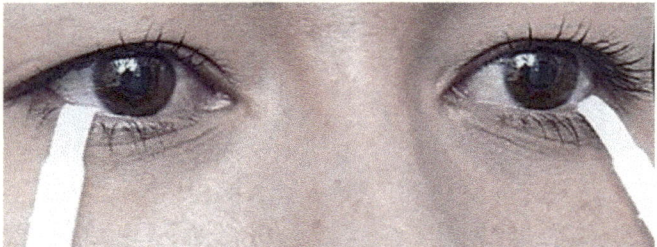

   a. Epiphora
   b. Dry eye
   c. Lacrimal pump failure
   d. Canaliculitis

6. A patient following severe reaction to a systemic drug presents with severe dry eye. The clinical photograph is given. Under which category of dry eye would you classify it?

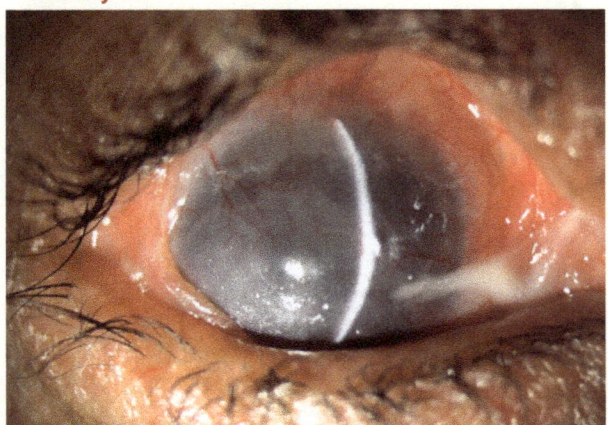

   a. Evaporative dry eye
   b. Aqueous layer deficiency dry eye
   c. Keratoconjunctivitis sicca
   d. Mucin layer deficiency dry eye

7. An elderly patient complains of continuous watering. The clinical photograph is given below. What is the diagnosis? *(NEET Pattern 2017)*

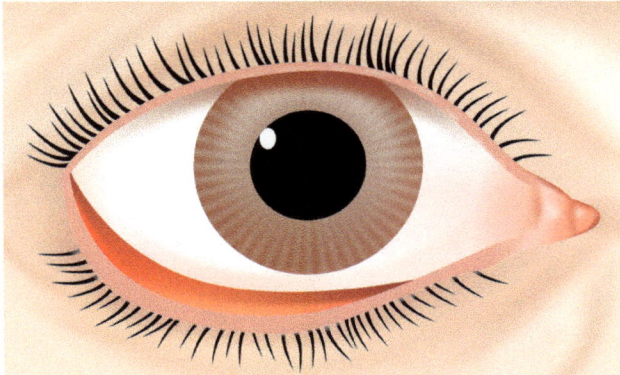

   a. Trichiasis
   b. Entropion
   c. Ectropion
   d. Distichiasis

8. A patient complains of irritation and foreign body sensation in the eye. The clinical photograph is given. Which of the following surgeries is most suitable for the patient?

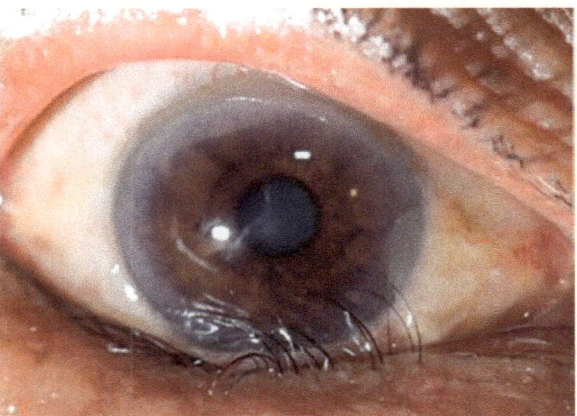

   a. Fasanella Servat
   b. Levator resection
   c. Fascia lata sling
   d. Jones' procedure

9. A 6-year-old child presents for evaluation to the OPD. The clinical photograph is given. Which is the surgery of choice for the patient?

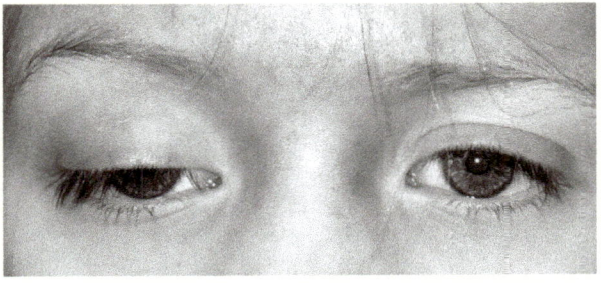

   a. Jones' procedure
   b. Tarsal fracture
   c. Levator resection
   d. Medial canthoplasty

10. From the picture what is the diagnosis?

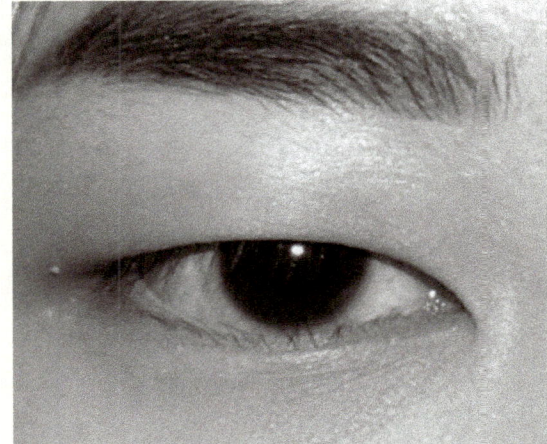

   a. Epicanthus inversus
   b. Epicanthus tarsalis
   c. Epicanthus palpebralis
   d. None of the above

Answer Key: 5. b   6. d   7. c   8. d   9. c   10. b

11. A patient with previous history of head trauma presents with complaint of redness in the right eye. The clinical picture is given. On examination a pulsation with thrill is felt on palpation of right eye which is abolished on pressing the ipsilateral carotid. What is the diagnosis?

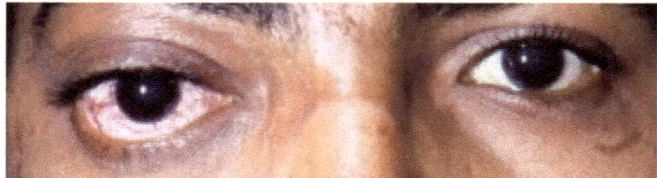

   a. Cavernous sinus thrombosis
   b. Carotido-cavernous fistula
   c. Blow out fracture of orbit
   d. Blow in fracture of the orbit

12. A patient with history of fist injury to the eye is brought for evaluation. From the X-ray, what is the diagnosis?

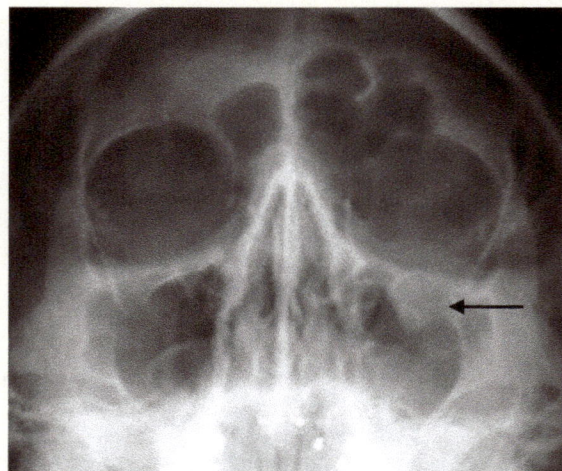

   a. Fracture of lateral orbital wall
   b. Blow out fracture of orbit
   c. Blow in fracture of the orbit
   d. Fracture of medial orbital wall

Answer Key: 11. b 12. b

ANSWERS AND EXPLANATIONS

1. **Answer c. Antibiotics followed by DCR after 4-6 weeks**
   (Ref: Yanoff & Duker 4th edition p 1349-1350)
   The clinical photograph shows Acute dacryocystitis, which is caused by acute purulent inflammation of the lacrimal sac secondary to obstruction of the nasolacrimal duct. The treatment is systemic antibiotics to aid in the resolution of acute stage followed by DCR after 4-6 weeks to bypass the obstruction of the nasolacrimal duct. Syringing and DCR are contraindicated in the acute stage.

2. **Answe c: Probing of the lacrimal drainage pathaway**
   The instrument shown in the picture is Bowman's lacrimal probe. They are available in different sizes and used for probing the lacrimal passage.

3. **Answer b. Nettleship's punctum dilator**
   This is used for dilating the puncta prior to probing of the lacrimal passage

4. **Answer a: Congenital dacryocystitis**
   (Ref.: Peyman's Principles and Practice of Ophthalmology. 2nd edition p 1794-95)
   The procedure shown in the picture is Crigglers's sac massage and it is the first line of management for congenital dacyocystitis

5. **Answer b: Dry eye**
   The test shown in the picture is Schirmer's test which is used for the evaluation of dry eye.

   > **Schirmer's I test**
   > - It is performed with Whatman's filter paper no 41
   > - The strips are about 35 mm in length. Each strip is folded at 5 mm and the folded strip is inserted into the lower fornix at the junction of medial two-third and lateral one-third of the eye.
   > - The patient is instructed to keep the eyes open and made to wait for 5 minutes in normal room temperature.
   > - The amount of wetting of the strip is noted at the end of 5 min. This denotes the total tear secretion, basal and reflex.
   > - Normal > 10 mm
   >   – Borderline 5-10 mm
   >   – Dry eye < 5 mm
   > - If the test is performed after instillation of local anesthetic drop, it denotes only the basal secretion. It is then called Schirmer's II test.

6. **Answer d: Mucin layer deficiency dry eye**
   (Ref:Peyman's Principles and Practice of Ophthalmology 2nd edition p 460-61)
   Severe drug reaction to a systemic drug may be indicative of Steven Johnson syndrome which is a cause of mucin layer deficiency dry eye.
   The picture shows conjunctival inflammation with corneal haze and vascularisation and loss of lustre of the ocular surface suggesting the same.

7. **Answer c: Ectropion**
   (Ref.: Peyman's Principles and Practice of Ophthalmology 2nd edition p 1807-1810)
   The picture shows outward turning of the lid margin, hence the answer is ectropion.

8. **Answer d: Jones' procedure**
   (Ref.: Peyman's Principles and Practice of Ophthalmology. 2nd edition p 1807-1810)
   The picture shows inward turning of the lower lid margin with rubbing of the lashes on the cornea. So the clinical condition is entropion of the lower lid. The appropriate surgery for the same is Jones' procedure.
   The remaining options are names of ptosis surgeries.

9. **Answer c: Levator resection**
   (Ref.: Peyman's Principles and Practice of Ophthalmology 2nd edition p 1807-1810)
   The picture shows moderate ptosis on the right side with absent lid crease and overaction of frontalis muscle. So it is a case of congenital ptosis. Hence the answer is levator resection.

10. **Answer b: Epicanthus tarsalis**
    (Ref.: Peyman's Principles and Practice of Ophthalmology 2nd edition p 1808-1809)
    Epicanthal folds are congenital anomalies where eyelid skin folds cover the medial canthus. They are of the following types.
    - *Epicanthus tarsalis:* Fold of skin extending from upper eyelid across the medial canthus
    - *Epicanthus inversus:* Fold of skin extending from lower eyelid across the medial canthus

    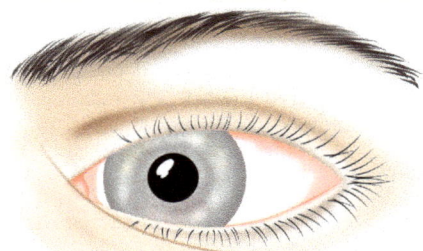

    - *Epicanthus palpebralis:* Fold of skin extending across medial canthus to both eyelids.

11. **Answer b: Carotido-cavernous fistula**
    The picture shows proptosis with dilated episcleral vessesls on the right side. This, along with the other features given in the question is typical of carotido-cavernous fistula.

12. **Answer b: Blow-out fracture of the orbit**
    The picture shows the classical **"tear drop sign"** caused by herniation of the inferior orbital fat into the maxillary sinus through the fractured orbital floor. (indicated by arrow)

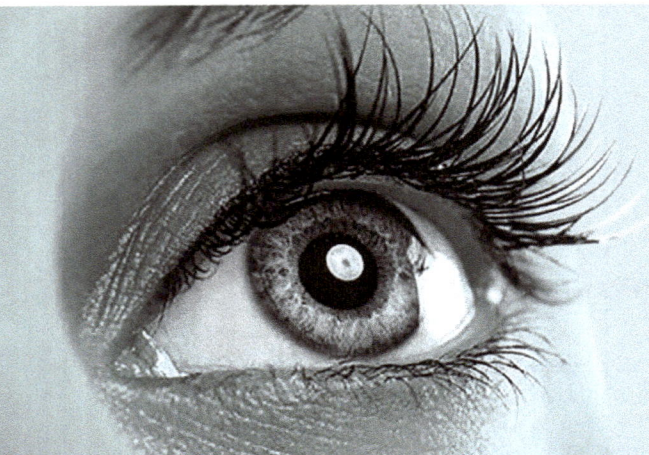

12
Assessment of Visual Function

Assessment of visual function involves the following aspects
- Visual acuity
- Color vision
- Contrast sensitivity
- Field of vision

VISUAL ACUITY

Visual acuity is a measure of form sense and it is the spatial discrimination capacity of the visual system. It is of two main types:
- *Minimum visible:* The ability to determine whether an object is present or not
- *Minimum resolvable:* The minimum distance between two points which can be discriminated by the visual system as two is the minimum resolvable visual acuity. This is the function of the fovea centralis and is commonly termed as visual acuity. It is defined as the reciprocal of the minimum resolvable visual angle expressed in minutes of arc

Visual angle: It is the angle subtended by the physical dimensions of an object at the nodal point of the eye. Two points can be discriminated as separate only if they subtend a visual angle of **1 min**^{Q} or more.

Tests for Visual Acuity

- *Snellen's chart:* This is used for testing distance visual acuity and consists of lines of black capital letters on a white blackboard. The letters in each line become progressively smaller in size:
    - The chart is to be read from a distance of 6 meters or 20 feet
    - From top to bottom for each line read by the patient, the visual acuity is expressed as 6/60 (20/200), 6/36 (20/120), 6/24(20/80), 6/18(20/60), 6/12 (20/40), 6/9(20/30) and 6/6(20/20)

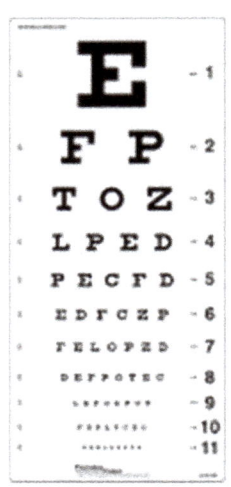

- **When viewed from a distance of 6 m, each letter on the 6/6 line subtends a visual angle of 5 min at the nodal point and each part of the letter subtends an angle of 1 min at the nodal point**^{Q}. Thus normal visual acuity when tested from 6 m distance should be 6/6
- **When viewed from a distance of 60 m, the letter on 6/60 line subtends a visual angle of 5 min at the nodal point and each part of the letter subtends an angle of 1 min at the nodal point.**
- **When viewed from a distance of 6 m, the letter on the 6/60 line subtends an angle of 50 min at the nodal point and each part of the letter subtends an angle of 10 min**
- *Snellen's E chart/Landolt's C chart*: The principle is the same as Snellen's chart but it is used for illiterates
- *ETDRS chart*
    - Testing is done from a distance of 4 metres
    - The main advantage with respect to Snellen's chart is that there are equal number of letters in each line and equal spacing between the letters
    - Visual acuity is expressed in logMAR units.

Assessment of Visual Function

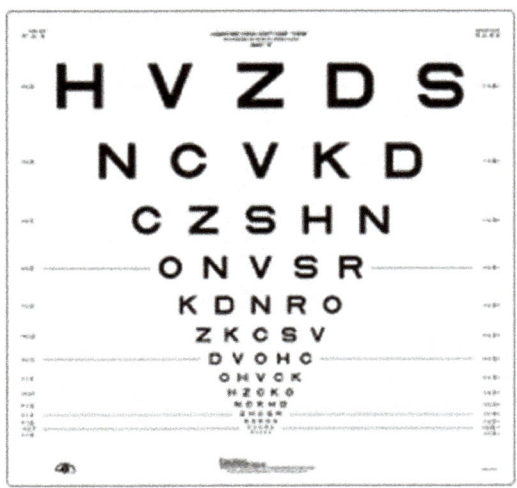

COLOR VISION

Color vision is the ability of the eye to discriminate between colors excited by light of different wavelengths. It is a function of the **cones**[Q] and hence best appreciated under **photopic conditions**[Q].

Transmission of Color Vision Signal

The pathway for transmission is as follows:
- *Photoreceptors:* The centre of the fovea is blue blind. Trichromatic color vision, i.e appreciation of all three primary colors: red, green and blue extends between **20–30 degrees of fixation**[Q]. Beyond 30 degrees red and green cannot be distinguished. In the extreme periphery all color sense is lost.
- Bipolar and horizontal cells
- *Ganglion and amacrine cells:* The **X type of ganglion cells**[Q] are involved in this transmission
- *Lateral geniculate body:* **The parvocellular part of the LGB**[Q] is involved in this function
- Layer IVc of the striate cortex (Area 17)
- Blobs in the layers II and III
- Specialized color detection area located in the **lingual and fusiform gyri of the occipital lobe**[Q].

Color Blindness

Color vision defects may be of two types: Congenital and Acquired.

Congenital Color Vision Defect
- *Achromatopsia:* In this condition there is no color perception due to absence of cones. It is a very rare condition.
- *Monochromacy:* In this condition, only one of the three primary colors, red, blue or green can be appreciated.
- *Dichromacy:* In this condition two primary colors are appreciated. The subtypes are
  - *Protanopia*[Q]: Red color is not perceived
  - *Deuteranopia*[Q]: Green color is not perceived
  - *Tritanopia*[Q]: Blue color cannot be perceived
- *Trichromacy:* In this condition all the three primary colors are appreciated but one of them is defective. So it is a color deficiency rather that color blindness.
  - *Protanomaly*[Q]: Red color perception is defective.
  - *Deuteranomaly*[Q]: Green color perception is defective.
  - *Tritanomaly*[Q]: Blue color perception is defective

Gene	Location	Defect	Inheritance
OPN1LW	X chromosome	Protan (red)	X-linked recessive
OPN1MW	X chromosome	Deuteran (green)	X-linked recessive
OPN1SW	Chromosome 7	Tritan (blue)	Autosomal dominant

Congenital color defects mainly have a sex-linked inheritance and are **more commonly seen in males**[Q].

Acquired Color Vision Defect

This type of defect may be unilateral or bilateral depending on whether the pathology leading to the color deficiency is unilateral or bilateral. The types are:
- *Red green deficiency:* This is seen in **optic nerve diseases**[Q] like optic neuritis, compressive, toxic, traumatic or congenital optic neuropathies
- *Blue deficiency:* This is usually seen in **retinal diseases**[Q] like macular edema, central serous retinopathy and retinal vascular disorders. It is also seen in **glaucoma**[Q].

Tests for Color Vision

- *Ishihara's pseudo-isochromatic chart:* There are **38 plates**[Q] which should be read at 75 cm under good illumination.
  - *Demonstration plate:* It is the testing plate used to identify **malingerers** since it can be seen by all patients even if they are color blind
  - *Transformation plates:* A particular number is seen on the plate by a color normal person whereas a different number is seen by a color deficient person
  - *Vanishing plates:* A number is seen by a color normal person but not seen by a color deficient person

- *Hidden plates:* A number is seen by a color blind person but not a color normal person
- *Diagnostic plates:* These plates are used to differentiate protan and deuteron defect. **The main drawback of this test is that it cannot detect tritan or blue color defect**
- Hardy-Rand-Rittler test
- City University test
- Holmgren's wool test
- Farnsworth-Munsell 100 hue test
- Farnsworth-Munsell D-15/Lanthony D-15/Adams D-15
- Naegel's anomaloscope
- *Occupational tests[Q]:* These tests are used to assess medical fitness in professionals like drivers, pilots, etc where color vision is of special importance. The common tests are Edridge Green lantern test, Farnsworth lantern test and Holmes-Wright lantern test.

CONTRAST SENSITIVITY

It is the ability to perceive slight change in luminance between regions which are not demarcated by sharp borders. The different tests used are
- **Pelli-Robson contrast sensitivity chart[Q]**
  - The chart consists of letters which subtend an angle of 3 degrees from a distance of 1 m
  - The chart is read from a **distance of 1 m[Q]** with full distance correction
  - Each line of the chart contains two triplets of letters and the contrast decreases from one triplet to the next. If two of the three letters in a triplet are identified then that is taken as the contrast sensitivity for the patient.
  - It is expressed in log units

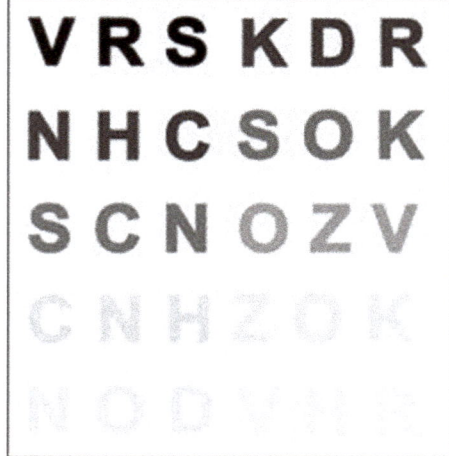

- Arden's gratings
- Cambridge low contrast gratings.

Assessment of Visual Function

QUESTIONS

1. What is the angle subtended by the largest letter on the Snellen's chart in the eye of a person who is viewing it from a distance of 6m? *(AIIMS 2016)*
   a. 50 min
   b. 10 min
   c. 5 min
   d. 1 min

2. Color vision is checked by which one of the following? *(Kerala PG 2015)*
   a. Snellen's chart
   b. Goldman's three mirror lens
   c. Slit lamp
   d. Ishihara's isochromatic charts

3. Holmgren's wool matching is used for assessment of: *(Bihar PG 2014)*
   a. Visual field
   b. Visual acuity
   c. Color vision
   d. Refraction

ANSWERS AND EXPLANATIONS

1. a. **50 min** *(Ref: Kanski 6th edition p 15-16)*
   The largest letter on the Snellen's chart is the 6/60 letter.
   When viewed from a distance of 60 m, it subtends an angle of 5 min at the nodal point of the eye
   When viewed from a distance of 6 m, it subtends an angle of 50 min at the nodal point of the eye

2. d. **Ishihara's isochromatic chart** *(Ref: Kanski 6th edition p 20-21)*

3. c. **Color vision** *(Ref: Kanski 6th edition p 20-21)*

13 Ocular Manifestations of Systemic Diseases

NEUROFIBROMATOSIS

Neurofibromatosis I	Neurofibromatosis II
Plexiform neurofibromas on the eyelids (S-shaped eyelid) **Enlarged corneal nerves**[Q] Congenital glaucoma Congenital ectropion uveae **Lisch nodules**[Q] Choroidal naevus Retinal astrocytoma **Optic nerve glioma**[Q] Spheno-orbital encephalocoele	Posterior subcapsular cataract Hamartomas of retinal pigment epithelium and retina

OTHER PHAKOMATOSES

Sturge Weber syndrome	Tuberous sclerosis	Von-Hippel–Lindau syndrome
Episcleral haemangioma Iris heterochromia[Q] Ipsilateral glaucoma	Atypical iris coloboma Iris hypopigmentation Retinal astrocytoma	Retinal haemangiomas Optic nerve haemangioma

Myasthenia Gravis

➢ Bilateral ptosis
➢ Extraocular muscle weakness leading to diplopia
➢ Nystagmoid movements

Myotonic Dystrophy

➢ Bilateral ptosis
➢ Pupillary light near dissociation
➢ **Presenile cataract (Christmas tree cataract)**[Q]
➢ Pigmentary retinopathy
➢ Low pressure

Multiple Sclerosis

➢ **Retrobulbar neuritis**[Q]
➢ **Internuclear ophthalmoplegia**[Q]
➢ Nystagmus
➢ Extraocular muscle palsies
➢ **Intermediate uveitis**[Q]

Marfan Syndrome

- High myopia
- Megalocornea
- Keratoconus[Q]
- Cornea plana
- Angle anomaly and glaucoma
- Ectopia lentis[Q]
- Microspherophakia[Q]
- Retinal detachment

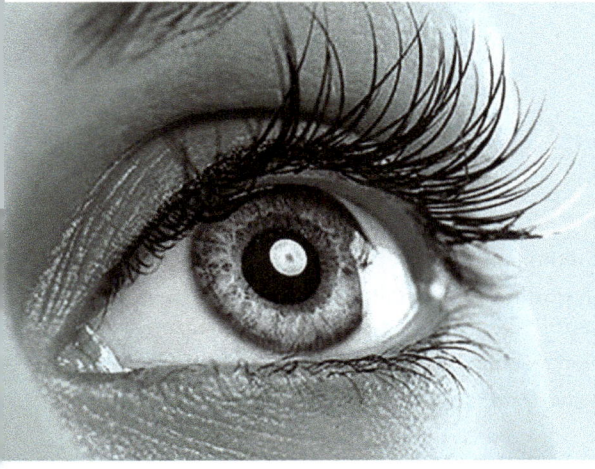

14
Miscellaneous

BLINDNESS

The definition of blindness is given according to Best Corrected Visual Acuity (BCVA) in the better eye.
Thus according to **WHO, definition of blindness** is:
- **BCVA in the better eye less than 3/60 which means inability to count fingers under good illumination at 3 meters**[Q]
- **Visual field, less than 10 degrees in the better eye**[Q].

According to **National Program for Control of Blindness (NPCB), the definition of blindness** was
- **BCVA in the better eye, less than 6/60 (Snellen's chart)**[Q]
- **Visual field, less than 20 degrees in the better eye**[Q].

In 2018, the nomenclature NPCB has been changed to **National Program for Control of Blindness and Visual Impairment** and the definition of blindness has also been modified. Thus the definition of blindness given by the national scheme now is the same as given by WHO:
- BCVA in the better eye, less than 3/60 which means inability to count fingers under good illumination at 3 meters[Q]
- Visual field less than 10 degrees in the better eye[Q].

BCVA in the better eye less than 6/18 is known as visual impairment or low vision
Most common cause of blindness in India: Cataract[Q]
Most common cause of low vision or ocular morbidity in India: Refractive errors[Q].

VISION 2020

Vision 2020: Right to Sight is a global initiative by the WHO to eliminate avoidable blindness.
It was launched at Geneva in 1999. The important global partners are:
- International Agency for the Prevention of Blindness
- Christoffel-Blinden mission
- Hellen Keller International
- Sight Savers International
- ORBIS International
- Rotary International
  - International Organization against Trachoma
  - International Association of Lions' Club
  - International Council of Ophthalmology
  - World Council of Optometry
- The diseases targeted globally under Vision 2020 are:
  - **Cataract**[Q]
  - **Refractive errors**[Q]
  - **Onchocerciasis**[Q]
  - **Childhood blindness**[Q]
  - **Trachoma**[Q]
- The Indian Chapter of Vision 2020 was launched at Goa in 2001. The diseases targeted under Vision 2020 India are
  - Cataract
  - Refractive errors
  - Childhood blindness
  - Trachoma
  - **Glaucoma**[Q]
  - **Diabetic retinopathy**[Q]

CAUSES OF LOSS OF VISION

Causes of sudden painful loss of vision
• Trauma
• Acute keratitis
• Acute angle closure glaucoma
• Acute iridocyclitis

Causes of sudden painless loss of vision
• Vitreous hemorrhage
• Central retinal artery obstruction (CRAO)
• Branch retinal artery obstruction (BRAO)
• Central retinal vein obstruction (CRVO)
• Branch retinal vein obstruction (BRVO)
• Retinal detachment
• Central serous retinopathy
• Optic neuritis (pain usually only on ocular movements)
• Cortical blindness

Causes of gradual painless loss of vision
• Refractive errors
• Pterygium
• Keratoconus
• Corneal dystrophies/ degenerations
• Open angle glaucoma
• Cataract
• Diabetic retinopathy
• Retinal dystrophies like Retinitis Pigmentosa, Stargardt's disease, etc
• Age-related macular degeneration (ARMD)
• Compressive lesions in the brain

Miscellaneous

QUESTIONS

1. Which of the following is not included under global Vision 2020 program? *(AIIMS)*
   a. Cataract
   b. Refractive error
   c. Trachoma
   d. Glaucoma

2. The visual acuity used as cut off for school screening program is: *(AIIMS)*
   a. 6/12
   b. 6/9
   c. 6/6
   d. 6/18

3. Most common cause of ocular morbidity in India: *(AIPG)*
   a. Cataract
   b. Refractive error
   c. Trachoma
   d. Vitamin A deficiency

4. WHO criteria for blindness means visual acuity less than: *(AIIMS)*
   a. 6/18
   b. 6/60
   c. 3/60
   d. 1/60

ANSWERS AND EXPLANATIONS

1. d. Glaucoma
2. b. 6/9
   Children with visual acuity less than 6/9 are referred for further evaluation. The initial screening is done by the school teachers and then referred to the Para Medical Ophthalmic Assistants (PMOA) at the upgraded PHC.
3. b. Refractive error
4. c. 3/60

IMAGE BASED QUESTIONS

1. Which visual function may be assessed from the test whose picture is given?

   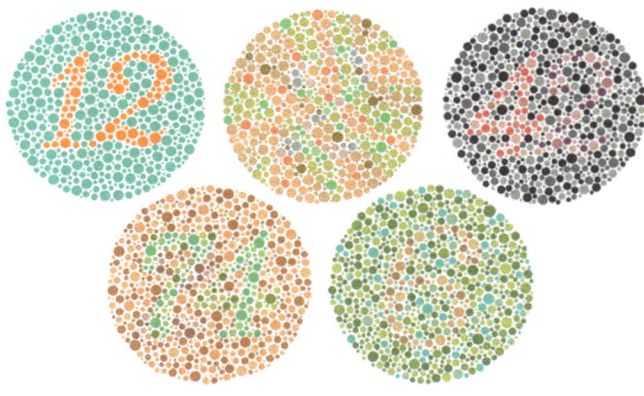

   a. Visual acuity
   b. Contrast sensitivity
   c. Colour vision
   d. Visual field

2. This is the anterior segment photograph of a 6 year old boy presenting with decreased vision in both eyes, intolerance to bright light since early childhood. The child has diffuse hypopigmentation of skin and hair all throughout the body. One other sibling has the same history. Which of the following features about the condition is false?

   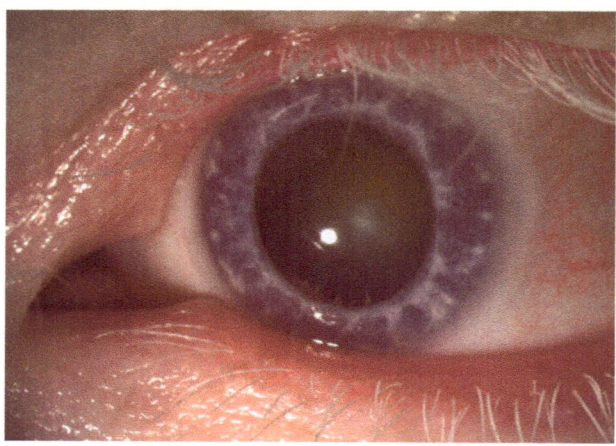

   a. Translucent iris
   b. Foveal hypoplasia
   c. Good stereopsis
   d. Nystagmus

3. This is the anterior segment photograph of a 12-year-old boy who presented with history of tennis ball injury to the right eye. What does the arrow in the photograph indicate?

   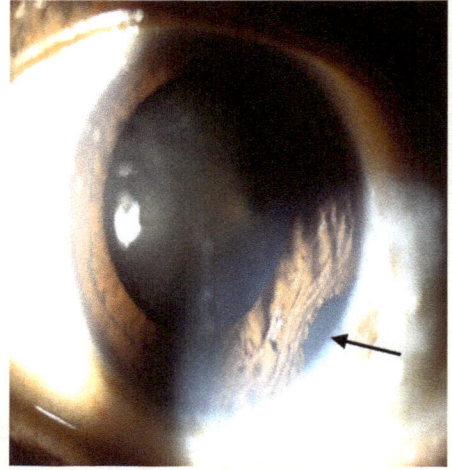

   a. Iris hole
   b. Iridodialysis
   c. Sphincter tear
   d. Multiple pupil

4. From the photograph, what is the diagnosis?

   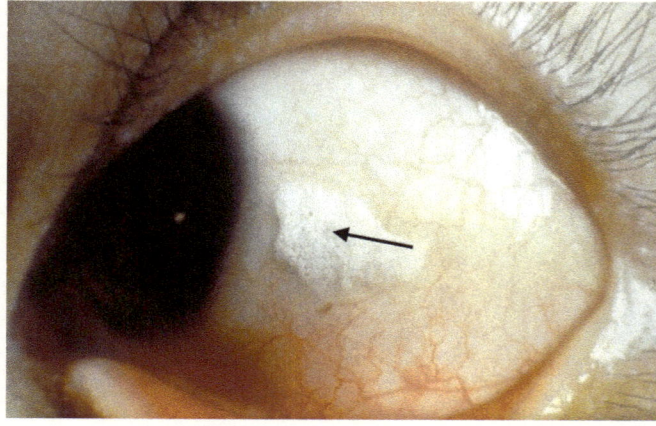

   a. Pinguecula
   b. Pterygium
   c. Bitot's spot
   d. Phlycten

Answer Key: 1. c   2. c   3. b   4. c

Miscellaneous

5. From the photograph, what is the diagnosis?

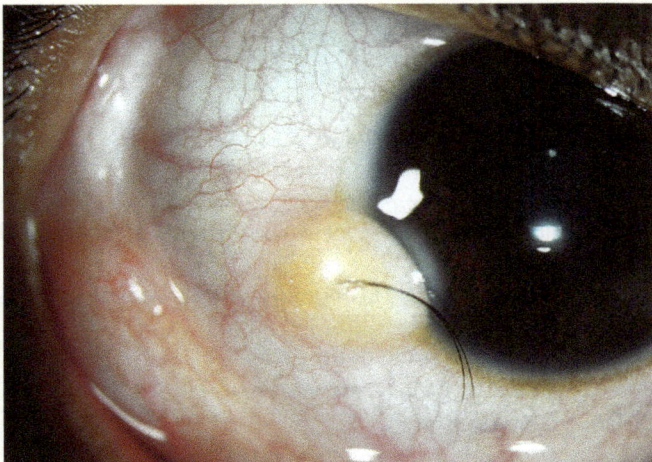

   a. Pinguecula
   b. Limbal dermoid
   c. Phlycten
   d. Pterygium

6. The anterior segment photograph of a patient is given. Which of the following is likely to be an association?

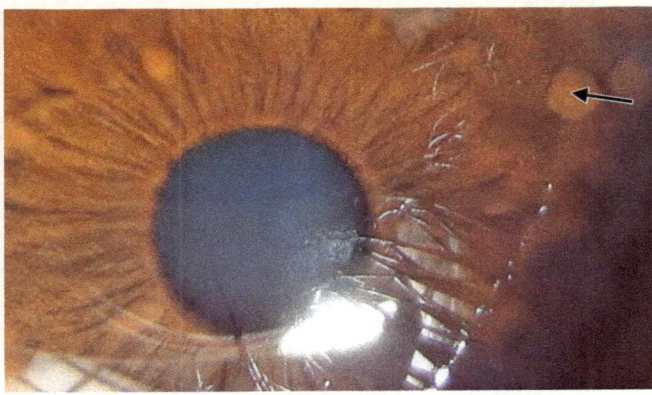

   a. Sturge Weber syndrome
   b. Neurofibromatosis I
   c. Myotonic dystrophy
   d. Marfan syndrome

7. What is the commonest cause of the condition shown in the photograph?

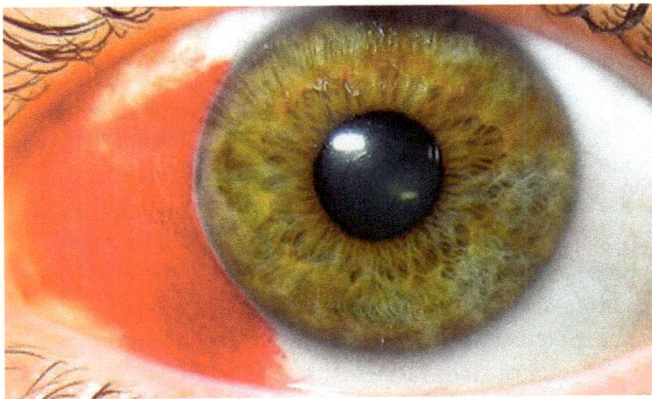

   a. Bleeding disorders
   b. Viral conjunctivitis
   c. Fingernail trauma
   d. Hypertension

Answer Key: 5. b   6. b   7. c

ANSWERS AND EXPLANATIONS

1. **Answer: c. Colour vision**
   The photograph depicts Ishihara's pseudoisochromatic test which is used to identify red-green colour deficiency

2. **Answer: c. Good stereopsis**
   The diagnosis is Oculocutaneous albinism
   Albinism is a disorder of melanin synthesis which may affect either the eye alone (ocular albinism) or the eyes, hair and skin (oculocutaneous albinism)
   Oculocutaneous albinism is of two types:
   - Tyrosinase negative or complete albinos-
     The features are:
     – Autosomal recessive inheritance
     – **Translucent iris** giving rise to pink eye appearance. This leads to light intolerance
     – Nystagmus
     – Hypopigmented fundus with **foveal hypoplasia**^{Q}
     – **Absence of stereopsis**^{Q}
     – Optic chiasma has very few uncrossed fibers
     – Strabismus may also be present
   - Tyrosinase positive or incomplete albinos-
     The feature are:
     – Less common
     – Autosomal recessive
     – Similar features but with less severity
     – Associated with syndromes like **Chediak-Higashi, Hermanasky-Pudlak**

3. **Answer: b. Iridodialysis**
   Iridodialysis means tearing of the iris from its root.

   Features of blunt trauma in the eye
   - Lid ecchymosis
   - Conjunctival laceration, subconjunctival hemorrhage
   - Corneal abrasion, corneal epithelial defect
   - *Hyphema*^{Q}: Blood in the anterior chamber
   - *Angle recession*^{Q}: Trauma to the angle leads to angle recession and **glaucoma**
   - Iridocyclitis or traumatic uveitis
   - *Iridodialysis:* Tearing of iris from its root. It may give rise to **D-shaped pupil**^{Q}.
   - Traumatic mydriasis
   - Sphincter tear leading to irregular pupil
   - Lens: **Vossius ring**^{Q}, **Rosette cataract**^{Q}
   - *Cyclodialysis:* Tearing of ciliary body from its root
   - Vitreous hemorrhage
   - Choroiditis, choroidal rupture
   - *Berlin's edema*^{Q}: Concussion edema of the nerve fibre layer of the retina which presents as **cherry red spot**^{Q}
   - Retinal tears and **rhegmatogenous retinal detachment**
   - **Traumatic optic neuropathy**^{Q}
   - **Avulsion of the optic nerve**^{Q}
   - **Globe rupture**
   - **Blow-out fracture of the orbit**

4. **Answer: c. Bitot's spot**
   This is a classical photograph of Bitot's spot seen in Vitamin A deficiency.

5. **Answer: b. Limbal dermoid**
   Limbal dermoid is a choristoma, usually seen in the **inferotemporal limbus.**
   It may be associated with Goldenhar syndrome.

Goldenhar syndrome
• Limbal dermoid
• Pre-auricular tags
• Microtia
• Mandibular hypoplasia
• Vertebral anomalies
• Cleft lip, Cleft palate

6. **Answer: b. Neurofibromatosis I**
   The photograph shows multiple nodular lesions on the iris (indicated by arrow). These are **Lisch nodules**, typical to Neurofibromatosis I

7. **Answer: c. Fingernail trauma**
   The condition shown in the photograph is subconjunctival hemorrhage

Causes of subconjunctival hemorrhage are:
• **Trauma**^{Q} (most commonly fingernail trauma)
• Foreign body
• **Hypertension**^{Q}
• Pertussis or severe cough due to any cause
• Bleeding disorders
• Pneumococcus
• **Hemorrhagic viral conjunctivitis**^{Q}

EU GSPR Authorised Reprsentative
Logos Europe, 9 rue Nicolas Poussin
1700, La Rochelle, France
Phone: +33 (0) 6 67 93 73 78
E-mail: contact@logoseurope.eu